Eye of the Heart

WILLIAM F. SULLIVAN

Eye of the Heart
*Knowing the Human Good in the
Euthanasia Debate*

UNIVERSITY OF TORONTO PRESS
Toronto   Buffalo   London

© University of Toronto Press 2005
Toronto Buffalo London
Printed in Canada

ISBN 0-8020-3923-5

Printed on acid-free paper

Lonergan Studies

National Library of Canada Cataloguing in Publication

Sullivan, William, F. 1959–
Eye of the heart : knowing the human good in the euthanasia
debate / William F. Sullivan.

(Lonergan studies)
Includes bibliographical references and index.
ISBN 0-8020-3923-5

1. Euthanasia – Moral and ethical aspects.   2. Lonergan, Bernard
J.F. (Bernard Joseph Francis), 1904–1984.   I. Title.   II. Series.

R726.S858 2005   179.7   C2004-902515-5

This volume was published with the aid of grants from the Canadian
Catholic Bioethics Institute, St Michael's Family Medicine Associates,
Department of Community and Family Medicine, St Michael's Hospital
(Toronto), and the Connie Heng Memorial Ethics Research Fund.

University of Toronto Press acknowledges the financial assistance to
its publishing program of the Canada Council for the Arts and the
Ontario Arts Council.

University of Toronto Press acknowledges the financial support for its
publishing activities of the Government of Canada through the Book
Publishing Industry Development Program (BPIDP).

Contents

Abbreviated Titles

The notes in this work make frequent reference to certain works of Bernard Lonergan. Standardized abbreviations, along with complete bibliographical information on each of these works, are listed below. Some of Lonergan's works, such as *Method in Theology* and *A Third Collection*, have not yet been published in the Collected Works of Bernard Lonergan (CWL), so naturally they are not cited as part of his Collected Works. In any given chapter, the first reference to a work gives the author, full title, full bibliographic information, and the page(s) referred to. Subsequent references give just the author and the abbreviated title, and the page(s) referred to.

Collection, CWL 4
Collection: Papers by Bernard Lonergan, S.J. Ed. Frederick E. Crowe. New York: Herder and Herder; London: Darton, Longman & Todd, 1967. 2nd ed. published in Collected Works of Bernard Lonergan, Vol. 4. Ed. Frederick E. Crowe and Robert M. Doran. Toronto: University of Toronto Press, 1988.

Insight, CWL 3
Insight: A Study of Human Understanding. London: Longmans, Green; New York: Philosophical Library, 1957. 2nd ed., 1958. 3rd ed., 1970. 4th ed., San Francisco: Harper & Row, 1978. 5th ed., published in Collected Works of Bernard Lonergan, Vol. 3. Ed. Frederick E. Crowe and Robert M. Doran. Toronto: University of Toronto Press, 1992.

Method
Method in Theology. London: Darton, Longman & Todd; New York: Herder and Herder, 1972.

Phil. and
Theol. Papers,
CWL 6
　　　　　Philosophical and Theological Papers 1958–1964. First pub-
　　　　　lished together in Collected Works of Bernard Lonergan,
　　　　　Vol. 6. Ed. Robert C. Croken, Frederick E. Crowe, and
　　　　　Robert M. Doran. Toronto: University of Toronto Press,
　　　　　1996.

Phen and
Logic, CWL 18
　　　　　Phenomenology and Logic: The Boston College Lectures on
　　　　　Mathematical Logic and Existentialism. Collected Works of
　　　　　Bernard Lonergan, Vol. 18. Ed. Philip J. McShane.
　　　　　Toronto: University of Toronto Press, 2001.

Second
Collection
　　　　　A Second Collection: Papers by Bernard Lonergan, S.J. Ed.
　　　　　William F. Ryan and Bernard J. Tyrrell. London: Darton,
　　　　　Longman & Todd; Philadelphia: Westminster, 1974. 2nd
　　　　　ed., Toronto: University of Toronto Press, 1996.

Third
Collection
　　　　　A Third Collection: Papers by Bernard Lonergan, S.J. Ed. Fred-
　　　　　erick E. Crowe. New York: Paulist Press; London: Geoffrey
　　　　　Chapman, 1985.

Topics in
Education,
CWL 10
　　　　　Topics in Education: The Cincinnati Lectures of 1959 on the
　　　　　Philosophy of Education. Unpublished text prepared by
　　　　　James Quinn and John Quinn. First published in Col-
　　　　　lected Works of Bernard Lonergan, Vol. 10. Ed. Robert M.
　　　　　Doran and Frederick E. Crowe. Toronto: University of
　　　　　Toronto Press, 1990.

Understanding
and Being,
CWL 5
　　　　　Understanding and Being: An Introduction and Companion to
　　　　　'Insight.' Ed. Elizabeth A. Morelli and Mark D. Morelli.
　　　　　New York and Toronto: Edwin Mellen, 1980. 2nd ed.
　　　　　published in Collected Works of Bernard Lonergan,
　　　　　Vol. 5. Ed. Frederick E. Crowe, Elizabeth A. Morelli,
　　　　　Mark D. Morelli, Robert M. Doran, and Thomas V. Daly.
　　　　　Toronto: University of Toronto Press, 1990.

Verbum,
CWL 2
　　　　　Verbum: Word and Idea in Aquinas. Ed. David B. Burrell.
　　　　　Notre Dame: University of Notre Dame, 1967. 2nd ed.
　　　　　published in Collected Works of Bernard Lonergan,
　　　　　Vol. 2. Ed. Frederick E. Crowe and Robert M. Doran.
　　　　　Toronto: University of Toronto Press, 1997.

Acknowledgments

I would like gratefully to acknowledge the assistance I received from several colleagues in writing this book. Michael Vertin, Joseph Boyle, Barry Brown, John Heng, Danny Monsour, Ken Melchin, Michael Stebbins, and Margaret Sullivan read the whole book in draft. All made helpful suggestions.

It is also a pleasure to thank all those who assisted with the editing and delivery of this book, including Anthony Palma, Jo-Anne Jackson-Thorne, Patricia Murphy, Ron Schoeffel, and the staff at the University of Toronto Press.

Finally, I should also like to thank those many friends and patients who have taught me so much about the reasons of the heart, in particular my late wife Connie and my late father, John Sullivan.

Foreword

1 Functional Specialization

In a book that he published in 1972, Canadian philosopher and theologian Bernard Lonergan proposed a technique for managing and even profiting from the complexity that invariably bedevils advanced studies. He labelled the technique 'functional specialization.' Though he developed it for the discipline of theology in particular, Lonergan envisioned functional specialization as potentially fruitful for any scholarly or scientific discipline, as well as for the complete set of such disciplines.[1]

Essentially, functional specialization is a particular way of organizing an investigative enterprise. We can illuminate it by comparing it with two other approaches. *Field* specialization organizes the investigation in terms of the *data* with which it begins. Thus, for example, biology can be divided into botany, the study of plants, and zoology, the study of animals. Historiography regularly is segmented according to the periods it regards, such as ancient, medieval, modern, and postmodern. Religious studies frequently is split into the study of eastern religions and the study of western religions. *Subject* specialization, by contrast, organizes the investigation in terms of the *results* it reaches, with different arrangements sometimes emerging because of basic theoretical differences between investigators. Thus, for example, religious studies often is partitioned into psychology of religion, sociology of religion, philosophy of religion, and so forth. Historiography can subscribe to linear, cyclical, or chaotic models. Biology can be structured along Darwinian or creationist lines.[2]

By contrast with both of the foregoing, *functional* specialization organizes the investigation in terms of the concrete *process* that, at their best, investigators actually go through in moving from data to results. It envisages that process as comprising eight distinct but interrelated sets of specialized operations or 'functional specialties.' While it is beyond the scope of this preface to present the functional specialties in detail, three points are especially pertinent for us here.

First, functional specialization takes it as indisputable that in any area of investigation, from subatomic physics to Trinitarian theology, valid conclusions are valid *judgments* – at least judgments of fact, and sometimes also judgments of value. Moreover, reaching a valid judgment is always a *process* of three or four steps: *attending to data, forming a hypothesis* about the intelligible unity of those data, *affirming the reality* of that intelligible unity (or denying it), and – where pertinent – *affirming the goodness* of that reality (or denying it). If any step of the pertinent process is omitted or poorly made, the judgment will be suspect.

Second, functional specialization distinguishes sharply between the judgments deemed valid by *other* persons and communities, whether past or present, and the judgments deemed valid by *oneself* and *one's own* community. Moreover, it holds that the ultimate goal of an investigation is to reach judgments that satisfy the most authentic of one's own aspirations, but that careful study of others' judgments is commonly an important step in properly pursuing that goal.

Third, functional specialization also distinguishes sharply between what one *encounters only in* a particular investigative situation, the situation's *empirical* features, and what one *brings to* that situation, the situation's *pre-empirical* features. The empirical features stand to the pre-empirical features like the respective lower and upper blades of scissors; and the forward movement of the investigation is like the closing of the scissors' blades. The most basic elements of what one brings – the radically pre-empirical features of the situation – are one's philosophical presuppositions, one's operative (if not always explicit) answers to three basic philosophical questions. (1) What acts do I experience myself performing whenever I am at least *apparently* knowing? (2) Why, if at all, does performing those acts constitute *valid* knowing? (3) What is the basic character of reality (including value, real goodness), namely, whatever does or would become manifest to me insofar as I validly know? Differences between various investigators' operative answers to these three basic questions commonly constitute a fundamental, though often overlooked, part of their disagreements about particular investigative conclusions.

2   The Advantages of Functional Specialization

Functional specialization has three significant potential advantages. First, by carefully *distinguishing* the various elements of the investigative process itself, functional specialization counters both oversimplification, the neglect of certain tasks, and confusion, the blurring of distinct tasks. Gathering data differs from formulating a hypothesis, both differ from affirming reality, and all three differ from affirming value. Again, it is one thing to learn that others have judged X to be Y, and it is quite another to judge for oneself that X is Y. Further, discovering the explicit import of another's judgment is different from discovering the philosophical presuppositions that inevitably shape that judgment's integral import, and both are different from determining one's own agreement or disagreement with those presuppositions.

Second, by carefully *relating* what it has distinguished, functional specialization displays the diverse investigative tasks as mutually complementary contributions to a common enterprise. Gathering data, formulating hypotheses, affirming reality, affirming value, discovering others' judgments, assessing others' judgments, elucidating philosophical presuppositions, assessing philosophical presuppositions – functional specialization lays out just how these different operations fit together. And thus it both restrains exaggerated ambitions and encourages appropriate exertions. It makes clear that no task that is actually just part of the total investigative enterprise can expect to satisfy the requirements of the whole. But it makes equally clear that the flourishing of the total enterprise requires the contribution of every part.

Third, and following from the preceding, functional specialization provides a way of meeting a twofold challenge that is becoming increasingly common in advanced studies, namely, relevant *data* that are far too extensive for any individual to address, and requisite *skills* that are far too diverse for any individual to master. Recognizing that an adequate investigation in such circumstances can only be a communal enterprise, functional specialization articulates a technique of effective collaboration for the community of investigators. Organizing the enterprise in terms of neither initial data nor terminal results but rather the investigative operations themselves, functional specialization encourages individual investigators to devote themselves to one or another functional specialty, but explicitly to envision their practice of that specialty as contributing to a common effort. It delineates precisely the matters on which they should listen to others and expect to learn from them, and the matters on which they should speak to others and attempt to teach them. And it gives them solid grounds for anticipating collective progress toward an investigative outcome that notably transcends what any one of them is capable of achieving on her own.

3   The Moral Status of Euthanasia: The Structure of Valid Judgments about It

William Sullivan's book illustrates something of functional specialization and the advantages it brings to a narrowly focused inquiry. For at one level the book may indeed be characterized as regarding a very specific matter, namely, the moral status of euthanasia; and as thus characterized, it clearly manifests several of functional specialization's beneficial features. Its fundamental organization emerges from sequentially considering cognitional operations, rather than cognitional data or cognitional results. Moreover, it begins by carefully elucidating the various accounts that other persons provide regarding their own cognitional operations, and only subsequently does it present the account that Sullivan himself, measuring it against the best of his own concrete cognitional practices, reckons to be the correct one. Furthermore, it clearly expounds and centrally employs the distinction between what one encounters only in a particular investigative situation, the empirical features of one's cognitional operations and objects, and what one brings to that situation, the pre-empirical features of one's cognitional operations and objects.

More amply, after recounting the overall pattern of cognitional operations, Sullivan devotes himself primarily to considering judgments of value. His focal interest is the role played by one's feelings in the process of making valid judgments of value. He addresses this issue in two main phases. In the *first* phase, he articulates the opposed stances on the issue that in his view are present explicitly or at least implicitly in an 'ascending' series of contexts. The first and most restricted context is that of the expressions of persons who in one way or another address *the moral value of euthanasia.* As extended examples in this context, Sullivan retraces the end-of-life stories told (through their ghost writers) by Sue Rodriguez and Dennis Kaye, two recent Canadian victims of amyotrophic lateral sclerosis (ALS). The second context, somewhat broader, is that of the expressions of persons who in one way or another take stances on *moral value as such* (and not just the moral value of euthanasia). The third and broadest context is that of the expressions of persons who in one way or another take stances on utterly general or *transcategorial value as such* (and not just specifically moral value).[3]

In the *second* phase of his investigation, Sullivan reverses the order of his considerations, now 'descending' through the previous series of contexts. In the first and broadest context, he affirms as correct both the stance of Bernard Lonergan regarding one's knowing of reality as such, and what he proposes as a 'Lonerganian' account of the role played by feelings in one's valid judgments about *transcategorial value as such.* In the second and somewhat more restricted context, he complements his previous step by taking explicit account of relevant special pre-empirical structures, thus arriving at what he claims is the correct account of the role played by feelings in one's valid judgments about *specifically moral value.* Finally, in the third and most restricted context, he complements his previous step by situating its results in the field of the relevant empirical determinations taken as determinate, thus arriving at what he maintains is the correct account of the role played by feelings in one's valid judgments about *the moral value of euthanasia*.[4]

It remains that Sullivan himself makes no definitive finding that the moral value of euthanasia in this or that particular instance is positive, or that it is negative. For his investigation is essentially just a philosophical one. His principal goal is simply to clarify the criteria of definitive findings, whether positive or negative. Like Lonergan, he maintains that at least implicitly holding a correct stance on the pre-empirical features of a valid judgment is a necessary but not sufficient condition of actually making a valid judgment; and he largely limits himself to spelling out the pre-empirical features of valid judgments regarding euthanasia's moral status, not their further, empirical features. That is to say, he is mainly concerned with just the 'upper blade' of the 'scissors' of methodical seeking and finding, not also the 'lower blade.' He aims to objectify the constant dynamic investigative structure that, in his view, the authentic inquirer brings to her study of euthanasia's moral status in every particular instance; but he refrains from the further steps of ascertaining and assessing the variable determinations of that structure that emerge as fully determinate only in this or that particular instance.

And thus even within his third and most restricted 'descending' context, the only decisive conclusion Sullivan reaches about the end-of-life stories of Sue Rodriguez and Dennis Kay is that, as regards the *pre-empirical* features of a valid judgment on the moral value of euthanasia, the stance implicit in Kaye's story is superior to that implicit in Rodriguez's story.[5] If he wished to go further and, for example, assess the validity of Kaye's implicit judgment that the moral value of taking his own life would be negative, Sullivan envisions that he would need to ascertain and assess a crucial set of *empirical* factors, namely, Kaye's actual reasons for making that judgment. But making such ascertainments and assessments are additional tasks – in effect, work proper to other functional specializations, work which in his present investigation Sullivan does not undertake.[6]

4   The Dynamic Structure of Ethical Studies

When viewed as regarding the moral status of euthanasia, Sullivan's book illustrates some of the clarificational and organizational advantages that functional specialization brings to a narrowly focused inquiry. However, it may also be viewed as illustrating some benefits that functional specialization brings to a somewhat more broadly focused inquiry. For at the level of the intermediate context in which it proceeds, the book is concerned to articulate and resolve the principal disputes about the character of moral value as such. The procedures by which it addresses this task constitute a model[7] of how to structure the integral enterprise of ethical studies both clearly and systematically.

First, Sullivan's model fosters the *clarity* of ethical studies. For example, by distinguishing between the empirical data that characterize this or that situation of moral inquiry and the basic moral presuppositions that one brings to any such situation, it counteracts the common tendency to confuse what one makes moral judgments about and the criteria in terms of which one makes them. Again, by distinguishing between basic moral presuppositions and moral conclusions, it counteracts the common tendency to blur the concrete heuristic universality of one's basic moral presuppositions, a universality which is certain,[8] and the abstract cognitional universality of generalizations of one's concrete moral conclusions, a universality which at best is just highly probable.[9] Further, by distinguishing between a first phase of moral inquiry, in which one delineates various conflicting moral conclusions and presuppositions, and a second phase, in which one determines which of those presuppositions and conclusions are correct and which are incorrect, it counteracts the common tendency to conflate the role of the human community and the role of oneself in the generation of moral judgments. Still further, by distinguishing between empirical instances of euthanasia, empirical instances of other human deeds that also regard organic human life (such as abortion, producing embryos for research, and cloning), and empirical instances of yet other human deeds (such as polluting the environment, cheating one's customers, lying to one's electors, and betraying the confidences of one's legal clients), it provides unambiguous grounds for differentiating the ethical study of euthanasia, the more inclusive study that is bioethics, and the endeavour of ethical studies in its completeness (which also includes environmental ethics, business ethics, political ethics, legal ethics, and so forth).[10]

Second, Sullivan's model fosters the *unity* of ethical studies. For it not only draws distinctions, it also spells out relations. Thus, for example, it affirms the relations between the objects and the criteria of moral judgments, between one's concretely universal basic moral presuppositions and one's abstractly universal moral generalizations, between the respective roles of the community and oneself in the emergence of moral judgments, and between the ethical study of euthanasia, bioethics, and the integral enterprise of ethical studies. Further, it presents the fundamental relations not as static but as dynamic, such that the integral enterprise of ethical studies is an internally unified process that tends toward both highlighting and eliminating disagreements over moral judgments and anticipating and achieving advances in moral knowledge. Still further, it envisions the diverse steps of that process not simply as distinct and related *tasks* but as distinct and related *specialties* at which different practitioners can become proficient. In other words, on the model Sullivan provides, the internally unified process that constitutes ethical studies can become the efficacious communal process of diverse but methodically collaborating ethical specialists, rather than remaining just the individual process of an overextended ethical generalist or the inefficacious communal process of a mere collection of such generalists.[11]

5 The Dynamic Structure of Transcategorial Valuative Studies

Thus far I have suggested that Sullivan's book illustrates some of the clarificational and organizational advantages that functional specialization brings to a narrowly focused investigative effort, such as studying the moral value of euthanasia, and also to a somewhat more broadly focused effort, such as studying moral value as such. I now suggest a third and final respect in which it very usefully illustrates benefits of functional specialization. For at the level of the broadest context in which it proceeds, the book is concerned to articulate and resolve the principal disputes about the character of utterly general or transcategorial value as such (and not just specifically moral value). The procedures by which it addresses this task constitute a model[12] of how to structure the integral enterprise of transcategorial valuative studies (and not just specifically ethical studies) in clear and systematic fashion. (The following observations partly just generalize and partly contrast with those made in the previous section. Moreover, let me apologize in advance for frequent use of the expression 'transcategorial valuative.' Though cumbersome, it provides the requisite clarity of contrast with 'ethical' or 'moral.')

First, Sullivan's model fosters the *clarity* of transcategorial valuative studies. For example, by distinguishing between the empirical data that characterize this or that situation of transcategorial valuative inquiry and the basic transcategorial valuative presuppositions that one brings to any such situation, it counteracts the common tendency to confuse what one makes transcategorial value judgments about and the criteria in terms of which one makes them. Again, by distinguishing between basic transcategorial valuative presuppositions and transcategorial valuative conclusions, it counteracts the common tendency to blur the concrete heuristic universality of one's basic transcategorial valuative presuppositions, a universality which is certain,[13] and the abstract cognitional universality of generalizations of one's concrete transcategorial valuative conclusions, a universality which at best is just highly probable.[14] Further, by distinguishing between a first phase of transcategorial valuative inquiry, in which one delineates various conflicting transcategorial valuative conclusions and presuppositions, and a second phase, in which one determines which of those presuppositions and conclusions are correct and which are incorrect, it counteracts the common tendency to conflate the role of the human community and the role of oneself in the generation of transcategorial value judgments. Still further, by distinguishing between questions about *moral* value in its characteristic specificity and *transcategorial* value in its characteristic generality, it provides unambiguous grounds for differentiating the specific endeavour that is ethical studies and the general endeavour that is transcategorial valuative studies.[15]

Second, Sullivan's model fosters the *unity* of transcategorial valuative studies. For it articulates relations as well as making distinctions. Thus, for example, it affirms the relations between the objects and the criteria of transcategorial value judgments, between one's concretely universal basic transcategorial valuative presuppositions and one's abstractly universal transcategorial valuative generalizations, between the respective roles of the community and oneself in the emergence of transcategorial value judgments, and between the specific enterprise of ethical studies and the general enterprise of transcategorial valuative studies. Further, it portrays the fundamental relations not as static but as dynamic, such that the integral enterprise of transcategorial valuative studies is an internally unified process that tends toward both highlighting and eliminating disagreements over transcategorial value judgments and anticipating and achieving advances in transcategorial valuative knowledge. Still further, it envisions the diverse steps of that process not simply as distinct and related *tasks* but as distinct and related *specialties* at which different practitioners can become proficient. That is to say, on Sullivan's model the internally unified process that constitutes transcategorial valuative studies can become the efficacious communal process of diverse but methodically collaborating transcategorial valuative specialists, rather than remaining just the individual process of an overextended transcategorial valuative generalist or the inefficacious communal process of a mere collection of such generalists.[16]

The preceding remarks indicate my high estimate of William Sullivan's book. Let me conclude by expressing my hope that it gets the excellent reception I judge it to deserve.

Michael Vertin
Philosophy, Religion, and Theology
St Michael's College, University of Toronto

Introduction

The Euthanasia Debate and the Problem of a Philosophy of Heart: Questions, Context, and Arguments

In 'Insight' the good was the intelligent and reasonable. In 'Method' the good is a distinct notion. It is intended in questions for deliberation: Is this worthwhile? Is it truly or only apparently good? It is aspired to in the intentional response of feeling to values. It is known in judgments of value made by a virtuous or authentic person with a good conscience. It is brought about by deciding and living up to one's decisions.

Bernard Lonergan, '*Insight* Revisited'

1   The Cognitive Role of Affectivity: Two Focal Questions

Two questions have motivated my research for this work. First, what role does affect or 'heart' play in evaluations or value judgments?[1] Second, what are some of the ramifications of the stance taken on this question by the Canadian philosopher and theologian Bernard Lonergan for the euthanasia debate?[2] In response to the first question, I will set forth and critically reflect upon Lonergan's contention that 'apprehensions [of values] are given in feelings.'[3] Subsequently, I will critically affirm the accuracy of Lonergan's account and use it to provide a detailed analysis of my own performance as a physician in making fact and value judgments. In response to the second question, I will highlight some of the ramifications of Lonergan's stance for understanding and assessing two cases that have been important to the euthanasia debate in Canada. This understanding and assessment, I will argue, has further ramifications for the entire euthanasia debate.

Broadly stated, the central aim of the discussion is to articulate a connection between psychology and philosophy by developing an account of value judgments that does justice to the facts of one's moral psychology. I will argue that particular value judgments that underpin bioethical issues such as the euthanasia debate presuppose some stance on the issue of the relation between psychology and philosophy. Moreover, I will argue that if Lonergan's account of the role of affect in value judgments is correct, then his position can be developed to make important and original contributions not only to this particular debate, but also to the broader enterprise of bioethics.

The two questions motivating the discussion direct attention to a reflective and a practical task that I will take up. The reflective task is to set forth Lonergan's critical-realist value theory. Lonergan's stance takes cognitional theory as foundational to any claim to know the good, and his cognitional theory includes some role for certain affective acts in evaluations. The practical task is to show that theoretical differences on this global philosophical issue have important implications for concrete medico-ethical judgments.

These distinct theoretical and practical tasks correspond to my background and interest in the interdisciplinary nature of bioethics. I intend that this discussion illustrate the need for those engaging in bioethics to have some expertise both in philosophy and in the concrete realities of medicine, and as well have as a grasp of the connections between the two. In order to meet the challenges that all bioethicists must face, I will be making use of my training and experience in both philosophy and medicine. As one trained in philosophy and specializing in medical ethics, I will engage key features of the contemporary discussion of methodological issues among bioethicists. In so doing, I will highlight some important and original contributions Lonergan's thought can make to this debate. As a physician with training in the areas of family medicine, geriatric medicine, psychiatry, developmental disabilities, and palliative care, my focal concerns have to do with the relevance of philosophy to medicine. In particular, I will be concerned with the issue of how philosophy really helps one to understand and respond to such human issues as the deep desolation some persons experience and express in a cry for suicide. The underlying and unifying theme of the discussion is that Lonergan's philosophical contributions can actually make an important difference on the practical level of ethical disputes, such as the euthanasia debate, and on how one operates as a caregiver.[4]

My interest in the cognitive role of feelings is motivated in part by my clinical interest in working with persons who have a cognitive impairment or developmental disability. If persons with a condition such as Down Syndrome illustrate a cognitive disability that is predominantly intellectual, other conditions exist that illustrate predominantly affective or emotional impairments. For instance, individuals with Asperger Syndrome illustrate a condition characterized by severe impairments in reciprocal social interactions, including features such as a lack of appreciation of social cues, or socially and emotionally inappropriate behaviour.[5] My particular interest is to highlight the importance of accounting for 'affective' cognitive abilities in assessing a person's medical decision-making capacity.[6] Because certain feelings play a cognitive role in value judgments, they must be taken seriously when assessing someone's decision-making capacity. This is especially true when caregivers call cognitive capacity into question because someone has an 'intellectual' cognitive impairment. Even more important is the failure to recognize the impaired decision-making capacity of those individuals who have a specifically affective-cognitive disability. This particular developmental disability provides, I think, the strongest empirical evidence for the cognitive role of feelings. The practical implication of Lonergan's theoretical view, then, has made me more attentive to the feelings of persons with various cognitive impairments.

My emphasis on the importance of feelings for decision-making enjoys some empirical support from psychologists who work with persons with a cognitive disability. Typically, psychologists distinguish between a cognitive impairment that affects intellectual tasks (e.g., doing mathematics) and an impairment that is affective in nature (e.g., one creating problems with interpersonal and social skills). Someone might be 'mildly mentally retarded,' based on an intelligence quotient or IQ score (e.g., an IQ of 50–69 corresponds to mental age of 9–12 years). Given such a score, someone who views medical decisions as strictly 'intellectual' judgments might regard such individuals as incapable of making medical decisions for themselves. But these same individuals can have more highly developed affective skills, which would make their emotional or affective 'mental age' much more advanced than their intellectual mental age – a situation which, in fact, is not uncommon. In such cases a person might be quite capable of making medical evaluations, given appropriate assistance in understanding the relevant medical facts and options. These psychological findings provide further empirical evidence to support Lonergan's claim that human cognition involves distinct intellectual and affective processes. In addition, this is an instance where a practical matter of determining decision-making capacity might hinge on one's global philosophical view of the elements that go to constitute a decision.

Some orienting remarks regarding some of the key methodological commitments that will shape this discussion are in order. The approach I will take follows from three main methodological commitments. I intend (1) to base my analysis on particular, concrete life stories, and on first-person claims based on these stories, rather than on general principles or policies; (2) to begin with an analysis of the phenomena of making a medical-fact judgment prior to addressing more difficult and subsequent questions such as the phenomena of value judgments and the epistemic status of one's knowledge of facts or values; and (3) to ground my assessment of Lonergan's claims in an autobiographical analysis rather than one that is subject- or person-neutral. Let me expand briefly on each of these methodological commitments.

The first pattern that will shape the discussion is suggested by the metaphors of 'bottom-up' and 'top-down.' I would characterize this pattern as one that begins with particular life stories, moves to address global philosophical issues, and then returns back to the particular stories. In chapter 2, for instance, I begin with two stories that seem to illustrate the relevance of affectivity in end-of-life decisions. Sue Rodriguez and Dennis Kaye both suffered from amyotrophic lateral sclerosis or ALS (Lou Gehrig's disease). Prior to their deaths, each wrote about their experience of living with ALS. On the basis of their stories, it seems apparent that certain feelings were cognitively relevant to their experiences and evaluations. If one agrees that certain feelings are cognitively relevant for value judgments, however, more difficult questions inevitably arise, such as: 'Which feelings are cognitively relevant?' 'How precisely do they function?' 'How is knowing values different from knowing facts and from deciding?' and 'Is my value knowledge ever more than just subjective?' In the story of Sue Rodriguez, for example, was her feeling that her life under certain restricted conditions would not be worth living a necessary and/or sufficient grounds for her negative self-evaluation? What was the relation between this evaluation and subsequent decisions to forgo active medical treatments, or directly to end her life by means of physician-assisted suicide? Was her self-evaluation strictly personal, and therefore had no legitimate interpersonal relevance for others such as Dennis Kaye, whose life was similarly restricted?

In the central chapters, I focus on the global issue of the role of affect in evaluations. And in the last part of the discussion I return to the previously treated stories in order to highlight some ramifications of Lonergan's stance on the role of affect in evaluations for these stories, and also for the related ethical and public-policy debate regarding euthanasia. By following this procedure, I hope to illustrate a methodological approach to bioethical questions that undercuts the particularist/generalist methodological divide, on either side of which some thinkers have attempted to situate all contemporary bioethicists.[7] I hope to show how concrete particular and global philosophical features of bioethical questions are complementary. Indeed, I will argue that it is possible, and even desirable, to attend both to the complexity and nuance of concrete particular stories and also to attend to more global philosophical considerations and conclusions that bear upon them.

One advantage of an approach that begins with particular cases is that it highlights the complexities of the circumstances in which philosophical and ethical issues arise. Underpinning this starting point is the view that what we are aiming at in ethical deliberations is some value that is a concrete actuality or a real possibility, rather than an abstract or unrealizable good. By adopting a 'bottom-up' approach that begins with cases, one has the advantage of ensuring that one is connecting to the questions and concerns with which individuals are actually struggling. Even if one's answers are challenged at the end of such an analysis, at least one cannot be accused of missing entirely the *real* issues and questions. The disadvantage of this approach, of course, is that one can easily become enmeshed in the particularities of stories, in the polemics of the debate, and in a number of other secondary issues that tend to obscure rather than clarify key philosophical issues. Although I will begin with the actual accounts of where feelings entered into the evaluations of two persons with a terminal illness, I will end with an articulation of the role of affect in evaluations and specify how differences on this question underpin many if not all of the different stances that have been taken in the euthanasia debate. At the end, therefore, I will proceed in a 'top-down' manner and illustrate by means of the euthanasia debate several important ramifications Lonergan's account has for ethics.

A second pattern that will serve as an organizing principle for this discussion is Lonergan's ordering of what he calls the 'three basic questions for philosophy.' In order of methodological priority, the first is the *phenomenological* question, 'What am I doing when knowing values?' The second is the *epistemological* question, 'How is doing this valid knowing?' The third is the *metaphysical* question, 'What is the structure of the real?' In chapters 4 and 6 I will compare and contrast Lonergan's answers to the phenomenological questions of how one makes fact and value judgments. And in chapters 5 and 7 I will explain Lonergan's answer to the epistemological questions of how one's purported knowledge of facts or values is genuine. As a methodological ordering principle, then, I will be following Lonergan's insistence that phenomenological issues are prior to epistemological and metaphysical ones. This places cognitional theory at the centre of his philosophy. Moreover, I will also follow the order of operations in his cognitional theory, which places fact judgments before value judgments or evaluations. And I will critically assess these methodological commitments in my own name in chapter 8.

An image Lonergan provides is useful for thinking about the relation between the concrete medico-ethical questions in the euthanasia debate and the global, philosophical question regarding where affectivity enters into evaluations. This is the image of a pair of 'scissors' cutting through paper at the point of contact between its two blades. One can imagine the lower blade of the pair of scissors 'picking up' concrete data and circumstances of life stories from which arise certain questions at the end of life, such as questions regarding the meaning and value of one's life in the context of suffering and declining health. In philosophical terms that will become clearer in chapter 9, this lower blade represents the *empirical* or a posteriori content of one's knowing. The upper blade of this metaphorical scissors represents the *philosophical, purely structural, heuristic,* or a priori features of one's knowing. These are the cognitive operations that one brings to any concrete issue, such as the operations of experiencing, understanding, judging, and evaluating. I will be focusing primarily on how affectivity enters into these upper- and lower-blade operations when it comes to evaluating. This analysis, I hope, will illustrate something of the importance of Lonergan's position for this debate and for ethics in general.

The third methodological commitment is to an autobiographical or first-person point of view. This is in contrast to the 'person-neutral' or 'absent-subject' point of view common in much of the contemporary scientific and medical literature that typically favours the use of the passive voice. A first-person point of view is necessary when one seeks to answer the phenomenological question 'What am I doing when I am knowing?' The data on which I need to reflect are my own cognitive operations that emerge in my efforts to know anything, which I will bring to light using medical examples. Moreover, this approach also helps to undermine a view of 'objectivity' that considers objectivity to be something that obtains apart from subjects. I will be challenging this view throughout the discussion.

My approach, then, seeks to highlight the ultimate grounds on which the reader can judge the account of the evaluations Lonergan, or anyone else, proposes: does the reader discover that this account describes with some degree of accuracy and adequacy his or her own cognitive performance when they are operating and evaluating successfully? Perhaps this approach may strike some readers as being too personal or even self-centred. But I am not claiming that the account given here is my own, or that it is beyond challenge. My claim is merely that the account of value judgments that I will elaborate describes my own conscious performance as a moral agent. On this basis, I will invite readers to verify this account for themselves by going through a similar process of self-reflection on their own successful performance as knowers and evaluators.

As for the general tone of my argument, it will be mainly positive and constructive. I want to begin with the self-evident fact that persons sometimes make fact and value judgments. Although such a starting point might be problematic from certain philosophical perspectives, it is one that is readily accepted by most of my medical and ethical colleagues. This positive starting point does not commit me to the further claim that persons who make either fact or value judgments are usually successful in their efforts to know, nor that they are able to provide an account of their knowing with a high degree of nuance or accuracy. Neither will this starting point prevent me from critically assessing and challenging Lonergan's contributions or from acknowledging the merits of opposing accounts. However, because it is too great a task to consider whether Lonergan's position is true from every standpoint, I will follow a critical method only secondarily and in a limited manner. Since one of the main aims of my discussion is to expound and clarify Lonergan's position, one of the ways in which I can achieve this will be by contrasting his account with rival ones, and by pointing out what results for ethics from his account.

2   The State and Context of the Two Questions

2.1 The Euthanasia Question

Most commentators on the issue of euthanasia agree that it is one of the most important, controversial, and divisive medico-ethical questions of the day. Various answers to this question are being offered by a variety of thinkers, coming from a variety of backgrounds. The ethical, legal, and public-policy ramifications of these different answers are quite extensive.[8] Because of the extent of the present conflict regarding euthanasia, the importance to the health-care system of any public-policy changes in this area, and the interdisciplinary nature of this debate, these questions are ideally suited to the sort of philosophical discussion in medical ethics that I am envisioning. A philosophical perspective brings to this medico-ethical-legal question some important advantages over other perspectives. One particular advantage over the patient's or physician's perspective is that it can both attend to the questions and insights that they raise and yet go beyond their particular perspectives by linking them to a long and rich philosophical debate on these very questions.

In medical, bioethical, and legal circles, the current majority opinion or 'received view' is opposed to euthanasia. In chapter 2, I will report Richard McCormick's articulation of this received view. I will also point out that other thinkers, such as Tom Beauchamp, argue with some persuasive force against this received view. Indeed, thinkers such as Daniel Callahan, who have been following the evolving history of this debate, claim that Western societies are currently at a delicate point and that this received view could soon be reversed. For, courts in various countries are repeatedly being asked to give patients the right to obtain a lethal prescription.

Central to my contribution to the euthanasia debate is the contention that differing positions in that debate are related to the differing accounts given of cognitional and decisional subjectivity. I shall argue that the frequently overlooked reasons for different positions on euthanasia are the varying stances on underlying philosophical issues such as the role of feelings in evaluations. One indication of this link is given in Tom Beauchamp's view that it is 'the person in question' who is in the best position to determine whether his or her life is worth living. In other words, a key claim this proponent of euthanasia uses to justify his stance is a methodological one that claims that the particular evaluator is somehow crucial to the validity of the evaluation. The advantage of this first-person perspective seems to be that it allows one access to certain personal or 'subjective' elements, including 'feelings,' that enter into these evaluations in important ways. These personal cognitive elements are thought to confer on the 'person in question' some advantage over others, who might not have access to this first-person data, when deliberating on whether his or her life is worthwhile. I take this claim, which is both a methodological and epistemological one, to be an important and often overlooked link between the contemporary euthanasia debate and the historical discussion of the interrelation of reason and emotion.

2.2 The Question of the Role of Affect in Value Judgments

On the state of the general philosophical question of the role of affectivity in value judgments, it is worth noting that feelings are a prominent topic of study. One can readily find evidence for this claim by reviewing the titles of many of the most recent publications in philosophy and ethics. Typically, the discussions deal with the link between the disciplines of psychology and philosophy. At one end of the spectrum of views is the claim that feelings are strictly psychological phenomena and have no genuinely cognitive attributes. Such a view is compatible with what Milton Hunnex refers to as an 'axiological objectivist' view of values, in which one purports to know true values but denies that feelings play a cognitive role in achieving this knowledge.[9] At the other end of the spectrum of views are those that reduce value expressions to feeling expressions. Typically such views are compatible with an 'axiological subjectivist' value theory in which value claims are merely expressions of one's psychological disposition.[10]

A third view of the link between psychology and philosophy bridges this subjective/objective divide by insisting that the act of knowing values partly involves feelings. The knowledge that one achieves in this manner, however, is not merely psychological. That is, this view affirms a link between feelings and value judgments, as the axiological subjectivists do, but it also affirms the axiological objectivists' view that one can move beyond one's own psychological matrix and come to know real values. This is Lonergan's position. It is less common than either of the other main alternatives, and it is the position I will be exploring in depth.[11]

In chapter 3 I will give a more detailed elucidation of the history of these different views regarding the role of feelings in value judgments. What I do wish to point out here, however, is that Lonergan's view on the relation between feelings and value judgments is a matter of some debate and disagreement among Lonergan scholars. Indeed, there are diverse accounts among these scholars regarding what Lonergan's own views were on how precisely feelings enter into value judgments. What is clear to most Lonergan scholars, however, is that his position would fall into the third of the three positions just outlined. That is, he affirmed the 'axiological objectivist' value theory that views values as real properties of persons or objects. He also maintained, however, that one somehow grasps such values in, or by means of, feelings. That is, he affirmed that feelings play a psychological role in value judgments, as the axiological subjectivists would also insist, but that this role is also a cognitive one.

What is less clear among Lonergan scholars is the precise cognitive function of these affective responses. Although I will rely primarily on Michael Vertin's interpretation of Lonergan's position, this issue remains, as I have just said, a disputed question among Lonergan scholars. Accordingly, even though I will be arguing that the interpretation of Lonergan that I will be promoting is, for the most part, accurate, the precise details of this account have not yet become the received view among Lonergan scholars.

I take this dispute among Lonergan scholars to be a secondary matter. My primary aim is to make Lonergan's position less vulnerable to more fundamental misinterpretations by those who are not well acquainted with his work. As for the broader issues, such as the centrality of cognitional theory to Lonergan's philosophy and the main outlines of his theory of cognition, Lonergan's more basic position is not in serious doubt among Lonergan specialists.[12]

3   The Position I Will Be Defending

On the global philosophical issue of the role of affect in evaluations, I will be arguing that Lonergan contends that certain affects, namely those that characterize one's intentional responses to values, are a key part of the cognitive basis for making an evaluation. Their role is analogous to that of reflective insights in grasping facts. In addition, I will be arguing that Lonergan's position is that accepting that affect plays a role in evaluations does not commit one to the further view that all evaluations are just subjective. The position I will expound is that the epistemic objectivity of one's evaluations is importantly related to one's own authentic subjectivity, which involves not only moral uprightness, but also an integration of the affectivity of one's categorial responses to values and to one's intending of transcendental value. This position affirms the role of both intellectual and affective cognitive acts in the process of making an evaluation. I will also be arguing, in my own name, that this position is more adequate than either of the other two main alternative ways of conceiving the link between feelings and evaluations, the view that feelings entirely determine evaluations, and the view that they play no role at all. By emphasizing merely a part of moral knowing, either affective or intellectual, these contrary stances result in a distortion of the whole of moral knowing. Further, I will also be arguing that a stance on this general philosophical issue has important ramifications for ethics, and I will use the euthanasia debate to illustrate what some of those ramifications are. In particular, an adequate stance on this global philosophical question provides the grounds for one to assess critically those concrete evaluations that underpin decisions for or against euthanasia, both at the levels of concrete stories and at the related ethical and public-policy levels of this debate.

My own view is that many of the philosophical critiques of euthanasia and *rational suicide* have been ineffective or unpersuasive because they fail to identify the essentially affective source of the issue. So often such arguments aim at exposing some defect in logic or reasoning, when the real defect lies elsewhere. Besides identifying the defect in the position, one also needs to be prepared to articulate what, in the words of G.K. Chesterton, the 'sane affections' are, and how they are linked with what Chesterton also calls 'good judgment' – which I would understand as including judgments about the good.[13]

As I have already indicated, on this general philosophical issue I will be drawing on Lonergan's analysis, in which he argues that the relevant 'feelings' are intentional responses to values. These feeling or affective responses enter into one's grasp of values, and they are part of the grounds on which one makes evaluations. They are not to be understood as sensory experiences, nor are they responses to what is merely agreeable or disagreeable to a person. Rather, they are intentional responses that are characteristically affective. They function somewhat like 'insights' that grasp some unity in a diversity. They are the proximate grounds or evidential base for one's grasp of a value.[14]

A related, though distinct, issue is whether the content of the evaluation

I achieve is cognitionally true or epistemically objective. On the general philosophical question of the role of affect in evaluations, I shall argue that Michael Vertin's interpretation of Bernard Lonergan's stance on this issue adequately captures the link between psychological affective responses and the cognitive function of such responses in evaluations. In so doing, Lonergan provides a critical-realist analysis of evaluations, in which affect plays an important part. Further, this position also provides a critical, normative basis for assessing particular evaluations, including those that arise in the context of a terminal illness.

Taking this stance on this global philosophical issue, I will argue, has important ramifications for the euthanasia debate. In particular, such an analysis sets out the main lines for challenging other stances. As mentioned previously, the first stance denies that feelings have any cognitive role in evaluations (e.g., typical axiological objectivists). On this basis, the cognitive import of one's affective struggles and tensions are disregarded as irrelevant to moral discernment. Even if this view of the matter were correct, it overlooks or blocks out a huge part of the stories of persons who actually struggle with these issues. The second stance insists that evaluations are wholly determined by feelings. Supporters of this view typically overlook the intellectual acts of knowing and concede too much by admitting that evaluations are ultimately merely subjective and cannot be legitimately assessed or challenged by others (e.g., axiological subjectivism). I will compare and contrast the views of Sue Rodriguez and Dennis Kaye on these issues, as well as the views of proponents and opponents of euthanasia at the ethical and public-policy level of the debate.

Put positively, I will affirm the evaluation that Dennis Kaye made of the worthwhileness of his own life even in the context of a disease as devastating as ALS. His experience and conclusions affirm the wisdom of the community, as passed down in professional codes and laws through the centuries. Today this wisdom finds expression not only in those laws that aim to protect vulnerable members of our society, but also in positive duties of responding with care, compassion, and practical assistance to all those who are dying, even when death cannot be avoided.

Since Lonergan himself did not write on the issue of euthanasia, I will be extending his view of the role of affect in evaluations to this issue, in order to highlight several presuppositions that commonly held definitions of euthanasia express. One presupposition that underpins these definitions is the meaning and moral significance of 'competence.' Lonergan's emphasis is similarly on the autonomous subject, and especially on the importance of 'authentic' subjectivity. But the commonly held definitions suggest a rather restricted view of moral subjectivity, in which the necessary and sufficient condition for evaluative competence is merely being capable of 'understanding' the nature and consequences of a decision. For Lonergan, the relevant competence is an evaluative one; this competence implies the presence of those 'sane affections' to which Chesterton alluded.

Another presupposition has to do with the relation between the cognitive issues of value judging and the decisional issues that follow such judgments. The distinction between cognitive and decisional issues sheds light on the view expressed in the euthanasia debate that the moral issues involve merely decisional factors, such as the particular means to death (euthanasia or assisted suicide), or how death is brought about (culpable active intervention or culpable non-intervention). The central moral issue in this debate, I would argue, is the judgment of whether a life under certain circumstances is worthwhile. However this question is answered, Lonergan would insist that the decisions regarding acts of euthanasia rest on evaluations, and that such evaluations are not made in isolation, as individualism supposes. Nor can others collaborate with someone's decision without becoming morally implicated, to some extent, in affirming the underpinning evaluation.

4   How the Discussion Will Proceed

In explaining Lonergan's position on the role of affectivity in value judgments, I will begin by attending to the concrete experiences and accounts of two persons with a terminal illness. I will follow this with an extended analysis of the role Lonergan thinks affect plays in evaluating. In the final part of the discussion I will revisit the two stories I began with and also focus on the related ethical and legal debate surrounding euthanasia, using that debate to illustrate some important ramifications of Lonergan's analysis for ethics. Although this analysis will draw on Lonergan's insights, I will base my own assessment of his insights in an account of what I take myself to be doing when knowing anything, and more specifically, when knowing values.

My assessment of Lonergan's view, then, will be based on my own auto-biographical self-description of how I actually make fact and value judgments. I am quite aware that this personal level of argumentation differs notably from what typically goes forward in philosophy, particularly among those who proceed in the analytic tradition of purely logical or linguistic analysis. Even so, I would contend that argumentation conducted at the personal level best attends to those subjective cognitive acts that underpin one's claims to knowledge, and that objections to this way of proceeding frequently presuppose the very notion of objectivity that I aim to challenge.

This procedure of attending to my own acts of knowing is unavoidable if I am to give a sincere explanation of how I come to affirm Lonergan's position. Although my affirmation, and Lonergan's justification of his own position, is essentially autobiographical, I do not insist that this account is the final word. Rather, I invite others to verify these findings in the laboratory of themselves. Post-classical Western philosophy has been criticized for paying insufficient attention to the traditional notion of philosophy as the 'love of wisdom.' Such a view of philosophy involved wedding a self-reflective understanding of oneself with one's practical concerns. My effort here is to operate in fidelity to this traditional notion of philosophy. Far from not doing 'real' philosophy, I will argue that some self-reflection and self-knowledge is crucial to the practical concerns of living a good life. This conjunction between theory and practice is another underlying theme pervading my entire discussion.[15]

As the recurring focus of the present discussion is the operation of value judging, and particularly the role of affect in such judgments, my approach to clarifying this role will be to follow the series of questions that Lonergan regards as the three basic questions for philosophy. In answering the phenomenological question, 'What am I doing when I am knowing anything?' the first of his three basic questions for philosophy, Lonergan articulates his cognitional theory, which is at the core of his philosophical contributions. He distinguishes and relates a series of four cognitive operations of experiencing, understanding, judging, and evaluating. Although I will focus in this discussion primarily on the last operation in this series, I will also need to address some of the prior operations in order to avoid distorting the account of the whole spontaneous process. This is precisely the sort of distortion I am arguing against.

Despite my focus on the role of affect in value judgments, I will also need to provide some account of Lonergan's answer to the two subsequent basic questions for philosophy, the *epistemological* and the *metaphysical* questions. Lonergan's answer to the epistemological question, 'How does doing this yield valid knowledge?' is important because it addresses a central concern about the status of one's knowledge of the good or values. A pivotal question for thinkers on both sides of this issue is whether evaluations that are based in part on feelings can be true or genuine. That is, if such feelings play a role in my value judgments, are these judgments therefore merely subjective? As previously mentioned, I shall argue that one's answer to the epistemological question not only shapes one's view of the epistemic status of moral knowledge generally, but also influences one's view of the role of feelings in value judgments.

Finally, I will briefly explore Lonergan's answer to the third basic question for philosophy, the metaphysical question, 'What do I know?' Here I will focus on Lonergan's view of the structure of the human good and on his stance on the value or moral status of human life. This is important because behind the euthanasia debate are opposing views on such meta-

physical issues as the grounds and absoluteness of moral norms, the relation between the individual and the social good, and the meaning or value
of human life in the context of suffering.

My argument will be structured into four parts and nine chapters.[16] In
the first part, I summarize the accounts that Sue Rodriguez and Dennis
Kaye give of their experience of the illness of ALS, and report opposing
views on the issue of euthanasia among ethicists and legislators.[17] The point
of beginning with the stories of Sue and Dennis is to highlight the relevance of feelings for their evaluations and decisions, which I take to be the
most fundamental level of debate. I will do this by concentrating on those
parts of their account of their illness in which feelings and evaluations are
especially prominent. By comparing their stories, I will draw out some of
the factors that influenced the different evaluations Sue and Dennis each
reached regarding whether their life with ALS was worthwhile, and if so, up
to what point. This contrast aims to shed light on some of the factors that
influence certain individuals to request assisted suicide. Another benefit of
comparing the stories of Sue and Dennis is that this comparison highlights
the fact that, despite the differing evaluations of their own lives with ALS,
they both demonstrated the sort of personal growth and communal contributions that one might achieve even in the context of an extremely debili-
tating illness. This prospect of growth and achievement at the end of life
underlines the very issue that I will be claiming is at the heart of the moral
debate about euthanasia. For both stories attest to the worthwhileness of
this phase of their lives, even in the midst of their losses and suffering.
Finally, concrete stories such as those of Sue and Dennis provide a context
from which ethical reflections and public-policy proposals can go forward,
and from which they can ultimately be assessed.[18]

In the second part, I outline the historical question of the relevance of
feelings for value judgments in the main Western philosophical traditions. I
sketch out some historically prominent views on the global issue of the
relevance of affectivity or *heart*, to value judgments. By means of this
historical review I hope to establish a connection between certain classic
philosophical positions and some of the more prominent contemporary
ethical theories. I also hope to show that Lonergan's position is located
firmly within the Aristotelian-Thomist tradition, and then indicate a number of important developments in this tradition, all of which provide a
context for understanding Lonergan's contributions.

Chapters 4, 5, 6, and 7 constitute part 3 of the discussion. In these
chapters I treat the distinct functions of *mind* and *heart*. The two chapters
on *mind*, and the following two chapters on *heart*, are structured to emphasize two related but distinct issues. In each case the initial discussion is of
the phenomenal activities of making fact or value judgments. This is fol-

lowed by a discussion of the epistemic status of these judgments. The core issue in part 3, however, is to provide an exposition and elucidation of Lonergan's position on the role of affect in evaluations.

I begin in chapter 4 with an explication of those cognitional operations that are prior and more evident, that is, fact judgments. I then proceed, in chapter 6, to analyse those cognitional operations that are subsequent and more difficult to express, that is, value judgments. Chapter 4 provides a phenomenal analysis of fact judgments. I attempt a self-descriptive reflection on my own cognitive performance as a physician who seeks to arrive at a diagnosis of the cause of someone's chest pain. In chapter 6 I extend this phenomenological analysis of a fact judgment that someone is having a heart attack, to provide a parallel, phenomenological analysis of a value judgment. As before, I proceed by self-descriptive reflection on my cognitive performance in evaluating the fact that someone is undergoing a life-threatening medical condition and deciding to implement certain actions. The point of both these analyses is to answer Lonergan's first question, 'What am I doing when I am knowing facts or values?' This will allow me to compare and contrast fact and value judgments and to distinguish clearly in each case the prior phenomenological issues (chapters 4 and 6) from the subsequent epistemological ones (chapters 5 and 7).

In chapter 5 I focus on Lonergan's account of the epistemic objectivity of fact judgments. In a parallel fashion, in chapter 7 I proceed from the conclusions of the phenomenological analysis of evaluations in chapter 6 to provide an exposition of Lonergan's epistemological analysis of these evaluations. In both cases, the question being addressed is 'How is doing whatever I say I am doing when knowing facts or values valid or epistemically objective?' My strategy here is to address this question by considering a variety of ways that I might fail to make epistemically objective fact or value judgments. Having presented Lonergan's account of the role of affect in evaluations in chapter 6, in chapter 7 I examine Lonergan's account of the objectivity of such evaluations. Moreover, in the final part of chapter 7 I provide a brief sketch of Lonergan's metaphysics of values, which he bases on his cognitional theory. There, I explain his view of the structure of the human good.

Chapters 8, 9, and 10 make up part 4 of this discussion. In chapter 8 I summarize Lonergan's answers to six core questions that regard his view of the role of affect in evaluations and indicate what results from this view. My aim here is to affirm critically Lonergan's core claims on the basis of my own self-description of making evaluations. I also respond to some important objections I anticipate others might raise in response to Lonergan's account.

In chapter 9 I return from the global philosophical question of the role of affect in evaluations to highlight some important ramifications of Lonergan's position for ethics, using the euthanasia debate as an illustration. My procedure is to compare and contrast what I take to be the positions of Sue Rodriguez and Dennis Kaye on six core questions that I posed with respect to Lonergan's position in chapter 8. I make similar comparisons and contrasts of opposing positions on the ethical and public-policy levels of the debate. This allows me to compare the philosophical grounds of these positions with Lonergan's. It will also allow me to distinguish their philosophical positions from their stances on what I would call an empirical issue. Finally, I hope to illustrate by means of these comparisons the frequently overlooked philosophical basis for the differences among disputants and to highlight the need for greater attention to concrete stories by disputants operating on subsequent levels of the debate.

Chapter 10 concludes the discussion. In this chapter, I articulate my own response to the euthanasia question. Besides contrasting positions on the basis of the philosophical stance Lonergan has articulated, and judging the debate on these grounds, this chapter includes a proposal for a comprehensive research program to address the necessary empirical issues that arise in this debate but which are not currently being addressed in a systematic or coordinated manner. I take this proposal, which focuses on distinct questions that need to be related, as a further and very important ramification of Lonergan's position for the euthanasia debate. Finally, I conclude the discussion on a more personal note with some reflections on Lonergan's contributions to my own self-understanding, mentioning in particular how his account of the role that affect plays in evaluations has heightened my awareness of the moral importance of my own affectivity and how this has enhanced my performance both as a physician and as an ethicist.

5   Why Lonergan?

Since some readers may be unfamiliar with the works of Bernard Lonergan (1904–1984), a few words of introduction and justification for drawing on him in this discussion are in order.[19] A philosopher, theologian, and methodologist, Lonergan has been described as 'a brilliant and original thinker of the highest rank.'[20] He was a professor at the Gregorian University, Rome (1953–65), Harvard (1971–72), and Boston College (1975–83). His honours include some twenty-one honorary doctorates, Companion of the Order of Canada, and Fellow of the British Academy. His legacy includes the establishment of ten Lonergan Research Centres around the world by the time of his death, and a commitment by the University of Toronto Press to publish over twenty volumes of his Collected Works and a companion series on applications of his work in various fields. A further indicator of the growing interest in his work is the number of translations of his works. Both of Lonergan's major works, *Insight: A Study of Human Understanding* (originally published in 1957) and *Method in Theology* (1972), have been translated into a number of different languages, including French, German, Italian, Spanish, and Polish. Furthermore, in 1995 Frederick Crowe, the past director of the Lonergan Research Institute in Toronto, reported that various articles have been translated and published in languages which include Japanese, Chinese, Danish, and Flemish. A further barometer of the interest in Lonergan's work among the next generation of scholars is suggested by the fact that over 200 doctoral dissertations have been completed on Lonergan's thought and works.

There are a number of reasons why I have chosen to explore Lonergan's philosophy on the question of the relation between affect and values. I will mention three.

The first has to do with Lonergan himself. I agree with William Fennell's assessment that Lonergan was a 'brilliant and original thinker.' Paradoxically, what I find most 'brilliant' about his work is the simplicity of his core insights on human knowing in general, which have a unifying effect on the whole of his life's work. And what I find most fascinating about the 'originality' of his work is the fact that he himself did not consider his core contributions to be original. Rather, he understands himself to be providing a contemporary expression and application of a long tradition of thought that proceeds from Aristotle, through Thomas Aquinas, to modern times.[21]

The second reason has to do with Lonergan's own shift on the issue of the relation between affect and value judgments. During the earlier phase of his career, Lonergan's cognitional theory can aptly be described as 'intellectualist.' In the later phase, he expressly incorporated affectivity into this cognitional theory and understood it to play a crucial role in apprehending values. As dramatic as this shift might appear, there is an important continuity between the positions of the earlier and later Lonergan, for in both phases he maintains an objectivist theory of values. This makes Lonergan an especially helpful thinker to explore on the issue of the relation of affect and value judgments, since he held in tension in himself the concerns of thinkers on both sides of the question. For those thinkers who want to articulate a theory of values that is consistent with their own moral experience, Lonergan agrees that affectivity is relevant to this experience. For those thinkers who are concerned to defend reason against the view that the achievements of moral deliberations are merely subjective, Lonergan also insists with them on the importance of employing 'right reason' in order to know epistemically objective values.

The third reason for my use of Lonergan has to do with his relevance to the concerns and issues of contemporary bioethicists engaging in discussions concerned with the nature of bioethics itself as a normative discipline. In the seminar series at the University of Toronto, which was subsequently published as *Philosophical Perspectives on Bioethics*, a broad range of contemporary bioethicists addressed the particularist/generalist issue. A pivotal question in that discussion was the extent to which general ethical claims, such as principles or normative theories, are either necessary or useful for resolving problems in bioethics (e.g., Tom Beauchamp's principles of autonomy, beneficence, non-maleficence, and justice). An alternative model proposed was to begin instead with particular cases and work toward identifying similarities among such cases as a basis for generalizing particular conclusions. A conclusion that the editors of the proceedings drew from this series was that 'the hard-line generalist or particularist is nowadays a largely mythical creature (or caricature). The question remains whether the generalist/particularist distinction is any longer a useful analytical device for identifying basic methodological differences.'[22]

In addition, the editors pointed out that despite their effort to invite participants who would represent the range of views in bioethics, 'nearly all [of them] reject foundationalism in favor of a version of reflective equilibrium.'[23] In light of this discussion about the nature of bioethics, I hope to employ Lonergan's thought to offer bioethicists a more useful analytic device for identifying basic methodological differences among contemporary positions. And one consequence of Lonergan's analysis will be to highlight the methodological significance of certain 'foundationalist' alternatives that Lonergan's own analysis would partly support, such as that of R.M. Hare.[24]

6   Scope of the Discussion and Its Envisaged Audience

The context and scope of the present discussion is suggested by Bertrand Russell's disjunction between intellectual and moral defects, and especially by his consequent insistence that philosophers can only address intellectual deficiencies with any efficacy:

> The evils of the world are due to moral defects quite as much as to lack of intelligence. But the human race has not hitherto discovered any method of eradicating moral defects ... Intelligence, on the contrary, is easily improved by methods known to every competent educator. Therefore, until some method of teaching virtue has been discovered, progress will have to be sought by improvement of intelligence rather than morals.[25]

My aim here is to begin to explore those specifically 'moral' defects to which Russell refers, namely, those cognitive errors arising in value judging that stem from the role of affect. This would be a far too grand undertaking unless I put strict limitations on what I will here attempt to achieve. In order for me to avoid disappointing certain expectations that readers might bring to this topic, then, it is necessary that I be clear about what I will not do, about what lies beyond the scope of the discussion, and about where and to what extent I will need to rely on other sources without attempting to defend those sources myself.

As mentioned previously, I begin my discussion of the euthanasia and assisted-suicide debate by reviewing Sue Rodriguez's case. I have taken the bulk of this information from her own account of her experience, as related in a book she co-authored with Lisa Hobbs Birnie. Although I have no reason to suspect that her public account of her experience (or, for that matter, Dennis Kaye's account of his experience) is at odds with the facts, I take no responsibility for the veracity of these accounts. In fact, I concede the possibility that other materials might come to light that will cast into question their versions of the events.[26]

Another difficulty of beginning with an analysis of the stories of Sue and Dennis is to connect this analysis with the larger public-policy debate on euthanasia. I will avoid attempting to generalize the conclusions of my analysis of these two cases to the policy debate on euthanasia.[27] And in order to keep my focus on the global philosophical issues, I will also avoid entering into a number of issues that are also relevant to the public-policy questions that the euthanasia debate raises. For instance, there are other important and revealing cases that have arisen in the Canadian context that I omit to discuss, such as the involuntary euthanasia of Tracy Latimer.[28] There is also a large collection of psychological, medical, and legal litera-ture that relates to euthanasia. Because my focus is on the ethical and philosophical issues connected with euthanasia, I do not discuss this body of literature. This was a particularly difficult omission in the case of the important research that has been done in palliative care, which is one of my personal interests and which originally motivated me to study the issue of euthanasia. Again, my main goal in addressing the euthanasia debate is merely to highlight some aspects of this debate for which Lonergan's account of moral knowing is relevant, in particular his stance on the role of affect in value judgments.

As regards locating Lonergan's position on the relation of affect to values in the history of Western thought, which I attempt in chapter 3, I make no claim to be offering a novel historical interpretation. Rather, I will rely mainly on standard historical accounts of the various thinkers and issues with whom I deal. What is perhaps somewhat novel is my grouping of thinkers according to what I take to be their presupposed views of knowing. Nor does this survey pretend to be exhaustive. My main aim is merely to locate Lonergan's position within a historical tradition of thought, to contrast this tradition with some noteworthy alternatives, and to suggest some connections between stances on this global philosophical issue and some prominent contemporary ethical theories.

Finally, I take responsibility for three key moves in the discussion: first, for analyzing the accounts of Sue Rodriguez and Dennis Kaye of their illness experience; second, for illustrating Lonergan's position on knowing facts and values in an extended analysis of a medical example; third, for sketching some ramifications of Lonergan's account of fact and value judgments for the euthanasia debate. As for the main lines of the interpretation of the later Lonergan's position that I will be illustrating and applying, I am most indebted to Michael Vertin. His interpretation of Lonergan's mature position on the role of feelings in value judgments does justice, I think, to what the later Lonergan wrote and said on this issue. Vertin's interpretation also emphasizes, correctly I think, the substantial continuity between the earlier and the later Lonergan's position. In his own published work on this issue, Vertin also adds some terminological clarifications to Lonergan's accounts and suggests certain terms that Lonergan himself did not use, such as 'deliberative' insight and 'transcendental affectivity.' I will employ Vertin's terminological suggestions and notional clarifications when I judge them to foster clarity of expression. I take no credit for these terms myself, nor do I want to give the reader the impression that I think Lonergan used this terminology or that Vertin's interpretation of Lonergan is the final word among Lonergan scholars.

The main audience to whom I address the present discussion is my philosophical colleagues. I am particularly concerned to address certain meta-ethical issues, such as those that the group that attended the previously mentioned seminar series on 'Philosophical Perspectives in Bioethics' addressed. Key issues of concern to this group include identifying important and fundamental methodological differences among thinkers. I wish to address this issue by offering Lonergan's views as providing analytical tools for identifying and critiquing methodologically distinct positions and thinkers. Lonergan also illustrates a foundationalist position that challenges the majority non-foundationalist views of contemporary bioethicists. The chapters that will be of greatest interest to this group, I think, are chapters 3, 4, 5, 6, 7, and 8. In addition, I wish to challenge this group of philosophers with a medical analysis of some of the complexity of particular cases that one commonly encounters in medicine. Chapter 2 reports some of the complexities associated with the stories of Sue Rodriguez and Dennis Kaye, and chapters 9 and 10 illustrate how I think a philosophical analysis can bring to light cognitive and decisional issues that are frequently over-looked by non-philosophical analyses.[29]

Another audience that I hope to address is medical practitioners. These are the persons who, at the end of the day, will be charged with the primary responsibility of helping those for whom they care to make prudent and responsible judgments and decisions.[30] An important advantage that this group has is extensive experience and facility at making practical judgments. This, I think, is an ideal starting point for philosophy. My concern is to acknowledge some of the philosophical complexity of the judgments they routinely make and to affirm their practical cognitional and decisional skills in this area. But I also want to challenge them to reflect on some of the philosophical stances on knowing that their own performance presupposes. On this basis, I want to help them discover something that Lonergan's thought has helped me to clarify, namely, what it means to be a knower and a responsible caregiver. By bringing philosophy to bear in a concrete way on their own medical knowing and performance, I hope to make philosophical and ethical issues much more concrete and relevant to caregivers. In turn, these same caregivers will then be in a better position to facilitate the deliberations of others in their care.[31] For the sake of this audience, I have tried in chapters 4 to 7 to provide an exposition of Lonergan's philosophy by illustrating it in terms of common medical judgments, evaluations, and decisions. For those readers who are interested primarily in the practical ramifications of Lonergan's philosophical contributions for the euthanasia debate, however, it would be sufficient for them to read chapters 2, 8, 9, and 10.

The third audience I hope to address is members of the public who have no specialized knowledge of medicine or philosophy. I realize that much of the discussion may require some familiarity with the specialized terminology and notions of medicine and philosophy. Still, I think that this 'intellectual' disadvantage is overcome when the discussion turns to the central issue of 'feelings.' On this issue, I have found members of this third audience to be most receptive to my argument, even to the point where they are surprised that anyone seriously doubts the cognitive function of feelings.

The discussion, then, can be read as an introduction into some of the main features of Bernard Lonergan's thought. It can also be read as a framework for rethinking the euthanasia issue on the basis of a critical affirmation of the role that feelings play in evaluations. Finally, it can be read as an illustration of one possible model for the interdisciplinary specialty of bioethics, one that is capable of bringing the insights of philosophy to the practical questions of medicine and also of learning from that interchange.

PART ONE

The Relevance of Emotions to the Euthanasia Debate

Affective Elements of
Two End-of-Life Stories
and the Euthanasia Debate

The disinterestedness of morality is fully compatible with the passionateness of being. For that passionateness has a dimension all its own: it underpins and accompanies and reaches beyond the subject as experientially, intelligently, rationally, morally conscious ... As it underpins, so too it accompanies the subject's conscious and intentional operations. There it is the mass and momentum of our lives, the color and tone and power of feeling, that fleshes out and gives substance to what would otherwise be no more than a Shakespearian 'pale cast of thought.'

Bernard Lonergan, 'Mission and the Spirit' (*A Third Collection*)

1   Dying in North America at the End of the Twentieth Century

At the heart of the euthanasia debate are stories of particular individuals who have personally faced the question of whether they should intentionally end their lives by some active means, that is, by some form of active voluntary euthanasia. My hypothesis is that a key insight into different conclusions persons might reach on the personal question of euthanasia is that those conclusions are correlated with differences regarding the affective elements that underpin them. Moreover, I will argue later that the divided public view of this matter also, at least in part, correlates with different views regarding the relevance and role of affectivity in value judgments generally.[1]

The goal of this chapter is to examine the relevance and role of affectivity in value judgments by focusing on the stories of Sue Rodriguez and Dennis Kaye. Their stories are helpful because in each case the question of euthanasia was a personal one for them that arose in the context of their experience of a terminal neurological illness known as amyotrophic lateral sclerosis. I will attend to those elements of their stories that enable one to understand better how a person experiences an illness, and how this experience conditions his or her medical and moral judgments. I will focus on the affective elements that enter into their evaluations of euthanasia, particularly feeling responses of anger, fear, and hope. Sue's experience will be explored first; I will then juxtapose her experience with Dennis's experience of the same illness. Before focusing on these two stories, however, I shall attempt to locate them within the broader Canadian and North American context of caring for dying patients.

1.1 Images of the Modern Medical Context of Dying

In September 1991 Bill Wenman, MP, introduced Bill C-203 to the Canadian legislature in the hope of redressing some of the problems of those Canadians who die in the modern medical context. The image he painted of such a death was certainly disturbing, as he spoke of people 'dying connected to machines and strapped to their hospital bed, rotting and suffering until all or most of their body parts are gone.'[2] The aim of his proposed act was to amend the Canadian Criminal Code in favour of allowing physicians intentionally to end a patient's life.

In order to begin to explore the prudence of such legislative initiatives, I need to locate some key issues for those who are dying in the current Canadian and North American medical and social context. In particular, the questions I need to address here include: Who are the dying in Canada and similarly developed countries? What sort of symptoms or reasons might lead persons who are dying to request euthanasia? How effective are caregivers and the medical system at responding to their needs?

According to Statistics Canada, roughly 215,700 individuals die each year in Canada, which is about one-half the annual Canadian birth rate, and one-tenth the number of annual deaths in the United States. In a report entitled *Good Care of the Dying Patient*, the Council on Scientific Affairs of the American Medical Association reviewed what is known about who the dying are in America, and how the American health-care system actually serves persons who are dying.[3] Many of the council's findings are applicable to the Canadian situation. Like our American counterparts, Canadians typically die in their seventies. In contrast to the pattern of dying at the turn of the century, when most North Americans died at home, most now die in hospitals, although the actual rates are not known. The illnesses that shape the dying experience now are mostly degenerative diseases, such as cancer, heart and vascular disease, other organ failures, and central nervous system dysfunctions.[4] Since our populations are aging, there is an increasing incidence of these diseases. The time course of these diseases is usually many years from onset to death, but again there is inadequate knowledge about the actual course of particular diseases and the intermediate markers that could signal progression. The concerns and needs of persons will vary, depending on factors such as the type of illness one is facing, one's stage in the life cycle, and one's personal, social, and spiritual resources.[5]

How frequent are persistent preferences for illegal forms of assisted suicide, and what are some symptoms of dying that might lead one to consider suicide? To put this discussion in context, it is worth noting that suicides represent about 4–5 per cent of all deaths in Canada, or about 3700 individuals. Among Americans between 11 and 24 years of age, suicides are the third leading cause of death, following motor-vehicle-related and other unintentional injuries, and then homicides.[6]

Among persons with a terminal illness such as cancer, some experts have reported that persistent requests for assisted suicide in the context of supportive systems of excellent care are rare (e.g., under 0.2% and 5%).[7] In a Canadian study of the desire for death among terminally ill patients, about 8.5 per cent (17 of 200 individuals) reported an apparent sincere wish to die. When 6 of the 17 patients who expressed a wish for death were reviewed two weeks later, in 4 cases the desire to die had decreased. These initial findings are comparable with 1995 figures in the Netherlands, where about 6–7 per cent of patients with advanced cancer eventually choose to die with physician assistance.[8]

The kind of case that has captured public attention as providing reasons for making assistance in dying legal include those with severe pain or other physical suffering, weariness of life, the absence of a sense of self-worth when not productive, and a desire not to burden family members.[9] In the previously mentioned Canadian study, the main factors that correlated best with the desire for death were depression, pain, and a low level of family support.[10] Other studies report additional reasons for requesting euthanasia and assisted suicide, such as a desire to maintain personal control, fear of being dependent on others, and concerns about being a burden to loved ones.[11] Hence, the majority of those with a terminal illness desire to carry on with life. Although many terminally ill patients experience a transient desire for death, a small number do have a persistent desire for death. Among the latter patients, some of the main reasons behind this desire, such as depression, poorly controlled pain, and a lack of social supports, represent needs that could potentially be met by caregivers.

A further question is how well these needs are currently being met. One assessment of the effectiveness of the Canadian health-care system in responding to the needs of the dying has come from a Special Senate Committee report on this issue.[12] The committee noted that although expertise in palliative care has been developing in Canada since 1975, 'the demand for palliative care is still greater than available services.'[13] Consequently, the committee recommended that the needs of dying patients could be better met by making palliative-care programs and training in pain control a top priority in the restructuring of the health-care system.[14]

1.2 Diverse Psychological Responses to the Experience of Dying

When speaking of the effectiveness of those who provide care for the dying, it is important to be mindful of the differing psychological patient responses to dying that might influence the effectiveness of care. For instance, Harvey Chochinov's study helpfully contrasts two patients who were identified as having a persistent desire for death. One patient was a seventy-two-year-old married man with prostate cancer who indicated that he was in severe pain. He met the diagnostic criteria for a major depressive illness and had a past history of depression. In addition, his wife had herself recently been diagnosed with a major illness that prevented her from visiting. The authors report that this man frequently prayed that his suffering would end by death, and that he was the only patient in the study to request euthanasia. The symptoms of pain, depression, and lack of social supports that underpinned this man's request for euthanasia are all issues that effective palliative care could successfully address.

The other case of a persistent desire for death that Chochinov identified in his study presents challenges that might well have exceeded the goals of symptom control that is the mandate of palliative care. This involved a married woman aged sixty-one years who had lung cancer. She had good palliative symptom control and experienced no pain. She was not depressed and had no psychiatric history of depression or other psychiatric disorders. Her desire for death was in the context of the recognition that her life was coming to an end. She hoped to die while she still remained mentally competent, with reasonable bodily control, and what she thought was an acceptable level of dignity.

The authors suggest that these two cases could help frame the terms of reference for the euthanasia debate. They do not dispute the claim that good palliative care can ameliorate the symptoms that most commonly distress dying persons, such as fear of pain, loss of control, indignity, and being a burden to one's family.[15] Still, these authors speculate that even the best system of palliative care will probably not meet everyone's needs. This is because there will always be some patients who, though psychologically stable, will nevertheless be determined to end their struggle with a terminal illness through euthanasia.[16]

2   Sue Rodriguez's Story

Sue Rodriguez's public life as an advocate of physician-assisted suicide began with her request to the Supreme Court of British Columbia that the law allow her the right to enlist the aid of a physician to assist her to commit suicide at a time of her choosing. She made this request as a forty-two-year-old recently separated mother with a seven-year-old son. Eight months prior to this request she had been told that she had a paralysing terminal illness called amyotrophic lateral sclerosis (ALS). With the aid of an unnamed physician, she carried out her plan to commit suicide roughly two years later. Behind Sue's decision to commit suicide lay a number of significant personal and historical issues that provide insight into the context and basis of her judgment. I will now sketch some of these issues.[17]

One important issue that sets the context of Sue's affective life and response to the stresses of her illness concerns her social attachments. I will sketch some features of Sue's story that provide glimpses of difficulties she experienced in forming attachments and being included in her community at various stages of her life. These include experiences in her family of origin (e.g., emotionally unavailable parents), childhood and adolescent tendencies of rejecting others (e.g., her sense of privilege and superiority), and also experiences of alienation and social isolation (e.g., her teenage rebellious behaviour toward her parents, which resulted in her parents sending her to a boarding school). Sue's early life was also punctuated by some significant losses (e.g., the death of her father when she was a teenager). These themes of attachment and social inclusion continued to set the context for many of Sue's adult relationships. So, although the focus of Sue's request was legal and political, I will be attending here more to the human, contextual elements that illustrate the relevance of her affective responses to her evaluations and decisions.

For most Canadians, Sue Rodriguez is remembered as the woman who 'almost succeeded in persuading the Supreme Court [of Canada] to strike down as unconstitutional the law against assisted suicide.'[18] Also, following the Supreme Court decision, the issues that Sue's case raised led to the appointment, in February 1994, of a Special Senate Committee charged by the Canadian parliament to 'examine and report upon the legal, social, and ethical issues relating to euthanasia and assisted suicide.'[19] After more than one year of deliberations, this committee forwarded a series of recommendations to Parliament. This Senate committee report was, in part, a response to Sue Rodriguez's request for physician-assisted suicide. Still, the committee's own deliberations, as well as those of the lower courts that

heard her case, avoided any exploration of Sue's experiences and deliberations that might have led to her request.[20]

One recommendation that the Senate committee did make was that
more research be done to understand why persons request euthanasia.
Since Sue's death, Lisa Hobbs Birnie has published a book, co-authored by
Sue, that provides some insight into Sue's personal and affective life. One
purpose of the book is to help others understand better Sue's request for
physician-assisted suicide. It does this by offering some glimpses into the
emotional road that Sue travelled, and so gives us a sense of the context of
her end-of-life decisions. Drawing on this text, I will begin by highlighting
some important affective features of Sue's story. Then, in the next section,
I will compare Sue's affective story with that of Dennis Kaye, another
Canadian with ALS who also published a book to help us understand better
the emotional road that persons with ALS travel.[21]

2.1 Medical and Legal Facts of Sue Rodriguez's Story

When Sue Rodriguez submitted her request for physician-assisted suicide to
the courts, she had been experiencing, over a period of several months, a
progressive loss of her ability to move. This had reached a point where she
was unable to walk, feed herself, or care for herself without assistance. Sue's
physicians had already diagnosed her condition as amyotrophic lateral
sclerosis, a fatal degenerative neurological disease affecting the motor
neurons of the brain and spinal cord. At the time of her application to the
courts for the right to physician-assisted suicide, Sue's physicians expected
her to live for another two to twelve months. This fact added some urgency
to the legal deliberations.

Medical experts described the terminal phase of this disease to the
British Columbia courts as follows:

> [I]n ALS, these nerve cells die in an inexorably progressive fashion.
> As the nerve cells die, the muscle units controlled by these cells
> weaken and shrink or atrophy. Other parts of the brain system, such
> as those governing sensation and intellectual abilities, are not affected
> by this disease ... Terminally, these patients are likely to be completely
> paralysed in all of their limbs, and they become unable to support
> even the weight of their head. They must be suctioned for secretions
> and they become dependent on assistance from caregivers to turn
> and move them to prevent pressure sores. They also require help in
> managing their urinary and bowel care. Often, they require tubes in
> to their stomach for feeding and tracheostomy tubes for breathing.
> Eventually, breathing machines or respirators are required.[22]

Soon after attending a meeting with other ALS patients, many of whom were at more advanced stages of the illness, Sue decided that a time would come when her life would no longer be joyful. Thinking ahead to this point, Sue projected that she would prefer to die quickly and painlessly by means of physician-assisted suicide. She asserted that only such a death would allow her to die with her dignity and spirit intact.[23] Knowing that counselling suicide is a criminal offence under subsection 241(a) of the Criminal Code, she realized that anyone who helped her could face legal difficulties for assisting in her suicide, including a maximum penalty of imprisonment for up to fourteen years. To avoid these legal complications she would need either to commit suicide unaided or to change the law. To commit suicide without assistance was an unattractive prospect to Sue, because she would have to act before she became too physically incapacitated by her illness, that is, at a stage when she might still be enjoying her life and not wish to end it.

In May of 1993, twenty-one months following her diagnosis, Sue asked the Supreme Court of Canada to allow her physician-assisted suicide. Her plan was to instruct a physician to connect her to a lethal dose of drugs to be infused into a vein on her request. A panel of nine judges deliberated about her request for four months. On 30 September 1993, a majority of five judges voted against permitting her physician-assisted suicide. This decision supported a lower-court ruling that 'the state's interest in protecting life's sanctity takes precedence over the right to a dignified death.'[24]

In the end, Sue not only challenged the law by taking her case to the Supreme Court of Canada; she also carried out her plan, despite the court's ruling. On 12 February 1994, almost three and a half years after her diagnosis, Sue died by physician-assisted suicide. Legal authorities failed to identify the physician who aided her suicide, and that person has escaped any legal scrutiny or sanctions. Hence, although Sue was unsuccessful in changing the law on physician-assisted suicide, she did win much public support for her position, and she carried out her original plan of dying in the manner and at the time of her choosing, unimpeded by legal sanctions.[25]

In their book titled *Uncommon Will: The Death and Life of Sue Rodriguez,* co-authors Lisa Hobbs Burnie and Sue Rodriguez chronicle some of the key events, thoughts, and feelings in Sue's life. From the first chapter, they point out a number of affective themes in Sue's personal and family life that conditioned her experience of, or response to, her illness. The most prominent emotion in Sue's story, for instance, was her anger toward others. Related to this anger was a life-long pattern of critical and controlling behaviour that undermined many of her relationships, so that, in the end, Sue was involved in no long-term, intimate relationships. Although these feelings seem to have been relevant to her value judgments, whether in fact they were relevant and precisely what role they played in Sue's deliberations are philosophical issues that I will pursue in chapter 9. Here, I will merely highlight some affective elements of Sue's end-of-life experience and deliberations, namely her feelings of anger and fear.[26]

2.2 From Alienation to Anger

One account of Sue's affective life comes from her psychotherapist, Dr Sandra Elder. Elder, a PhD in psychology, was working as a registered grief counsellor with the Association for Death Education when she met Sue. Hobbs Birnie recommends Elder in her book as the person who was better able to understand Sue's emotional state than anyone else. It is somewhat surprising to learn that, in Elder's assessment, anger was central to Sue's personality:

> Sue had an aching soul, and never had internal peace. She wouldn't let love in, and when you are starved for love, you sabotage any attempts people make to give it to you. There's a sort of attitude: love me, leave me alone. If you love, you can forgive and let go of the anger. I can say goodbye without a terrible resentment. But anger was Sue's foundation. Her identity was based on it.[27]

Sue knew that Elder would portray her as a deeply angry woman because they had discussed this theme on several occasions. Nevertheless, Sue insisted that Hobbs Birnie include an interview with Elder in her biography. When Hobbes Birnie asked Elder why she thought Sue had insisted on including an interview with her in her book, Elder replied:

> All I know is that Sue wanted me to talk to you [Hobbes Birnie], and she must have known what I would say, because we had discussed these matters together. Perhaps she felt a total picture should come out. She was a very honest and courageous woman. She was not afraid of the truth or of reality. Perhaps she felt, as I do, that her accomplishments were of such significance that the rest paled beside it.[28]

Examples of this anger were evident in Sue's relations with her caregivers at the time of her diagnosis. She described the physicians who performed her initial investigations as leaving her without 'any idea of what was going on,' and hence she felt totally unprepared for the bad news.[29] Sue's ALS specialist, Dr Andrew Eisen, who first told her of her diagnosis, also sensed her anger at the time.[30] In a televised interview a year later, Sue characterized Eisen as cold and insensitive. Recalling the events at the time of her diagnosis, she described the responses of her physicians and nurses as 'awkward,' 'embarrassed,' and 'lacking in kindness.' She recalled, for example, that no one attempted to speak to her, hold her, or comfort her. Moreover, Sue concluded that Eisen was 'indifferent' to her fate and 'unaware or unconcerned' about her safety. This was because Eisen did not raise any concerns about the risks to Sue's safety when she told him, shortly after learning about her diagnosis, that she was leaving hospital.[31] Sue also generalized her anger beyond those who told her the bad news of her diagnosis. Anger had also permeated her relationships with family members from the time she was young. Hobbs Birnie concludes that, to the end, Sue remained bitter toward her husband and distant from her siblings.[32]

Two people who escaped Sue's anger were her grandparents. It was largely their influence that shaped her early development and attitudes. Sue's maiden name was Shipley; she was a descendant of Adam Shipley of Yorkshire, England, who landed in Annapolis, Maryland, in 1688. The Shipleys were one of America's founding families, a fact of which Sue was deeply proud. She was especially proud of her paternal grandparents, Howard and Virginia Shipley. Howard was a wealthy man, educated at the Virginia Military Institute (to which he left his large estate following his death).[33] Sue describes her grandmother, Virginia (Gigi), as 'an elegant, articulate and slightly eccentric woman who lived life to the hilt.'[34] Howard's holdings included the Canadian Ice Machine Company, a refrigeration and air-conditioning supplier located in Toronto. Both Sue's father, Tom, and her uncle worked for Howard Shipley's company. The Shipley's family motto reads: 'My soul is not content with quiet idleness.' When Sue discovered the family motto sometime during her struggles with the paralysing effects of ALS, she was struck by the irony that the motto of her unknown ancestors so well expressed her own sentiments.[35]

Howard Shipley's one visible 'soft spot,' apart from his wife Gigi, was his 'spunky, long-limbed granddaughter' Sue. Of him, Sue recalls: 'I loved my grandfather. There was nobody like him. I was the only one who could see through his facade. He had a very sweet side which he didn't show to everyone ... I valued him, although he was a hard one to understand and I don't accept the way he treated his family.'[36] Of Gigi, Sue reports: 'She was my mentor, teaching me the importance of reading, of grooming myself physically and mentally. She was an inspirational person for me, very clever, in control but she had to do it cleverly. When grandfather criticized his own children, she took part in it, she sided with him.'[37]

Sue was the second of five children born over a period of ten years. She believed that she had a privileged childhood. Sue and her sisters were given a variety of 'extras' from her wealthy grandparents: expensive summer camps, dancing lessons, piano lessons. Sue said that these extras, and the annual trip to the family's summer cottage (owned, incidentally, not by her own father, but by Howard), added to a feeling that she already had 'of being different and somehow "special."'[38]

In her biography, Sue relates three incidents that occurred during her childhood that help to explain the anger Elder saw as foundational to her personality. The first incident involved an intergenerational conflict between Sue's parents and her wealthy and controlling grandparents.

On Sue's thirteenth birthday, her family was gathered at their lakeside cottage. Sue's father, Tom senior, had organized a local regatta. During the day, Tom Sr became intoxicated on alcohol (four years later he died of alcohol-induced cirrhosis of the liver). When he returned home late and found Sue and her younger brother, Tom Jr, still running around outside, he became angry at them. Tom Sr subsequently scolded Sue and Tom Jr and sent them to bed. But instead of obeying their father, Sue and Tom Jr rowed across the lake to their grandparents' cottage. Howard and Gigi supported Sue and Tom Jr's rebellion against their parents and kept them for two weeks, despite protests from Sue's parents. Recalling this event, Sue reports: 'We'd hidden in the bushes. I didn't know what I'd done wrong when father scolded me. My feelings were hurt. It was my birthday and I'd gotten no attention because of the regatta. So we rowed over to my grandparents. That started a quarrel between my parents and grandparents and it was decided we'd stay.'[39]

Although Sue saw that her grandparents controlled the family, and sided with them against her parents, her grandparents did not consistently support and include Sue or her siblings in their busy lives. As her mother recalled this event, Howard and Gigi returned Tom and Sue to their parents two weeks later because 'they grew tired of having them around.'[40]

The second incident occurred when Sue was fifteen. By this time she had become a rebellious teenager. She shocked her parents by experimenting with marijuana. Following this discovery, Sue's grandparents financed sending her to a Mennonite boarding school in a different city. The aim of this move was to address Sue's misbehaviour by keeping her 'out of trouble' and enable her to develop better study habits. Sue resented this move to her dying day. She describes that year as follows: 'It turned out there wasn't room for me to live at the school so I was boarded out with a private family. Their living style was not at all what I was used to. I spent my entire time begging my parents to let me come home.'[41]

It was during these turbulent and vulnerable adolescent years, when Sue was seventeen, that her father died. Although her memories of her grandfather remained vivid and powerful to the end of Sue's life, Hobbes Birnie reports that those of her own father were 'gray and tenuous.'[42] Tom Sr had been sick for a year; weak, wasted, and dependent on others. As he grew more ill, he moved out of his home and returned to his mother, Gigi, to be nursed by her and to die. This was apparently done by the family for two reasons, to 'spare the family suffering, ... [and because] Gigi was more of a caregiver [than Sue's mother Dorothea].' Sue recalled to Hobbs Birnie frightful images of her father 'reduced to skin and bones, coughing up blood, with sorrow in his eyes.'[43] Sue later admitted that the feelings these images evoked in her, feelings which affected her when she faced the prospect of living with ALS, also shaped her thinking about her own dying. Sue maintained that it was not the fact of her father's death that most affected her; rather, it was 'his dying.' Repeatedly, Sue recalled to Hobbes Birnie: 'it was the memories of his illness that preceded [his death] and the embarrassment of everyone's staring at her at his funeral.'[44]

Sue's mother and siblings add a qualifying perspective to Sue's memories and evaluations, especially concerning the effect of Sue's grandparents on the family. Sue's mother Dorothea, or Doe, recalls, for example, feeling resentful and demeaned by the way Howard and Gigi controlled her adult children's lives: 'It was horrible. Tom was belittled and I was powerless. His parents controlled their entire family with their money. They'd cut us out of the will if we didn't do this, or wouldn't do that. Tom's father was a tyrant, a bitter man, very conscious of his money. Sue saw a different side, her relationship was special. She loved him.'[45]

Like his mother, Tom Jr, Sue's younger sibling by fourteen months (and the only family member to keep in regular touch with Sue from the onset of her illness), also describes his grandparents in negative terms:

> Our grandparents wanted to raise us. My grandfather would stomp on people to get what he wanted. Sue had the qualities of both my grandparents except she was gentle and smooth at the same time ... I don't want to blame everything on my grandfather and grandmother but they certainly had a long-term effect on my family.[46]

Sue's anger, then, becomes a somewhat more understandable part of her character given even this brief sketch of some of the alienation from others she suffered as a child. This was due, in part, to the intergenerational family conflicts between her parents and grandparents, which left her with a sense of disdain toward her own parents, whom she perceived as losers. Added to this was the episodic nature of her grandparents' nurturing, which undermined many of her childhood attachments and relationships. Being the 'favourite' of her wealthy grandparents, Sue grew up feeling 'special,' and she received many of the material benefits of the Shipley family. But Sue also experienced the dark side of her family, particularly regarding control and boundary issues, which were made worse by the conflicts between her parents and grandparents and her father's alcoholism.[47] This context shaped Sue's affective development. Although she developed many strengths by modelling herself after her grandparents, this conflict, which arguably alienated her from her parents and siblings, was something she never overcame nor, probably, ever understood. Besides her responses of anger, which became even more apparent in the context of her experience of ALS, her responses of fear, over such things as a lack of control, also seem to have been relevant to her end-of-life conclusions. I will now trace the shift in Sue's responses to her illness from a period of hopeful vulnerability to one of despair.

2.3 From Vulnerability to Despair

One might expect fear to be part of anyone's response to a terminal illness. But it might not be immediately apparent what it is that one fears. In Sue's case, she describes the fear that ALS would rob her of the qualities of her life that she most treasured: her beauty, physical prowess, independence, and ability to communicate.[48] She especially dreaded losing control over her life, which would be signified by losing the ability to speak. In fact, the prospect of being unable to communicate by speaking so distressed her that she decided that when she lost her ability to speak, she would kill herself. But what becomes evident on reading Sue's story is that in the end these physical losses were less troublesome to her than the human losses she suffered.[49]

Sue initially expressed her desire for 'self-deliverance' as a response to the physical and aesthetic losses that she anticipated would occur as the ALS progressed. Her fear of these losses with the progress of ALS spurred her efforts to find a cure. When the practitioners of traditional medicine were unable to offer her realistic hopes of the cure she desired, she turned to practitioners of 'alternative' medicine. These alternatives, unfortunately, consumed not only her time and money, but also her hope. Sue describes some of the lengths to which she went in her ultimately frustrated efforts to find a cure for ALS:

> I spent a fortune on naturopathy, acupuncture. I spent $10,000.00
> travelling to Colorado to have my amalgam fillings removed. On any
> given day I was seeing three types of care givers. I'd have an appoint-
> ment with an acupuncturist in the morning, then a specialist in
> psychoimmunology, then a nutritionist. It just went on and on for
> weeks.[50]

It was after Sue's final attempt to find a cure for her illness that she decided to commit suicide. This idea came to her following an ALS Society meeting she attended shortly after returning from an American diagnostic centre where she had spent a significant amount of her dwindling finances in the hope of reversing the decline in her health. Hobbs Birnie describes the circumstances of Sue's decision as follows:

> When [Sue] attended a meeting [of the ALS Society] in April 1992, following her return from Colorado Springs, her mood had changed. With all hope of a cure gone, she could see her own future in the faces and voices of the 25 other members whose scooters and hi-tech wheelchairs crowded the room ... That night she decided to commit suicide. Sue made this decision without fuss, hesitation or moral argument. The idea came and she accepted it. It felt right. The dominant nature of her disease was now clear. It would rob her of everything that gave value to her life and then slowly, at its own leisure, kill her. She did not fear pain: drugs could take care of that. She feared a drugged-out twilight of total dependency and hopelessness. Slowly, Sue was moving toward the position that she would steadfastly and publicly maintain for the next two years – that the quality of life is the essence of life, and that a life deprived of quality was not worth living.[51]

Interestingly, Sue's fear of a loss of certain 'qualities' of her life (such as her functional capacities, like speaking) influenced her thinking more than her fears about the terminal physical aspects of dying. Still, in her testimony to the courts, she raised the issue of the cruel physical manner in which she expected to die as a result of ALS. She sought a humane active intervention that would hasten her death in order to avoid certain aspects of the dying process, such as dying by choking or suffocation, or having to have her respiration supported by a ventilator. As she reported to the B.C. court:

> I just feel an inner guidance tells me that [physician-assisted suicide is] the right thing for me to do and I should be allowed to do it. I would like that option because I feel that I don't want to die a gruesome death of trying to get air or to go into a choking spasm or starve. My muscles are slowly atrophying and the airway will close down. My muscles will be unable to push food down my throat. I will die of choking, asphyxiation or pneumonia.[52]

Dr Andrew Eisen, the renowned international specialist on ALS who originally diagnosed Sue, entered the legal fray to rebut some of the

negative images of dying with ALS with which the courts had been presented. In his statement to the British Columbia Court of Appeal hearing
Sue's case, Eisen addressed the misinformation that was being spread about
ALS, and claimed that '[i]t is virtually unheard of for someone with ALS to
choke to death. It just doesn't happen. The vast number die quietly and
peacefully in their sleep.' He added that although many patients do progress
to a stage at which a ventilator could be employed to assist their breathing
(especially at night, which is when most patients die), 'assisted suicide
becomes a "non-issue" at that point [when they are on a respirator] because
of the Nancy B. case.'[53] That is, given the legal precedent of the Nancy B.
case, where a fully conscious woman died after a respirator was removed,
there is no legal obligation for someone on a ventilator to continue to use
this type of support. Hence, withdrawing the respirator does not constitute
physician-assisted suicide.

Part of Sue's concern about being dependent on others was her fear that
those who cared for her would regard the provision of this care as
excessively burdensome. Sue resolved some of these initial fears during
the course of her illness. In an open letter to a newspaper, she described
her acceptance of her declining physical abilities. She realized, to the
surprise of herself and her friends, that she did not feel frustrated by her
diminishing ability to do things for herself. Reflecting on this discovery,
she concluded: 'I've made the transition of accepting my body the way it
is right now.'[54] Part of this acceptance of her own physical state was
expressed by a change in her attitude toward her dependency on others:
'I seem to have accepted having others help me with the day-to-day
physical necessities.'[55]

Even if Sue became more at ease with her dependency on some people,
she continued to sense and fear that she was burdensome to others: 'There
are times when I feel a tremendous amount of grief and pain, reflections of
what my loved ones – family and friends – are experiencing as they watch
me decline. It is their grief and pain that I find difficult to accept.'[56]

Even more disturbing than Sue's fears of 'being a burden,' of dependency or losing control, was her fear of isolation. By this time, most of her
care was provided by professionals, rather than family members or loved
ones. Despite the competence of this care, Hobbes Birnie highlights her
sense of isolation and loneliness even in the midst of these many caregivers:
'It is not as if there is someone waiting to embrace her, to say with love and
sincerity how happy they are she is still with them, to hear with genuine
interest how she spent the night, whether she slept or dreamed. Awakening
to the day, she awakes to loneliness.'[57]

Besides feeling that she had become a burden to her husband, Sue
recounts two incidents that provided her with convincing evidence that it

was time for her to die. The first incident occurred when Sue's mother Doe phoned to speak to Henry, Sue's husband. After Doe spoke briefly to Henry, he asked Doe if she would like to speak to Sue. Doe declined to say hello to Sue, even though Doe had not spoken with Sue for a couple of weeks. Sue was hurt by this apparent slight by her own mother, and took this incident to be 'further proof' that it was time for her to go, proof that she had already become a 'non-person' to others and that others had grown tired of, and indifferent to, her struggles.[58]

Sue's feeling that her mother no longer cared about her was compounded by her strained relationship with Henry and her son Cole. She interpreted their behaviour toward her as further evidence that she had become a non-person, or that, from their perspectives, she had already died. Sue's marital problems, however, predated her illness. Henry had left her prior to her diagnosis. After learning that she had ALS, Henry agreed to return to live with Sue 'for the sake of their son Cole.' Sue's illness further strained their relationship, and their arrangement was not a happy one. Now, not only did it seem to Sue that her mother preferred to speak to Henry rather than to her, but also that Henry preferred to spend his time with other women rather than with her. In fact, it was prior to Sue's decision that it was time to kill herself that Henry had told her that he was dating other women. Henry explained his behaviour as part of his effort to be more independent of Sue. As he put it, he wanted to free himself of the 'guilt and brainwashing' Sue was inflicting upon him. In addition, Sue's eight-year-old son, Cole, was also behaving badly toward his mother at that time. He had taken to shouting back at her, responding with anger at her increasing incapacity. An important part of Sue's role as mother to Cole was her own ability to influence (or control) his behaviour. To her, his misbehaviour signified that she was failing in this motherhood role, which would soon be over.[59]

A second incident that provided further proof for Sue that it was time to kill herself involved someone outside of her family. One of Sue's new friends offered to take Sue for a few days to her house. Sue looked forward to this event as a small holiday, a chance to be with one of her few friends, and a break from the routines of her home life. The friend, however, failed to follow through with her promise to Sue. Recalling these events, Sue concluded: 'I don't count like other people anymore. I'm a crumpling person.'[60] Her final conversation with Hobbs Birnie before her death reiterates these feelings of worthlessness and of being a burden to others:

> I feel for my family, for my mother, for Henry, for my son. I feel it has been going on for too long. Even the home-makers I have, I can sense it in the way in which people touch me. Maybe there should

be an endless supply of people with patience and commitment. But there isn't. That's the reality. I wish people, like the courts, would deal with these things and forget their theories.[61]

Sue's need for independence and control bears some relationship to her fear of 'not counting' in the eyes of others. Indeed, her self-controlled death poignantly symbolized this need for control. Just as her own experience of family as a child was characterized by power relationships and control by others, so also these themes of controlling others, or of being controlled, continued to dominate her relationships. This was particularly evident in her relationship with her son. Above everything, Sue wanted to secure Cole's enduring love and respect, something that neither of her parents were able to secure from her. She wished to stay with Cole for as long as possible. But she also wanted to avoid leaving him with disturbing images of a mother 'paralysed and drooling, unable to speak or hold her head up.' To prevent these images from haunting Cole into his old age, images that she thought would not only be psychologically traumatizing but would also undermine his love and respect of her, Sue believed that it would be best that she not stay around too long.[62] She acknowledged that there was a connection between her attitudes toward Cole and her own experiences with her parents. She feared Cole's 'disrespect for the loser' that she herself had felt toward her own mother. She also feared that her dying and physical state would embarrass Cole, just as she had felt socially embarrassed by her father's wasted physical appearance, his inability to speak or care for his simplest needs during the terminal phase of his life, and his death.[63]

An incident of Cole's misbehaviour illustrated Sue's fears and steeled her resolve to 'end it before she lost all control and before her son, Cole, suffered too much.'[64] Sue had developed a phobia about bugs and spiders, possibly because she was no longer able to flick them off her body. One day when Cole was pushing Sue in her wheelchair in the garden, he intentionally pushed her into a spiderweb. Sue cried out for him to stop, but, to her anger, he continued to push her right through the spider's web, which had a large spider right in the middle of it. Of this event, Sue said:

> It's a childlike thing; he thinks it's funny. And because of the way I react, it eggs him on to do it more. When he's away, I miss him terribly, and then he's back a couple of hours and I think what a little monster he is! I just feel so helpless. He wouldn't have gotten away with it before, but now I can't do a thing about it, just sit and see it. He's hurting terribly because he knows he's going to lose his mother, and he takes it out on me sometimes. It makes me think

about what it would be like if I waited until the end, the helplessness of it all.[65]

Sue's final statements before her suicide summarize her views and underlying concerns. She made these statements to Cole in a dictated letter, and to Henry in her will. She summarized her message to Cole as follows: 'I tried to help him understand why I was going to take my life. I finished my letter this way: "I have decided to leave now because my body is deteriorating and I don't want to suffer anymore, nor do I want you to have to watch me."'[66]

Sue's final message to Henry was delivered to him in her will, which she arranged to be read to him one month after her death. In it Henry was informed of changes Sue had made to her will two years earlier, changes that she had never discussed with him. These would allow Sue to maintain some control over Henry even after her death. The details of the changes involved Sue placing a set of restrictions on what Henry could do with the house. He could not rent it or cohabitate there with a spouse; he must sell it within three years, and Sue's share of the equity had to be put in a trust for Cole. This message, and the manner of its delivery, expressed some of the conflicts that Sue was experiencing and some of the interpersonal tensions with which Sue and Henry were struggling even before her decision to commit suicide. It also suggests something of the complexity of the human and family issues that underpinned her end-of-life decisions.

Some of the complexity of Sue's affective life was captured in the images of a recurring dream she first had in May 1993, the theme of which was being controlled by others. In this dream she was being held captive and was unable to escape. Sue described the dream as follows:

> I was attending a party where I had dressed up with shoulder pads
> that were made up of feathers and pearls – quite elaborate. Some-
> one drove me home but before we arrived he told me he liked me
> and would I go out with him sometime. I said yes, but didn't really
> want to go. And then in the next scene, he was taking me to his
> home where he held me prisoner for what seemed like years. While
> I had some freedom, any attempts to escape were unsuccessful.
> Other people were around who were either understanding or were
> being held captive as well.[67]

Sue did not interpret this dream in her biography. Still, it is interesting that the dream's themes of imprisonment and of control (e.g., actively by some physical power, or passively by being physically desirable) were prominent in her own story. Her interest in this dream suggests that she was beginning to appreciate some of the complexity of her own behaviour and decisions. Even if one concedes that Sue's decision for euthanasia was a strictly logical or 'intellectual' one and was unrelated to her affective life, it would still be difficult to maintain that her personal history and character did not condition her end-of-life decisions. These other factors surely shaped Sue's experience of ALS, and her affective life shaped her responses to it; and all of these find expression in her answer to what made her life worthwhile.

In summary, Sue's story highlights at least three points that are relevant to my argument regarding the role of feelings in value judgments. First, there is a distinction between the biological facts of an illness and one's psychological and moral responses to an illness, that is, the relation one adopts to the biological facts. Second, there is some connection between the psychological and the moral. Certain elements of one's response that are typically identified as psychological, such as one's fears, somehow are related to one's value judgments and decisions. Even so, there is evidence that Sue's psychological responses to various concerns developed and changed during the course of her illness. Again, one's psychological responses and value judgments have an important communal dimension or context. Sue's decision was an 'individual' one only in the sense that it was her idea and not a conclusion others were foisting upon her. Even so, her decision for assisted suicide cannot adequately be understood apart from her relationships with others, in particular the ones I have just sketched: her relationships with her grandparents, parents, husband, son, and friends. Recognizing this fact undermines the claim that these are strictly private issues. Attempts to understand these responses in isolation from one's personal history and psychological strengths and vulnerabilities, as well as one's community, therefore, are bound to be superficial.

I have focused on describing some affective features of Sue Rodriguez's story. In particular, I have highlighted two emotions that played a prominent role in Sue's story and decisions, her anger and her fear. But were these emotions really related to her value judgment and decision about euthanasia? Is an account of her affective life relevant to those who debate this issue? It seems plausible to answer both of these questions affirmatively. Far from being unintelligible, Sue's feelings are consistent with her core values and value judgments. Moreover, they are intelligibly related to Sue's life history, her moral development, and her experiences of family and community. As Hobbs Birnie points out, it was Sue's public image that made her such a powerful advocate for euthanasia. This image was of a woman who had a lovingly responsive and supportive family, of someone who was at peace with herself and her life, and who was not ambivalent about what she wanted and did not want at the end of her life. But her own account of her story undermines the message the media image suggests. It reveals a less obvious image of an isolated, lonely, vulnerable, and bitter woman who lacked any positive and intimate lifelong supports. In her story are hints of significant intrapsychic and interpersonal conflicts, such as her fear of loss of control over the dying process, or even of transferring this control to her medical caregivers. Sue's illness brought out character traits that were already well established. To highlight these points I will now contrast Sue's story with that of another person who also wrote about his experience of living with ALS, Dennis Kaye.

3   Dennis Kaye's Story

Dennis Kaye was one of Sue Rodriguez's peers. A fellow native of British Columbia, Dennis lived on Quadra Island and worked with his father as a logger from his youth. He later married, and raised a family of two daughters. He was thirty years old in 1985 when he developed neurological symptoms and was diagnosed with ALS. Between then and his death in 1996, Dennis also faced the many struggles that those with a terminal illness typically encounter.[68] Many Canadians came to know Dennis through his reflections on life with ALS. He shared these reflections with the public in his correspondence with the then Canadian Broadcasting Corporation's *Morningside* host, Peter Gzowski, and in his book, *Laugh, I Thought I'd Die*. Dennis includes in his book his correspondence with Sue Rodriguez, which is helpful for my present purpose of comparing and contrasting their experiences of ALS. Dennis's story chronicles emotional responses to difficulties, including anger and fear, that were similar to the ones Sue experienced. Despite these similarities, however, Dennis affirmed a different evaluation of his life, and he rejected the apparent solution of euthanasia.

Since my goal is to discern some relation between emotional responses and evaluations, I will now describe some of the affective features of Dennis Kaye's story. These features provide helpful data for subsequent analysis of this issue.

3.1 From Anger at Lost Abilities to Righteous Anger

Dennis announced in his book that his first goal was to 'smooth the emotional road' for those who might face, in themselves or a loved one, a terminal condition. The main emotion Dennis sought to smooth was anger, or resentment.[69] In contrasting Sue's experience of ALS with his own, Dennis reported that her disease 'struck with a vengeance.'[70] Within eight months of Sue's diagnosis of ALS she had lost the dexterity of her hands and the strength of her legs. This resulted in her experiencing several nasty falls. Although Dennis's illness had progressed further than Sue's at the time of their correspondence (e.g., he was already unable to speak), his losses had occurred more gradually.

Dennis supported Sue's efforts to take her concerns to the courts, and thereby to raise public awareness about ALS. But there was also a hint of resentment in Dennis's response to Sue's argument for physician-assisted suicide. He felt personally slighted by her argument that physician-assisted suicide was necessary in order to avoid the fate of advancing to what she called a 'merely biological existence.' Dennis considered himself to be living the very existence that Sue judged to be not worth living, a condition she sought to avoid by her suicide. Dennis countered the implication that his life was a mere biological existence by insisting that 'even though I have to type with a stupid-looking contraption on my head [i.e., a wand device], on good days, I like to think I'm more than that [living a merely biological life].'[71]

Dennis's response to Sue was consistent with those of other ALS sufferers. For instance, Anne Molloy, a lawyer for the Coalition of Provincial Organizations of the Handicapped (COPOH), argued in support of Sue Rodriguez at the Supreme Court. Nevertheless, a key point of her presentation was that the lives of those with handicaps are at risk of being devalued in our society. She explained the nuances of the Coalition's stance as follows:

> Most of our factum pointed out how vulnerable the disabled were and that they needed protection from their lives being devalued. We wanted safeguards there to make sure people are not taken advantage of or pressured into doing something they didn't want to do. People can be influenced by a doctor or relative saying: 'Don't live on a respirator, that would be sheer hell.' But how do they know, if they haven't done it themselves? Maybe it's better than being dead. Some in the medical profession, and some families, subtly encourage the disabled to quit fighting.[72]

Dennis also expressed his anger in response to injustices committed by able-bodied persons against those with handicaps similar to his own. For instance, he recounts the story of another ALS patient, Aleza, that 'touched a raw personal nerve.' Describing the contents of a letter Aleza's widowed husband sent him following her death, he reports:

> Unable to care for Aleza in the end stages of her illness, [her husband] grudgingly admitted defeat and checked her into the hospital. To his anger and disbelief, and despite pleas to the contrary, he repeatedly found the staff treating her as though she were

mentally retarded. Needless to say, his grief was compounded by an unwarranted sense of guilt over the institutional nightmare he had unwittingly inflicted on the woman he loved.[73]

Dennis tells us that his practical response to Aleza's experience was to add a central chapter to his book on the 'nuts and bolts' of caring for someone with ALS. The goal of this chapter was to educate at least some of his readers to be more sensitive to the vulnerabilities of other ALS patients who find themselves in Aleza's circumstances. Dennis's anger here expressed his own estimation of the value of others, such as Aleza, who are afflicted with ALS. This affirmation of the value of an individual despite their handicap with ALS is what motivated him to educate others about this condition. His anger also reflected his evaluation of his own life. Dennis's own experience of living with ALS provided him with the grounds for his empathy and compassion for others who were similarly afflicted. His righteous anger was directed not inward at himself, nor outward toward others who would not collaborate with suicidal plans (as in Sue's case), but toward those who slighted or devalued a person on the basis of the incapacities that resulted from their being afflicted with ALS.

3.2 From Vulnerability to Love

Like Sue, part of the 'rough emotional road' that Dennis travelled while living with ALS included struggling with feelings of fear. In his letters to Peter Gzowski, Dennis wrote about such things as 'Lifestyles of the Sick and Feeble,' and he signed his letters as 'The Incredible Shrinking Man.'[74] Behind his humour was a sense of the incongruity between what he had become (sick, feeble, and shrinking) and what he used to be (healthy, strong, and growing). Dennis admitted that the dark object of his humour was his attachment to, and pride in, his former physical self-image:

> I was never what you'd consider a Charles Atlas, but its safe to say that neither muscle nor stamina were things I needed more of. I never thought about it much back then, but I derive a kind of blue-collar pride from the fact that my fitness was the result not of working out, but of working ... If I was really bound for physical ruin, how long could I cling to this notion of masculinity? Day-to-day deterioration only fuelled feelings of inadequacy, and for a while, self-esteem fell to an all-time low.[75]

Dennis used humour and insight to challenge, reframe, and play with some of his responses to his illness. He was able to find humour, for instance, in his tendency to base his self-esteem on physical attributes. His humour allowed him to distance himself from fears that were part of his experience of ALS. His jokes about his outer weakness also revealed his growing inner strength. As he put it, 'Today I measure my strength, or lack of it, in terms of my ability to control things like resentment and frustration.'[76] Despite Dennis's best efforts, like Sue he found that his greatest challenge was to avoid fearing that he was merely a burden to others.[77] His greatest strength in opposing these negative feelings was his ability to find humour in his experiences and to share this humour, and other insights into life, with others.

Dennis relates a story from which came the title of his book. This story provides the context from which arose this 'change of heart' toward his illness. This change of heart was occasioned by an attempt at disrobing, which left him in a 'panting heap of arms, legs and underwear.'[78] But rather than slipping into self-pity, frustration, and anger, he was 'seized by the sweet slapstick of the situation.' His laughter woke his wife, who then joined the chorus. Based on his experiences of indulging in such foolery on many subsequent occasions, Dennis concluded that humour 'can not only make a seemingly unbearable situation bearable, but will, in the process, make life far more bearable for those around you.' He discovered in his insights and humour valued 'gifts' that he could offer to others. This gift of humour counterbalanced his overwhelming sense of only taking from, or 'burdening,' others.[79]

3.3 From Anger and Fear to Gratitude towards One's Community

Although Dennis certainly experienced the emotions of anger and fear as part of the experience of his illness, for him the more foundational emotion was a feeling of gratitude toward his community. It is important to include this aspect of Dennis's story because it highlights the communal dimension of his experience of ALS. It strikes me that this is a key issue underpinning the entire euthanasia debate; that is, how can a community best support those with a terminal illness, especially those who are overwhelmed by fears and anxieties? Dennis relates the story of an incident that captures a spirit of gratitude that might be at the heart of one's experiences of community. Although it occurred sometime in his youth, before he formed his own intimate community, it was a spirit that later animated his affective life and that of his family in a way that also shaped his, and his family's, experience of ALS. Reflecting on this experience, Dennis says that 'sometimes a seemingly insignificant event can determine the way we treat others for the rest of our lives.'[80]

This seemingly insignificant incident took place on the banks of the

Shannon River in Ireland, when the teenaged Dennis stopped for a rest during a cycling trip through the country. As he lay resting beside the beautiful river and countryside scene, an elderly woman appeared from a nearby dwelling carrying in her hands a tray burdened with a home-made lunch. She addressed Dennis in her heavy Irish brogue, saying: 'When I was young I used to cycle too, and ye build up an awful sweat, ye do. Once yer all filled up, just leave the tray on me gatepost, would ye?'[81] Dennis reports that as suddenly as she appeared, she was gone. Twenty years later he admits that 'as long as I live I'll never forget the sight of that little Irish woman. Her kindness is with me still.'[82]

Later, Dennis's family became an important object of gratitude for him. At those times when he worried about a premature death, his concerns centred on missing key events in the life of his family. As it turned out, Dennis lasted longer than his caregivers predicted, and he was able to be present for such important events as his daughter's first school play. Although the subtitle of Dennis's book is *My Life with ALS*, I think he would have better signified the content of his book by a title such as *Our Life with ALS*.[83] Indeed, whenever Dennis spoke about his life in his book, it was always in the context of others who accompanied him. Dennis's story played a central and defining part in the life-stories of others intimately connected to him, such as his wife, family, friends, and even animals (e.g., his dog). Dennis emphasized that these links were crucial to his sense of fulfilment and well-being. They provided him with an answer to the question of 'why' he should continue to live given all the restrictions that ALS had imposed on his life.

Dennis referred to his immediate family as the 'first and most critical link' in the chain of charity. He reflected on the possibility of having to face ALS without their support and quickly concluded, 'I don't think I'd be alive today.'[84] For him, they were truly his 'life-support system.' He was reminded of this fact each time his wife spoon-fed him.[85] Despite the effects that the biological decline of his physical condition with ALS had on him, Dennis noted how his experience also affected those closest to him. He concluded that everything one did, saw, felt, or even thought was, in some way or another, inseparably linked to one's primary caregiver.[86]

On this point, then, Dennis's experience of ALS contrasted sharply with Sue's. For Sue, the experience of dying was essentially one of increasing isolation from, and then resentment toward, her intimate community. Like Dennis, she also grew tremendously during her illness and was able to accomplish some important goals. This testifies to the fact that this time of illness was not simply one of unmitigated evil. The emotions that dominated Sue's experience, however, were anger and fear, as compared to humour and gratitude in Dennis's case. Finally, there seems to have been similar challenges in Sue's and Dennis's experiences of, and affective responses to, their illness, although their dominant affective responses and conclusions regarding euthanasia differed. Corresponding to differences in their communal supports, it is not surprising that Sue insisted, for instance, that the question of euthanasia was (and ought to be?) a strictly private one and Dennis did not.

I have highlighted some ways that emotions seem to have been relevant to different decisions about euthanasia by two persons with ALS. Sue Rodriguez and Dennis Kaye differed not only on this question, but more fundamentally on the question of whether they considered their lives with ALS to be worthwhile. By contrasting their stories I have identified some factors, including emotions, that entered into their evaluations and decisions. Their stories raise questions about the interrelation of reason and emotion, and they provide a concrete context for the bioethical and legal debate about euthanasia. Before turning, in chapter 3, to a historical review of some important views on the interrelation between reason and emotion, I will first sketch the views of some prominent proponents and opponents of euthanasia in the North American bioethical and legal discussions.

4   The Euthanasia Debate: Ethical and Public-Policy Perspectives

4.1   The Bioethical Debate: Tom Beauchamp and Richard McCormick

Most bioethicists identify at least two main concerns underpinning the question about euthanasia. The first concern regards the legitimacy of the traditional absolute prohibition against taking one's own life.[87] Against this prohibition, some persons advance the view that someone might rationally judge their life, under certain conditions of suffering, to be *not worth living*. Given such an evaluation, taking one's life could be a permissible (or even laudable) response to suffering since, on balance, it produces more value for the individual or society.[88] The key question here has to do not so much with the means one chooses to use to quit life, but with whether the evaluation that some life is no longer worthwhile ought to be affirmed and acted on.[89]

A second concern regards the more general notion of individual autonomy or freedom. The view here is that one ought to be self-determining and in control of one's life and death. On this view, the traditional wrongness of killing rests, in part, on the fact that to deprive someone of their life normally violates their autonomy. But this does not apply to those cases where someone wishes their life to be ended, as in voluntary euthanasia. In such cases, respect for a person's autonomy seems to require one to comply with their wishes, even though this act eliminates the capacity for future autonomous acts. If respect for personal autonomy is morally paramount, and such respect includes honouring a suicide wish, then the autonomous individual who judges that his or her life is *not worth living* ought to be supported by action in complaisance with this decision. This holds even if one implicates others by involving them in one's own suicide.[90] This interpretation of the main concerns that have given rise to the euthanasia debate have been articulated by several prominent bioethicists.[91] One particularly helpful articulation of the issues is given by Daniel Callahan.

Callahan, a medical ethicist and president of the Hastings Center, provides an overview of the current state of the euthanasia debate in his foreword to the book *Euthanasia Examined*.[92] His comments helpfully highlight the relation between this debate and some of the human concerns about dying that are prevalent today. He notes that historically the profession of medicine has condemned the practice of euthanasia from the time of Hippocrates. Although there have been periodic legal skirmishes over this issue, especially in the first half of this century in Great Britain and the United States, nothing much happened to the laws prohibiting such acts. Callahan reads the current agitation over this issue as being different in degree from any of the prior legal challenges. Public-opinion polls in both Canada and the United States indicate a growing willingness among physicians and lay persons to change the legal prohibition of euthanasia and physician-assisted suicide.[93] He also notes 'the considerable plausibility of some of the explanations and interpretations that proponents of euthanasia and physician-assisted suicide urge. Their 'kindly rationales' note 'the pervasive public fear of a bad death and the desire of people to have some final control over their life and fate in the face of unbearable and unredeemable suffering. The proponents hold out the promise of a more humane medicine, now able to go all the way in helping patients.'[94]

For Callahan, Western society has reached a critical moment on this issue. It is 'being asked whether in the name of mercy and self-determination one of the oldest of medicine's prohibitions should be overturned.'[95] He admits that euthanasia and assisted suicide are persuasive to members of the public because they are presented as possible solutions to the fear individuals have about living a life they no longer deem to be worth living, that is, a life of suffering that is 'unbearable and unredeemable.' Callahan concludes that what is at stake in this debate are questions of fundamental importance for Western society, such as what we value and how we understand life and death.[96]

A further curiosity about the state of the medical-ethical question of euthanasia is the disparity between the public's apparent acceptance of arguments favouring euthanasia and a much more critical view of the proposed reforms among many bioethicists. This discrepancy points to a possible pedagogical problem, namely, that for some reason these experts are failing to convince members of the public that allowing such reforms is truly unwise. Another possibility is that members of the public find those bioethicists who argue in favour of euthanasia to be particularly persuasive.

One example of a bioethicist who highlights the relation between this debate and more general ethical issues is Tom Beauchamp, a senior research scholar at the Kennedy Institute of Ethics and professor of philosophy at Georgetown University. Beauchamp agrees with Callahan's appraisal of the importance of this public-policy issue, and adds that the American debate has reached a watershed:

> We are at a delicate point in this evolving history [of the legal right of patients to control his or her death, or at least obtain a lethal prescription]. Neither in law nor in bioethics is the justification of physician assistance in suicide the received opinion at the present time, but support for physician assistance in dying could soon become the received opinion in both disciplines.[97]

The critical evaluative question Beauchamp poses is whether the act of assisting persons in bringing about their deaths 'causes them a loss or, rather, provides a benefit.'[98] In answering this question Beauchamp maintains that, as a matter of procedure, the *person in question* is best situated to make the evaluation that 'lingering in life is, on balance, worse than death.' Given that this *person in question* judges that they would be better off dead, Beauchamp contends that the various means that such a person might select to achieve the end of quitting life are morally indifferent. That is, '[t]he person in search of physician-assisted suicide, the person who seeks active euthanasia, and the person who forgoes life-sustaining treatment to end life are identically situated.'[99]

There are two general philosophical points that Beauchamp brings to his analysis of the euthanasia debate. I would like to highlight these because they serve as a point of entry for the contribution I would like to make to the debate. First, Beauchamp clearly distinguishes the *cognitive issues* of evaluating one's life from the *decisional issues* that follow from this evaluation. In so doing, he locates the key issue in this debate as a cognitive one, namely, one of making an evaluation. Second, on this key evaluative issue Beauchamp emphasizes the methodological point that the *person in question* is the one who is in the best position to make this evaluation properly. In so doing he grants an evaluative authority and epistemic objectivity to such an individual that challenges conventional notions of cognitional authority and objectivity, at least in matters of fact. Beauchamp elucidates neither the cognitive advantage such an individual has nor the cognitive acts in which he or she would need to engage in order to make this evaluation properly. Nevertheless, he admits the *possibility* of some people legitimately judging their death to be of greater value than their continued life. In so doing, he rejects an absolutist stance on this ethical question, and concludes in favour of a public policy that would allow euthanasia.[100]

If Beauchamp represents well the arguments of the proponents of euthanasia, a leading opponent is Richard McCormick. In a lecture delivered in 1997, McCormick addressed Beauchamp's position directly. He agreed with Beauchamp that the issue is an evaluative one regarding whether or not one's life is worthwhile, rather than primarily a decisional issue. But for him this does not mean that there is no difference between decisions to kill and to allow to die. On McCormick's analysis, one can be culpable for either decision. But only if I consider life to be an absolute good am I culpable in all cases of allowing persons to die. On the other hand, if I regard life as a basic good, I am not always culpable for allowing death to come, although I would be violating this basic good by killing.[101]

For McCormick, beyond the logical problems of Beauchamp's denial of the difference between killing and allowing to die are important cultural biases that shape his view, such as a certain North American pragmatism. He explained that for the pragmatic person, the only fact of these cases is the fact of death. After all, the pragmatist reasons that the manner in which death came about makes little difference once a person is dead. McCormick countered this view with the example of a husband and son who stayed with their dying wife and mother following a massive stroke that had left her unconscious. Their time was spent doing little things for her such as moistening her lips. Mostly it was spent just being with her during her hour of death. When they reflected later on this experience, they both readily admitted that their presence did not make any difference to their mother's survival, but it made a huge difference to themselves. Such a response might well be incomprehensible to the pragmatist.[102]

If the arguments of Beauchamp and McCormick fairly indicate some of the key ethical issues that underpin the current state of the euthanasia question, and if this question intersects with more general philosophical questions, then it would be helpful to enter this debate on these terms. One might do so by focusing on the cognitive issues connected with making evaluations, and further elucidate some of the normative features of these acts and, consequently, the contents achieved by means of them. That is, given the current consensus on the ethical issue underlying the euthanasia debate, it seems appropriate for this discussion to focus on the various factors involved in making evaluations. Such a focus will allow me to explore the role of individual feelings and conscience as a basis for more general public-policy decisions about euthanasia.

4.2   The Public-Policy Debate: Senate Committee Minority and Majority Members

Two key legal concerns in the North American euthanasia debate involve determining a person's capacity to consent to medical treatments and the legal status of those treatments that might hasten death. Other legal concerns include procedural questions, such as who makes this evaluation and who does what to whom. The dominant or received ethical and legal view in both Canada and the United States is that there is an important distinction between euthanasia and assisted suicide, on the one hand, and withdrawing life-sustaining treatments, on the other. Arthur Schafer, a Manitoba ethicist, points out that acts that intentionally hasten death are prohibited by the Canadian Criminal Code: '[D]octors can withdraw life support with the consent of the patient or a family member, if the patient is incapacitated ... It is illegal to do anything to hasten a patient's death, even 30 minutes, or five seconds earlier than if he would otherwise have died.'[103]

The sense that the Criminal Code of Canada is not keeping pace with developments in ethical thinking and medical practice has prompted much legal and legislative debate in Canada. In the previously mentioned Special Senate Committee Report on Euthanasia and Assisted Suicide, entitled *Of Life and Death*, the authors recommended their report as 'an initial step' in the long process ahead for Canadians attempting to find solutions to the legal, social, and ethical issues related to euthanasia and assisted suicide. Like Callahan, the authors of this report expressed their understanding of the call for euthanasia as stemming fundamentally from fears individuals have about the dying process. They stated in their introduction that, '[w]ith the advent of modern medical technology and the more common usage of artificial measures to prolong life, many people today are more fearful of the process of dying than of death itself.'[104] Because of its importance in the Canadian context, I will highlight some of the reasons this report was commissioned and its main conclusions.

This report can be understood as a response to Sue Rodriguez's 1993 legal challenge to the Canadian laws prohibiting assisted suicide. As the authors pointed out, this legal challenge focused the Canadian public debate of the issues of death and dying on questions about assisted suicide and euthanasia. Although Sue Rodriguez's case did not illustrate the use of invasive 'artificial technologies' to prolong life, it did persuade many members of the public, as well as the medical profession, to support the move to relax the legal prohibition of euthanasia. As evidence of this shift in opinion, the authors pointed to Canadian public-opinion polls that, in the wake of her case, indicated a growing support for the position that people should be able to take control of their dying processes. The authors also noted a shift toward a more permissive view on this issue among physicians. Although the Canadian Medical Association continues to uphold the position that members should not participate in euthanasia or assisted suicide, its membership has become divided in their views on this issue.[105] Evidently, Sue Rodriguez's case had a powerfully persuasive effect in the Canadian euthanasia debate. It is for this reason that I have chosen to examine her experience and conclusions more closely in my discussion.

At the end of their extensive study of this issue, the opinions of committee members diverged over the more difficult questions that the assisted suicide and euthanasia debate raises. The minority members of the Senate committee were persuaded that Sue Rodriguez's case illustrated the need some individuals have for physician-assisted suicide in order to secure a good death.[106] They recommended that 'the *Criminal Code* be amended to permit voluntary euthanasia for competent individuals who are physically incapable of committing assisted suicide.'[107] In explaining this recommendation they appealed to several ethical notions. For instance, they thought that if they allowed assisted suicide, they would also have to allow euthanasia in order not to violate the *equality* argument in section 15 of the Charter of Rights. They also appealed to the principle of *autonomy*, which they interpreted as justifying allowing the withholding and withdrawing of life-sustaining treatment. From this, they reasoned that the same principle justifies permitting voluntary euthanasia on the basis of competent patients' wishes, where competence involves meeting intellectual criteria. This is because they denied any ethically important distinction between the status of acts of providing treatment to alleviate suffering that may hasten death, on the one hand, and voluntary euthanasia, on the other. The relevant point of similarity between these two acts, for them, was the foreseeable consequence of the death of the patient.[108]

The majority view, by contrast, recommended to Parliament that there be no amendments to subsection 241(b) of the Criminal Code, which specifies that it is an offence to counsel suicide. Their view seemed to be that denying Sue Rodriguez physician-assisted suicide was denying her a benefit, but this was justified on the basis of the harm that this might bring to society.[109] What all members agreed to, however, was to recommend that 'research be undertaken into ... why it [assisted suicide or euthanasia] is being requested, and whether there are any alternatives that might be acceptable to those who are making the requests.'[110] In chapter 9, I will return to these opposing views in order to analyse them from the perspective of Lonergan's philosophy.

PART TWO

Historical Views on the Relevance of Emotions in the Moral Life

3

Historical Views on the Relevance and
Role of Emotions in the Moral Life

But if it is only in the palpable consequences which everyone can see that there can
be science, then there is no science of man, because the consequences of the really
profound human errors occur only fifty or a hundred years later, and then the span
of time is a bit too long for anyone to say that palpably this evil at this time is due to
that man's error being propagated a century ago.

Bernard Lonergan, *Topics in Education*

1   Overview of Historical Positions

The goal of this chapter is to highlight some of the historical discussion on
the relevance and role of affectivity in value judgments and to situate
Lonergan's position within this spectrum of views.

The issue is not new and has been raised by major thinkers within and
beyond Western philosophical traditions.[1] In this chapter I will sample a
range of historical positions answering the question 'What is an emotion?'
In each case I will indicate whether the thinker whose ideas I survey
considers emotions relevant to moral knowing, and if so, whether the
content of such knowing is ever epistemically objective. My aim here is,
first, to highlight some prominent views on the emotions that are common
in contemporary ethical discussions and are opposed to Lonergan's view;
second, to focus on a few thinkers from whose works Lonergan draws in
formulating his own positive view on the role of the emotions in value
judgments. This survey, although far from historically exhaustive, will be
sufficient to illustrate that there is significant disagreement on such basic
issues as what an 'emotion' is and what its function is in the cognitive

process. Moreover, it will show that there is even less agreement on what 'rational discourse' is.

In an effort to avoid becoming distracted from this goal by advancing my own, possibly controversial, historical interpretations, I will rely extensively upon the historical accounts argued for by others. I have selected a few secondary sources that I judge to provide relatively standard historical interpretations, or that elucidate the contemporary philosophical under-standing of certain terms and concepts. I will be drawing primarily on Cheshire Calhoun and Robert Solomon's book *What Is an Emotion?* for their review of the range of theories about what an emotion is.[2] Although Calhoun and Solomon's historical analysis is clear and plausible in its main lines, it proposes views on what an emotion is that differ significantly from Lonergan's position. Hence, by drawing on this interpretation of the his-tory of Western thinking regarding emotions, I hope to be less prone to the charge of historical anachronism, that is, of reading Lonergan's own views about the emotions into historical stances.

For conceptual and terminological issues, I will be drawing extensively upon two recent publications, *The Oxford Dictionary of Philosophy* and *The Oxford Companion to Philosophy*.[3] I will appeal to these sources mainly to specify how contemporary philosophers use certain terms. Again, the definitions set out here will simply serve as a common starting-point for a subsequent detailed analysis. Finally, I will draw on a few other second-ary sources, such as Frederick Copleston's standard *History of Philosophy*, to supplement Calhoun and Solomon's discussion of certain thinkers, especially those in the Aristotelian tradition whose contributions are particularly important for understanding Lonergan's position.

There are two main issues I hope to highlight in this chapter. First, in the historical survey of positions I will distinguish two main families of views on emotions as they relate to epistemically objective evaluations. The first family denies, in different ways, that emotions are relevant to such value judgments.[4] Within this family of views, there are two subsets. On one view the problem is emotions themselves, which some thinkers take to be essen-tially non-cognitive phenomena. According to them, feelings are incapable of yielding epistemically objective value judgments. Although they affirm that one can achieve such knowledge, they claim it is not by means of emotional responses. According to the second view, the problem is not emotions themselves, but rather human cognition generally. That is, value judgments are never epistemically objective. Although thinkers who hold this position affirm that emotions might play a key role in achieving 'appar-ent' knowledge of values, they consider such judgments, like fact judg-ments, to be merely epistemically subjective.

Contrasting with this first family of thinkers is a second in which all agree that emotions are cognitive in the strict sense of providing one with access to the real. For this family, not only are certain affective responses relevant to value judgments, but such emotions are a necessary condition for achieving epistemically objective evaluations. I will highlight the distinctiveness of these two families in sections 2 and 3, and argue that the second family is represented by the Aristotelian-Thomistic tradition's view of the cognitive role of emotions. I will also sketch a series of developments within the Aristotelian-Thomistic tradition that will be important for understanding the background of Lonergan's own position on the cognitive role of the emotions in value judgments.

The second main issue I hope to draw out is the distinction between the purported role of emotions in one's cognitive activities and the cognitive contents achieved by means of those activities. It is important to highlight this distinction in order to avoid confusing Lonergan's cognitive view of the emotions with non-cognitive positions, such as that of David Hume. For Hume, values are essentially expressions of emotional preferences. What he means by a 'value' is merely something that strikes one as agreeable, not something that is truly good or worthwhile. That is, Hume holds a subjective value theory. By contrast, Kant maintains a practically objective value theory but at the expense of rejecting the cognitive relevance of one's emotions or 'inclinations.' What I hope to argue is that the Aristotelian position in general, and Lonergan's stance in particular, differs from both of these views. Lonergan's position agrees with Hume's view that emotions are involved in the process by which we come to know values. But Lonergan maintains that there is an important distinction between emotional responses to objects as agreeable and as valuable or as goods. Hence, the contents of such knowledge are, at least sometimes, more than just epistemically subjective reports about what I find agreeable. That is, it makes sense for Lonergan to claim that I find something disagreeable but nevertheless judge it to be truly worthwhile. In section 3 I will begin to sketch some important contributions of the Aristotelian tradition to Lonergan's own views of the cognitive role of emotions in value judgments.

2   Some Accounts of Emotions as Irrelevant to Knowing Values

The understanding of emotions that various thinkers presuppose typically differs on the point of how emotions relate to human cognition.[5] Calhoun and Solomon explore the rich history of such theories in their book *What Is an Emotion?* They point out that emotion is an often neglected aspect in the history of ideas, and that one can learn much by reviewing and exploring what great thinkers in the Western traditions of thought had to say about the affective side of our psychology. These traditions have disagreed regarding the relation between reason and the passions.

> Many neglected [emotion] all together. Some treated the emotions with disdain, as the 'lower' part of the soul. It was in reaction to such attitudes and the exclusive celebration of reason that David Hume sounded the rebellion that still motivates much of the current controversies: 'reason is, and ought to be, the slave of the passions.'[6]

What, however, does this historical dispute have to do with contemporary ethical positions on topics such as euthanasia? One suggestion is that stances taken on this question shape ethical theories, which in turn provide the basis for the distinct positions taken on various particular moral issues. Thus, Richard Norman argues in his account of the history of moral philosophy in *The Oxford Companion to Philosophy* that the main ethical traditions of previous centuries that were developed by certain key thinkers are still, in one incarnation or another, alive and well.[7] On his reading, the main traditions still prominent in contemporary ethics emanate from specific thinkers. For instance, *utilitarianism* and *contractarian ethics* developed from Humean and Hobbesian accounts of moral knowing. These theories are closer to each other on the spectrum of positions regarding the connection between emotion and reason than they are to the other theories, even though Hume's and Hobbes's ideas are very different. *Rights-based theories* stemmed from Kant's philosophy. Finally, *virtue ethics* has its ancestry in Aristotle's ethics. In this chapter I will be pointing out the different ideas that Hume, Hobbes, Kant, and Aristotle had about the connection between emotions and reason. It should come as no surprise that there are corresponding differences in their ethical theories.

I begin the discussion with William James because he illustrates a position that is at one end of a spectrum of views on the relevance of emotions to moral knowing. I will, however, provide a more extensive review of the Aristotelian tradition from which comes virtue ethics. This position, at the other end of the spectrum of views I will highlight, is important for understanding Lonergan's intellectual roots.

2.1 William James (1843–1910): A Physiological Theory of the Emotions

According to Calhoun and Solomon, much of the modern debate regarding emotions falls between two theories, the still dominant Jamesian theory and the Aristotelian conception of the emotions. For James, an 'emotion' is a physiological reaction, and its sensory accompaniment is a 'feeling.'[8] On this account, there is no distinction between an emotion and the sensory perception of some physiological disturbance, such as the rumblings of one's stomach before a meal. Emotions *are* a special kind of perception; they are not distinct mental phenomena.[9] What is of interest to James is not so much the psychology of my experience of emotions, but their physiological basis.[10] James's account parallels Descartes's more antiquated mechanistic explanation of emotions such as fear.[11] Both Descartes and James sharply contrast 'rationality,' which for them involves conscious and interpretive activity, and 'emotions.' According to James, 'consciousness practically plays no part, either as partially constituting emotion or in generating and maintaining it.'[12] Descartes and James, then, articulate a position at one end of the spectrum of views on the relevance of emotions to value judgments. They maintain that emotions are irrelevant because they are not cognitive phenomena.

2.2 David Hume (1711–1776): A Sensory Theory of the Emotions

David Hume holds the position that emotional responses are entirely constitutive of *moral knowing*. That is, moral judgments and statements expressing them are simply utterances about how I feel in relation to some object or circumstance. In the end, such 'knowing' is never epistemically objective. Hume's account of the emotions illustrates what Calhoun and Solomon call a pure *sensation theory*. It also exemplifies a position moral philosophers refer to as *ethical subjectivism*. As noted previously, Richard Norman claims that Hume's position provides the philosophical foundations on which subsequent utilitarian and contractarian ethical theories were constructed.[13]

In contrast to Descartes and James, Hume ignores the associated physiological disturbances that accompany emotions. Instead, he focuses on the characteristic psychological or mental aspect of emotions. Hume did not believe that one could locate emotions in one's body, the way one can with merely physiological phenomena such as hunger pains. Attending to the psychological rather than to the physiological features of emotions allows Hume to distinguish between the calm and violent emotions, which is the central way he classified them. Calm emotions such as aesthetic enjoyment have merely a mental effect or *feel*. Violent emotions, like rage, generally involve physiological disturbances in addition to this mental feel. By contrast, an aesthetic experience according to James's physiological theory can only be called an emotion by stretching the theory to its limit, for example, by postulating very mild, almost indiscernible physiological disturbances.[14]

Historians commonly acknowledge Hume's ideas to be the high point in the tradition of the eighteenth-century British Moralists, who championed what is called *ethical naturalism.*[15] This tradition looked to the facts of human psychology as the 'natural' foundation for moral beliefs. Thomas Hobbes (1588–1679) began this tradition by suggesting that all human passions are manifestations of the desire for one's own good. On this view of human psychology Hobbes based his contractarian theory of morality. Subsequent British Moralists sought to answer Hobbes's egoistical theory by challenging his views on human nature, human passions, and affections. Hume's own moral theory followed earlier versions of 'moral sense' or 'moral sentiment' theories proposed by thinkers such as Lord Shaftesbury (1671–1713) and Francis Hutcheson (1694–1746/7). These thinkers maintained, against Hobbes, that besides the affection towards one's private good, humans also experience natural affections toward the public good; and these affections do not oppose one another.[16]

A natural affection that became key to Hume's moral philosophy was 'sympathy' or 'fellow-feeling.' This refers to the human capacity to experience another's feelings of happiness and misery. Hume maintained that our moral judgments stem from this sentiment rather than from reason. He thought, however, that reason was necessary to know the consequences of actions. Thus, Norman remarks: '[W]hen all the facts are known, some feeling or sentiment is necessary to lead us to a judgment of approbation or disapprobation.'[17] In this way, moral sentiment plays a decisive role in one's value judgments and the propositions that express one's knowledge of the apparent good.

Note that, on Hume's account, only certain feelings have this evaluative function. He considered what he calls 'ordinary' emotions, such as fear, resentment, and hope, to be more or less blind or irrational responses. He thought that only certain calm or 'intellectual' emotions, such as sympathy, are relevant to moral evaluations. But why did Hume take most 'ordinary' emotions to be irrational? Part of his reason has to do with the fact that ordinary emotional responses frequently are at odds with one's more considered approbation or disapprobation of things. For instance, I might initially respond with resentment toward something that was done, and only after further deliberation approve of it.[18]

Even when Hume accords some evaluative role to the emotions, as in the 'intellectual emotions,' we need to be cautious in interpreting what he calls a 'moral conclusion.' For him, these conclusions are, at best, merely empirical statements about what causes one to feel positively or negatively disposed to some object.[19] On this interpretation, even intellectual emotions are irredeemably subjective psychological phenomena. They provide a subjective report of a 'feel' that some object evokes. This is analogous to reporting that I feel cold when I jump into lake water. By this I might merely mean that the water causes me to feel cold, and I prescind from making any claim about the water really being cold.[20]

2.3 Immanuel Kant (1724–1804): Emotions as Non-evaluative Inclinations

Like Hume, Kant also juxtaposes reason, or rationality, and emotion. Emotions orient one in a world of likes or desires, but not in a world of meaning and value. In this regard, Kant grants emotions a greater cognitive role than does James, for whom they are entirely non-cognitive. But Kant withdraws from affirming Hume's view of emotions as being at the heart of ethics. Rather, Kant bases ethics on reason, in an effort to avoid Hume's subjective ethical conclusions. Since ethics is strictly a rational enterprise for Kant, reason supports 'practically' objective ethical conclusions. If his writing on this matter is interpreted in the framework of the *Critique of Pure Reason,* one cannot interpret Kant's view of the epistemic objectivity of values as anything more than a merely 'practical' objectivity. In that work, Kant specifies that all human knowledge is limited to mere appearances of things or phenomena, and cannot penetrate to a knowledge of what he called things-in-themselves or noumena.[21] In the light of this conclusion, then, Kant's reason grounds merely a practical morality, since our knowledge of values is also limited to mere appearances. Nevertheless, Kant regards this practical objectivity as superior to Hume's subjectivism, and so he regards all emotions, or what he generally calls 'inclinations,' as unnecessary conditions for value judgments.[22]

It is also worth observing that the most influential dimension of Kantian ethics is his assertion that all moral agents deserve our 'respect.' This assertion is one basis for subsequent rights-based theories.[23] Although Kant highlights 'respect' as fundamental to his view of the value of moral agency, he does not seem to think of this attitude as an emotion or mere inclination. Nevertheless, at least he admits the value of having passion in order to achieve 'great' things. In his lectures on history, for instance, he quoted approvingly the aphorism 'Nothing great has been done without passion.'[24]

What does Kant understand by *emotions,* and why does he consider them to be irrelevant to moral knowing? In his moral philosophy, Kant rejects the notion of the good in terms of utility and contractual arrangements that promote human desires. His most fundamental complaint against *ethical naturalism* is that it appeals to the facts of human psychology as the foundation for moral beliefs. In stark contrast to such natural inclinations, Kant maintains that the only thing that is good without qualification is a good will. This is the motivation to do one's duty for its own sake. Accordingly, Kant sought to determine the form of our moral duty without any reference to natural human feelings or to social or historical contexts. He does this by appealing to the universality of reason, which he expresses in his 'categorical imperative.'

Why does Kant consider emotions, such as compassion, to be inherently problematic guides for determining one's moral duty? Kant's reason has to do with the epistemic objectivity of value judgments based upon such emotions. Kant seeks to ground a rational and objective morality on something more stable than emotion. The contingencies of human affective tendencies and inclinations are too unstable to ground what he takes to be the necessary and universal claims that constitute a moral law. To the extent that one's actions are governed by one's moral maxim, which one can universalize without inconsistency, they will have moral worth.[25] Kant rejects the possibility of deriving such a principle of morality from the affective constitution of human nature:

> For duty is practical unconditional necessity of action; it must, therefore, hold for all rational beings (to which alone an imperative can apply), and only for that reason can it be a law for all human wills. Whatever is derived from the particular natural situation of man as such, or from certain feelings and propensities, or even from a particular tendency of the human reason which might not hold necessarily for the will of every rational being (if such a tendency is possible), can give a maxim valid for us but not a law; that is, it can give a subjective principle by which we might act only if we have the propensity and inclination, but not an objective principle by which we would be directed to act even if all our propensity, inclination, and natural tendency were opposed to it.[26]

Hence, emotions are too particular and unstable for Kant to provide a proper basis for the objective and universally valid moral law he seeks to ground.[27] In other words, they are irredeemably subjective and hence irrelevant for grounding epistemically objective value judgments.

Finally, according to R.S. Downie, the subsequent history of philosophy has minimized or even denied the possibility of Kant's category of a priori knowledge, and so also the rationalism that depends upon this category. Still, Kantian ideas emerge in several contemporary ethical thinkers. For instance, R.M. Hare's 'prescriptivism' develops a more moderate Kantian idea of universalizability, but departs from Kant by incorporating utilitarian considerations. John Rawls's theory of justice is influenced by the Kantian idea of mutually respecting autonomous rational wills. Other theories are simply influenced by Kantian ethics. Friedrich Nietzsche and Jean-Paul Sartre, for instance, are greatly influenced by Kant's autonomous will. For Kant, the autonomous will is free but constrained by its essentially rational nature. For Nietzsche and Sartre, however, the will is 'free' in as much as it is unconstrained, even by reason, and creates its own values in arbitrary free choice.[28]

3   Some Accounts of Emotions as Relevant to Knowing Values

The preceding historical examples illustrate different members of a family of views, all of which hold that emotions are not a necessary component of epistemically objective value judgments. Lonergan rejects the view, presupposed by all these thinkers, that there is an utter disparity between emotions and reason or cognition. His stance is in continuity with the Aristotelian and Thomistic tradition. It articulates an ethics that is *person-centred* instead of person-neutral, *particular* rather than general, and *epistemically objective* as opposed to merely subjective. For this tradition, emotions, like the virtues, are relevant to value judgments. I will provide some historical context for Lonergan's position by sketching out the contributions of four thinkers in the tradition from which he draws.

3.1 Aristotle (384–322 BC)

Aristotle's discussion of the emotions occurs principally in three works, *Rhetoric, On the Soul,* and the *Nicomachean Ethics.* This last work is generally regarded as his definitive lectures on ethics.[29] In all three books he discusses emotions in relation to both cognition and ethics. In the *Rhetoric*, for instance, Aristotle analyses the emotion 'anger' caused by strong moral beliefs about how others should behave. Moreover, the perceptions of being slighted and of impending danger are necessarily and properly mentioned in the essential definitions of anger and fear.[30] In *On the Soul*, Aristotle avoids Plato's sharp division between the rational and non-rational parts of the soul. Instead of arguing for the sharp division between intelligence and sensation, Aristotle's distinction is between the reasoning part and emotional responses.[31] He insists that these parts necessarily form a unity. In this way, he avoids many of the problems of more modern theories that presuppose a mind-body dualism.[32]

In the *Nicomachean Ethics,* Aristotle places emotions at the centre of his account of the virtues. He bases this account on what he takes to be the ultimate end of action, namely happiness (*eudemonia*). In order to know what our happiness consists in, we need to identify the distinctive function of human beings. Aristotle takes this function to be activity according to reason. The moral virtues are stable inclinations to perform such activities. Virtues such as courage or generosity are predominantly a matter of feeling the right way toward some object or situation. That is, they properly dispose one to the good and hence promote behaviour that is appropriate to the particular situation, behaviour that is neither excessive nor deficient to the circumstances. This enables one to find the *mean* that lies between extremes:[33] 'Hence, actions are called just or temperate when they are the sort that a just or temperate person would do. But the just and temperate person is not the one who [merely] does these actions, but the one who also does them in the way in which just or temperate people do them.'[34]

Several contributions Aristotle makes to the discussion of emotions are worth highlighting. First, for Aristotle the human good is concrete. On this view, ethics starts with the concrete choices and actions of persons, and then reflects on and criticizes these choices to inform future choices. If one considers the human good as a concrete object of choice, all of the elements that enter into this choice become ethically relevant. This makes the emotions relevant to ethics. Moreover, Aristotle's approach to ethics is empirical, and his conclusions are normative or prescriptive. In thinking about ethics he presupposes that there are virtuous persons and that such persons exemplify what the virtues entail concretely. His position holds us to the normative standard inherent in the judgments of virtuous persons, and to their dispositions that incline them to act in certain ways in whatever concrete circumstances they may face.

Second, Aristotle points out the importance of *habits* to ethics. He notes that the term *ethics* is cognate with the term *hexis*, which means habits. Ethics is about acquiring good or virtuous habits, which includes habitual ways not only of acting, but also of feeling and of being properly disposed toward certain activities. Since children respond primarily to feelings of pleasure and pain, the teacher must use pleasure and pain correctly to encourage in children good actions and a positive disposition toward such actions. Part of what it means to be a virtuous person is to be positively disposed toward good actions. Such a disposition enables one to understand and carry out what ought to be done in diverse circumstances. Aristotle concludes his discussion by stressing the importance of this correct habituation right from an early age: 'A state of [character] arises from [the repetition of] similar activities. Hence we must display the right activities, since differences in these imply corresponding differences in the states. It is not unimportant, then, to acquire one sort of habit or another, right from our youth; rather, it is very important, indeed all-important.'[35]

Third, Aristotle's psychology also offers a model for understanding the relationship of diverse cognitive processes, such as sensing and understanding. In his *On the Soul*, for instance, Aristotle points to the very process by which humans are capable of knowing forms or intelligible unities in a sensory image or representation.[36] Aristotle is referring to the cognitive correlative of the distinction between matter and form. The *matter* is what is given in the image. The *form* is the intelligibility of that image. An act of understanding involves grasping a form or intelligible unity in an image. For Lonergan, the accuracy with which Aristotle indicates his understanding of this act of understanding suggests his familiarity with the nature of human cognition. Moreover, in this passage Aristotle highlights the relation between sense and intellect, which Lonergan includes in the process that leads to the key cognitive act of having an insight. As I will note in chapter 6, Lonergan argues that there is an analogy between the operation of having an insight that leads to grasping some intelligible content and certain affective responses that grasp particular values.[37]

Like most of his contemporaries, Aristotle does not focus on justifying the human capacity to know reality. Most likely, the seriously sceptical questions about the human capacity to know reality simply did not occur to Aristotle or his contemporaries. Rather, Aristotle proceeds from the assumption that we can know real things. In *On the Soul*, he accounts for our knowledge of the real in his doctrine of cognitional identity between the knower and the known in the act of cognition: 'Knowledge when actively operative is identical with its object. In the individual potential knowledge has priority in time, but generally it is not prior even in time; for everything comes out of that which actually is.'[38]

Aristotle's starting-point is the real world. He is not concerned with the predominantly modern question of how, if at all, we achieve genuine knowledge of the real or the good. Aristotle's thought avoids many of the epistemological questions of modern and contemporary thinkers. Still, on the assumption that certain emotions, such as anger, have some relation to real injustice, Aristotle explores the relations between such emotions and certain beliefs. Hence, although Aristotle does not address more modern concerns about how we can know the real, Calhoun and Solomon nevertheless conclude that Aristotle's theory of the emotions stands up well to contemporary accounts, and avoids many of their problems.

One of Aristotle's legacies is the family of ethical theories referred to as 'virtue ethics.' Michael Slote points out that almost all systematic approaches to ethics say something about the traits that count as virtues and about the virtues as a whole.[39] A key difference among these theories is the degree of priority accorded to virtues in their accounts. Virtue ethicists hold that morality is to be understood most fundamentally in terms of inner traits or dispositions, known as virtues. Classically, there were four cardinal ethical virtues: temperance, justice, courage, and practical wisdom. To these, Christian thinkers added three theological virtues: faith, hope, and love. The moral virtues are primarily thought of as dispositions toward the good rather than as skills or capacities that allow one to take part in bringing about the good. The virtuous person, for Aristotle, is the one who is positively disposed to, or aims at, fine and right action.[40]

Aristotle's realist account of virtue ethics is only one of several versions. For him, the virtuous agent perceives what is the right or noble action in a situation on the basis of his or her virtuous disposition toward the good. This version of virtue ethics contrasts sharply with other versions, such as the one that, according to some interpreters, Plato defended and those defended by the Epicureans and the Stoics.

For Plato, the virtuous agent has independently admirable motives or other positive inner states. He takes these inner states themselves as of primary concern, rather than considering them merely as disposing the agent properly toward the good. For Plato, it is the expression of these inner motives or states in action that makes these actions right or admirable. That is, his concern with virtue is not understood primarily in relation to knowing and then doing what is right or noble. Rather, Plato's primary concern is to promote an inner disposition of harmony between the parts of the soul. One's acts are of secondary importance, for they derive their goodness or nobility from the fact that they proceed from an inner state of harmony and maintain or enhance it.[41]

The Epicureans and the Stoics shared Aristotle's concern with the relation between the virtues and happiness. In their ethics they introduced two influential concepts into the philosophical tradition that underlie positions taken in the euthanasia debate. Epicurean ethics was a form of hedonism, identifying the good and happiness with what is pleasurable. Although the term 'epicurean' has become a label for positions that promote the pursuit of sensuous pleasure, this is historically unwarranted. The pleasure that the Epicureans did advocate was principally mental tranquillity, akin to Plato's harmony among the parts of the soul. In fact, the Epicureans advocated the virtue of moderation in the pursuit of sensual pleasures, since without such moderation these pleasures were apt to disrupt tranquillity. Another way to this mental tranquillity was the employment of philosophy to argue against those beliefs that induce fear and mental distress, such as beliefs in the gods and the afterlife.

The Stoics also introduced the idea that happiness or the good life consists in living in accordance with 'nature,' 'the natural law,' or 'reason.' To live according to reason is to render oneself immune to the disturbances of the emotions. In practice, the ideal they sought was akin to the mental tranquillity of the Epicureans. Like Plato, the Epicureans and Stoics made certain mental states the primary aim of philosophy. This is what they meant by virtue and the good. Effecting positive changes in the world is 'good' only by association, as either flowing from or contributing to one's mental tranquillity or harmony. In contrast to Aristotle's objectivist position, these versions of virtue ethics are subjectivist.[42]

Aristotelian virtue ethics also downplays the importance of general moral rules. For Aristotle, the virtuous person perceives the good in concrete circumstances of daily life and is able to act fairly effortlessly upon what he perceives to be the unique moral requirements of the situation.[43] Virtue ethicists who speak of moral rules tend to understand them as general statements that follow from particular judgments about what is right or noble. This position is in stark contrast with Kantian and Utilitarian positions. For these modern theories, the virtues, at best, complement the main task of formulating ultimate principles or rules of ethics. For the Kantians, the virtues are tantamount to dispositions to obey or follow what these rules prescribe. For the Utilitarians, they are the dispositions whose existence furthers the goals specified in principles of right action.[44] The key difference is in the starting points of moral reasoning. For Aristotle, the good is concretely intelligible, and his ethics begins with reflections on the intelligibility of particular determinations of the good by the virtuous person. For the Utilitarian, the good is concretely experienced. This experience is good in as much as it is agreeable or pleasurable, but there is no need to reflect further on its intelligibility. For Kant, by contrast, the good is abstract and general. It is first grasped as a universal moral law, and then one invokes the law to decide particular cases.

3.2   Thomas Aquinas (1224/5–1274)

Aquinas advances Aristotle's virtue ethics. His is the most influential version of moral philosophy in medieval Christendom. This philosophy is born of an attempt to marry Christian morality and the contributions of Greek philosophy, mainly those derived from Aristotle.[45] An important idea which Aquinas takes from Aristotle is that to know what the end of human action consists in, one must identify the distinctive 'functions' of human beings. Aquinas understands these functions to be consistent with the end of human life, an end with which a divine creator endows humans. Like Aristotle, Aquinas holds that to understand this end, it is essential to understand human nature and to identify the natural purposes proper to human beings.[46] For Aquinas, this end is the fulfilment of our deepest desires in loving union with and possession of God, in this life and in the next. In this end, then, is the notion of a personal, loving relationship with God. Reflecting this end, Aquinas makes charity the principal virtue that sets the context for the practice of all the other virtues.[47] By supposing a different end of human life, Aquinas transposes Aristotelian virtue ethics into a new key. Thus, Aristotle's virtuous individual is the most independent of persons. For Aquinas, by contrast, the virtuous person is the most dependent in so far as he or she truly realizes and fully lives according to his or her relation of ultimate dependence on God.[48]

Besides the ultimate human dependence on God, Aquinas also recognizes our dependence on God-given natural human attributes, including those belonging to human psychology. The extent and place that the topic of the passions occupies in Aquinas's major work, the *Summa Theologiae* (*Summary of Theology*), gives evidence of the importance he ascribes to emotions. His treatise *De Passionibus Animae* (The Passions of the Soul) occupies the largest section of the *Prima Secundae* of the *Summa* (i.e., the first part of the second part of the *Summa Theologiae*). Here, the first 5 questions investigate the ultimate goal of human life, and the remaining 298 deal with human activity in so far as it bears on reaching this ultimate goal. Questions 6 to 48 study the acts themselves, and in questions 22 to 48 Aquinas addresses what he calls the *passiones animae*, or the passions.[49]

John Patrick Read is one Thomist scholar who argues that the emphasis of Aquinas on the passions is consistent with his view that all human functions are important for our ultimate end. This includes not only those functions that are specifically human, but also those we share with animals. Read believes that Aquinas scholarship pays too little attention to this fact. As a consequence, this scholarship typically ignores much of Aquinas's psychological writings, even though Aquinas believes a study of these functions to be intrinsic to any study of the moral and spiritual life. Although the passions Aquinas describes in this section of the *Summa* are not specifically human, nevertheless he understood them to be part of human nature. Unlike a substantial portion of the tradition that follows Aquinas, Read contends that Aquinas recognizes every asset humans enjoy and neglects nothing that pertains to human well-being and happiness.[50]

Aquinas uses several conceptual distinctions to systematize his treatment of the passions. For instance, he specifies each passion according to its object. The sensory *orexis* or appetitive faculty deems objects to be either good or evil. Aquinas speaks of good objects as those that evoke the emotion love and are sought after; evil objects are those that induce hatred and are avoided. Another basic distinction is between objects as present and as future. Future possible objects, for instance, might be easy or difficult to obtain if good, or to avoid if evil. Objects that are present and easy to obtain inspire concupiscible passions, such as joy. Those objects or entities that are future and difficult to obtain or avoid, that is, arduous goods or evils, induce irascible passions, such as hope or fear. This scheme is dynamic and changes depending on the relation between the agent and the various objects being sought or avoided. For example, in relation to an arduous good one might be (1) apprehending the object as desirable, or (2) in the process of striving for that which one desires, or (3) resting in the joy of its possession: 'Accordingly, the first change wrought in the appetite by the appetible object is called *love*, and is nothing else than complacency in that object; and from this complacency results a movement toward that same object, and this movement is *desire*; and lastly, there is rest which is *joy*.'[51]

The emotions an athlete might experience in his quest to win a competition illustrate some of these features of Aquinas's analysis. If winning is the object of the athlete's desire and this goal is difficult to obtain, then this goal would be an arduous good (i.e., in the future and difficult to obtain). The move from merely wanting this end to making some effort to attain it corresponds to a shift from the appetite as concupiscible to the appetite as irascible. If the athlete is progressing well toward this goal, he will be hopeful. If he estimates his likelihood of success in attaining his goal to be good, he will be filled with courage. If the reverse is true, he will be despairing and fearful. Anger might arise if he believes that someone unjustly undermined his chances of success. With his success at winning the competition, he experiences delight and rest in the possession of the object of his love. Hence, from the athlete's initial emotion of neediness, when he is without the good he desires, he ends in the state of joy with the possession of his prize. Conversely, if he fails to achieve his end, he moves from a state of neediness to one of sorrow.[52]

The above analysis illustrates several noteworthy features of Aquinas's view of the emotions and their relation to reason. First, he defines emotions by reference to their relation to objects, even when these objects are not materially present, for instance, as imagined future possibilities.[53] For him, terms such as wanting, hoping, courage, fear, joy, and sorrow are labels for experiences whose intelligibility is captured by reference to objects. The possession of an object might be perceived as good, and one's failure to possess it as evil. In this way, Aquinas's analysis is thoroughly intentional.

Second, the 'good' or 'evil' objects to which the sensory *orexis* or 'flesh' relates us are merely 'apparent' goods and evils. It is a further question for Aquinas whether these objects are truly good, that is, whether they are also good or evil objects from the vantage point of what he calls the intellectual appetite or the will. For Aquinas, a key distinction that underpins this whole discussion of the passions and acts common to man and animals is that between the appetites of the sense and intellectual faculties.[54]

Third, regarding the morality of the passions, Aquinas considers them in two ways. Considering them as merely natural acts, they are neither good nor evil. For in as much as natural acts are more akin to instincts and not matters of choice, moral considerations are irrelevant. Still, even as natural acts they might be subject to the command of the reason and will. To this extent they have moral relevance. The passions are considered voluntary either from being commanded by the will, or from the will not checking them.[55]

Aquinas acknowledges that emotions have their own bent. Still, he also recognizes that rational powers might control them indirectly. For instance, the angry man might decide to cool his anger with a cold shower (i.e., make deliberate use of a physiological mechanism to counter an emotion). Again, he could invoke an angry response to counter inappropriate lustful passions (i.e., deliberately fostering one emotion to counter another). The key difference between the goods grasped by sensitive appetites and those grasped by intellectual ones is that one knows the intellectual good through some judgment. In this way, Aquinas thinks that some emotions, such as sorrow, may be said to be morally good. For instance, the experience of sorrow after doing some evil act might be morally good because it provides some inducement for the person to avoid repeating this act.

Finally, the terms 'complacency' and 'connaturality' figure prominently in Aquinas's account. He speaks of complacency in an object that is connatural to the agent. If the object is connatural or fitting to the agent, that is, in keeping with his or her appetites, he or she 'adapts' to that object. Conversely, the agent may be said to apprehend the object as connatural through or by means of this experience of complacency or adaptation to the object. Following this sensory apprehension, the agent might initiate a move toward acquiring the object. In humans, an analogous pattern occurs at the intellectual level. Hence, Aquinas distinguishes among objects (e.g., good or evil, present or future, simple or arduous to obtain) and among emotions according to our relation to the possession of these objects (e.g., desire becomes joy with the possession of what was initially a future arduous good). Of key importance in this whole discussion, however, is the recognition of a moment of complacency that occurs prior to the grasp of, and subsequent move toward, the good. This moment of complacency is distinct from the emotion of joy, as it might occur in the mere apprehension of a good *in absentia*.[56]

Aquinas's psychological theory can accommodate cases in which the agent misapprehends objects of desire. Following Aristotle, Aquinas maintains that the correctness of such apprehensions is conditioned by the agent's moral character and habits. If he has a wicked habit, for instance, evil might appear to be good because 'to anyone that has a habit, whatever is befitting to him in respect of that habit, has the aspect of something loveable, since it thereby becomes, in a way, connatural to him, according as custom or habit are a second nature.'[57]

Quoting from Aristotle's *Nicomachean Ethics*, Aquinas concludes that 'the virtuous man judges aright of the end of virtue, because *such as a man is, such does the end seem to him (Nic. Ethics iii. 5).*'[58]

In chapter 6 I will indicate how Lonergan develops these notions, especially that of complacency. I will explore the apprehensive act that Aquinas seems to be highlighting in his discussion of complacency and ask how this act might be understood as an affective cognition and where it fits in relation to value judgments. For now, let me complete this brief survey of the Aristotelian-Thomistic tradition by summarizing some modern developments brought about by thinkers such as Max Scheler and Edith Stein.

3.3 Max Scheler (1874–1928)

Max Scheler, along with Edmund Husserl, whom Scheler met in 1901, founded the philosophical movement known as *phenomenology*.[59] Scheler was also a founder of philosophical anthropology and of sociology of knowledge, and the first to apply phenomenology practically to problems, for example, in ethics, culture, and religion.[60] A contemporary of Martin Heidegger, he was also preoccupied with the questions 'What is man?' and 'What is his position in Being?'[61]

Scheler held a position at the University of Munich between 1907 and 1910. There he met Franz Brentano and a number of Husserl's students, including Edith Stein. In 1916, after Scheler had left the University of Munich, he set out his views on feelings and value judgments in his major work in moral philosophy, *Formalism in Ethics and Non-Formal Ethics*. In this work, Scheler distinguishes between two types of feelings, those that are 'non-intentional' states or trends, and those that are 'intentional responses.'[62]

In *Formalism*, Scheler seeks to ground an ethical absolutism and value-objectivism in an emotional intuitionism.[63] He develops a distinctive theory about how we grasp values in persons, things, and acts, basing his theory on a phenomenological analysis of making evaluations. Scheler concludes that 'our original awareness of valuable features of the world around us occurs in our emotional responses to them.'[64] He refers to these emotional responses as 'value-feelings,' or 'feeling-functions.' These are intentional affective responses to values, and are a kind of 'intuition' or 'insight' into what is or is not valuable. Unlike Hume and Brentano, Scheler maintains that the 'value-facts' that we come to know by our feeling-functions are not thereby irredeemably subjective. When we say that a Van Gogh painting is beautiful, for instance, we are not simply saying that it evokes certain agreeable feelings, as perhaps Hume's analysis might suggest. Rather, it is through certain feeling responses that we first grasp the aesthetic value of such a painting. For Scheler, then, such feeling responses have a cognitive function in the strict sense of being an intrinsic part of the process by means of which we know values through value judgments. Although I might grasp the aesthetic value of one painting as superior to another through these psychological feeling-functions, for instance, I might nevertheless subsequently affirm the content of this value judgment as epistemically objective. Moreover, Scheler believes that these feeling-functions are a necessary part of the process of making an evaluation. As he puts it, if we were not emotional beings, our whole intellectual life would be restricted to knowing facts without ever evaluating them.[65]

Even though Scheler believes that humans know values through feelings, he is ready to admit that our feelings in relation to values might differ. He accounts for these differences by appealing to sociological and/or communal factors that influence the range of value-feelings one acquires. On his account, a person is essentially both individual (i.e., a concrete unity of acts) and a member of a community. In order to understand an individual, one needs to view him or her in the context of their community, and the community itself in the context of its history. The life-history of individuals and their communities differ, and these differences will condition the habits individuals acquire as well as their responses to values. Moreover, Scheler observes that, as a matter of sociological fact, many persons in modern societies lack feelings for higher values. Because of this, these persons are incapable of fully participating in the types of communities (e.g., political and religious) devoted to these higher values. Nevertheless, he thought that, as a matter of social policy, everyone should have adequate, perhaps equal, access to the values a community can offer them.[66]

Although Scheler begins his analysis by attending to such psychological phenomena as feeling-functions, he concludes his discussion by affirming an epistemically objective scale of value preferences. He argues that there must be a scale of distinct values to explain such things as the possibility of enjoying a glass of wine while being in an unhappy mood. He interprets this experience as providing evidence for the presence of at least two distinct values to which one might be responding affectively at the same time. In preferring one value to another, one relies on some ranking of these values. Although Scheler suggests six criteria for ranking values, he maintains that it is impossible to derive or deduce this scale of value preferences logically. His own ranking is as follows: pleasure-pain (values of sensible feeling); noble-vulgar (values of vital feeling); beautiful-ugly; just-unjust; pure knowledge of truth (spiritual values); and holy-unholy (religious values).[67]

Following Hume's earlier example, Scheler also takes 'sympathy' to be an important emotion to analyse, since it has great relevance to morality. In his work *The Nature of Sympathy*, Scheler analyses sympathy phenomenologically in order to address the philosophical problem of the apparent bridge between a subject and an object. As previously discussed, it is essentially this problem that leads Hume to reject the possibility of epistemically objective knowledge.

Later, Scheler would revise some of his conclusions regarding empathy under the influence of Edith Stein's philosophical dissertation on 'The

Problem of Empathy,' which Edmund Husserl supervised.[68] To her contribution to the discussion I now turn.

3.4 Edith Stein (1891–1942)

Edith Stein's influence on the thinking of both Scheler and Husserl in the area of the affective life make her contributions to this tradition worthy of highlighting. For Stein, as for the later Scheler, the exploration of emotional responses to another person is especially important to the philosophical debate regarding the capacity of a person to know some other person, which Stein refers to as a 'foreign consciousness.' By examining one's empathic feelings in relation to another person, one is thrown into the world of intersubjectivity. This phenomenon casts new light on the apparently impassable bridge between oneself and any non-self. This is precisely how emotions, for Stein, become a key to the intellectual puzzles of the mind/body duality or the bridge between the world of subjects and of objects. For Stein, it is by means of certain feeling-functions that humans have the capacity to understand other subjects, who in some sense are also objects. This occurs through one's capacity sometimes to grasp what another is feeling. In such 'empathic responses,' as she called them, one can experience feelings that are, in the first instance, the other person's. Stein indicates that the original source of the feelings is in the other person's experience, a fact that she highlights by calling them 'non-primordial' feelings. That is, I grasp another's feelings, and in some manner *experience* them, in my interpretation of the other. This interpretation is based on certain expressions that portray their emotional state, expressions that they might only inadvertently manifest.[69]

For Stein, genuine empathy is no mere projection of oneself into another. Nor does she interpret empathy to be merely a remembered experience of feelings similar to those the other is now experiencing. Although I never 'feel' what the other is experiencing, I might be able to identify, explicate, and objectify the other's experience. Indeed, Stein claims that such attention to the feeling-functions of another is a necessary condition for comprehending the psychic life of one's fellow humans.[70]

In comprehending persons through empathic responses, we have a basis for understanding both them and ourselves, and different scales of values.[71] Stein, like Scheler, believes that by means of such empathic encounters with another, one can grasp the 'kernel value' at the centre of the other's character. Just as one distinguishes among values and ranks them, so one can also distinguish among personality types based on their ranking of values preferences.[72] On this account, one's being able to share, in some way, the feelings of another, does not exhaust the meaning of compassion or empathy. Rather, compassion or empathy also involves some personal discernment, since it invites one to discover not only another's kernel values, but also one's own. This explains why a genuine empathic encounter with another is typically a personal challenge. It calls into question not merely the values the other holds, but also one's own.

The positions of Scheler and Stein on emotions, and their relevance to value judgments, are in stark contrast with some of the other moral philosophers previously mentioned. Against Hume, Scheler and Stein would counter that not everything psychic and spiritual can be derived from sense experience. Against the Utilitarians, they would condemn the subordination of the noble to the useful, attributing this to the industrial, business mentality. Against Kant, they would reject the reduction of all feelings to some precognitive level, thereby excluding the relevance of the emotions to anything cognitive, including ethics. Against Kant's formalism, Scheler would reject the supposition that the basic principles of ethics and values depend on logical axioms. Finally, as to Aristotle and Aquinas, they would reject the presupposition of a set of timeless, static goods and ends. Instead, they would highlight the importance of history and sociology in understanding what persons judge to be genuinely good.[73]

4   Some Terminological Clarifications

To round out this survey of some of the prominent notions concerning the relation between reason and emotion in the history of Western philosophy, I will now attend to some of the terminology I will be using in the subsequent sections of this discussion. Because there are diverse views on the relation between emotions and reason, I need to define some of my key terms in a way that will promote clarity of expression without committing me to a definitive stance on how emotions enter into reason, if at all. In this section, I will focus on three terms: *affect*, *evaluations*, and *euthanasia*. I will begin by establishing an initial understanding of the terms *affect* and *evaluation* that is consistent with Lonergan's usage. I will also discuss these terms in the context of their historical and contemporary philosophical usage. Finally, I will also define the term *euthanasia*, in order to highlight the relevance of key notions, such as *competence* and *voluntariness*, in the contemporary debate. A more precise meaning of these terms will become clear, I hope, as the discussion advances. What I am particularly concerned to avoid here are certain misunderstandings of these terms.

4.1 Affect

The term *affect* is roughly synonymous with terms such as 'feeling,' 'emotion,' or 'passion.' The long and convoluted history of the use of the term 'passion,' for instance, illustrates well the tendency, both inside and outside philosophy, to contrast passions, emotions, feelings, or affects, on the one hand, with reason, on the other hand. Robert Solomon points out that the ancient philosophers treated passion as a kind of madness, and the Stoics diagnosed passions as 'profound and often fatal misunderstandings.' Consistent with this view is that of those modern philosophers who treated the passions as 'confused perceptions and distorted judgments.' The dominant philosophical opinion was summed up by the Greek Aesop, who maintained that 'reason must be the master of the passions.' Against this long-standing advice is an equally long tradition of thought that sought to give the passions their due by challenging their unflattering contrast with reason. This opposing stance was summed up by David Hume when he announced that 'reason is and ought to be the slave of the passions.'[74] This dispute underpins the various definitions of emotions that I will briefly explore.

Lonergan uses the term *affect* when he speaks of the goal of moral development. That goal is a state where values are whatever one loves, and evils are whatever one hates; and if the goal is attained, 'affectivity is of a single piece.'[75] In the case of Lonergan's core claim that 'apprehensions of values are given in feelings,' he qualifies the more general term 'feelings' to denote those psychological elements of consciousness that have evaluative attributes.[76] The 'feelings' to which Lonergan is referring are those that are intentional affective responses that relate one consciously to objects that are values.[77] I will use the term *affect* in the subsequent discussion to denote this more restricted sense of 'feelings.' In this way, I hope to avoid certain misleading images and preconceptions that are now commonly attached to terms such as 'passions,' 'emotions,' or 'feelings.' Hence, by focusing on affect and its role in value judgments, I am referring to those feelings or emotional elements of one's moral psychology that are intentional, that is, directed to certain objects. These are the affective elements that Lonergan claims have a cognitive function, and they play some role in value judgments.[78]

In chapter 4 I will further clarify Lonergan's specialized understanding of 'feelings' by locating it within a range of views represented in the main traditions of Western philosophy. However, in order to provide a preliminary clarification of what Lonergan means by *affect*, it may be helpful at this point to compare and contrast his use with other contemporary definitions of this term.

In the *Oxford English Dictionary* (*OED*), the terms 'affect,' 'feeling,' 'emotion,' 'sentiment,' 'passion,' and 'appetite' are used synonymously and mutually define each other. The *OED* defines the term 'affect' in much the same way as 'feeling.' In its first sense, 'affect' is a mental disposition or constitution; a mood, feeling, desire, or intention. The *OED* further qualifies the meaning of 'affect' as referring to a disposition that is (1b) 'inward,' rather than an external manifestation or action, and (1c) 'a feeling, desire, or appetite, as opposed to reason.'[79] This definition of 'affect' is compatible with the sense in which I will be using the term to refer to emotional, feeling, sentimental, or passionate experiences of consciousness. Accordingly, I will not be using 'affects' to refer to certain somatic or physiological states or to non-cognitive psychological states.

The usage I am adopting is consistent with current usage in mainstream Western philosophy. For instance, Simon Blackburn defines 'affective' in his *Dictionary of Philosophy* as 'the feature of an experience which renders it pleasurable or desirable, or the reverse, or which gives it a distinctive emotional tone.'[80] He defines emotion as 'a state that can prompt some activities and interfere with others. These states have characteristic feelings, and they have characteristic bodily expressions. Unlike moods, they have objects: one grieves over some particular thing, or is angry at something.'[81]

Blackburn defines 'emotion' as having an object, unlike moods or affects. This definition suggests that although emotions are distinct from intellectual acts, they are nevertheless cognitive.[82] This view of emotions is roughly compatible with Lonergan's view of 'affective responses,' which are a subset of feelings that besides having physiological and psychological characteristics (i.e., pleasurable or desirable, or the reverse) also have a cognitive function. That is, certain affects not only are bodily and mental experiences, they also have a 'directed, cognitive side having a specific object.'[83]

A pithy allusion to the specifically evaluative cognitive function of an affective response is the sense of the term 'feeling' that Shakespeare used in *Richard II*, where he writes: 'the apprehension of the good, Gives but the greater feeling to the worse.'[84] Here, feeling is understood as a feature of one's apprehensive acts. It is by means of one's affective responses to some thing that some content is known – in this case, the worth or value of a thing. This usage suggests not only the apprehensive feature of certain feelings, but also a certain non-identity between the psychological quality of a feeling and the content that one grasps by means of it. That is, for Shakespeare the 'greater feeling' of approbation grasps the good or the greater value, even though this same thing might be 'worse' in the sense that it is less satisfying to oneself.

There are also several different uses of the term 'feeling' to be kept distinct from what I have in mind when using the term 'affect.' These uses typically presuppose some non-cognitive theory that sharply disjoins feelings/desires, on the one hand, and reason/beliefs, on the other. Consequently, they tend to define 'feelings' by emphasizing their psychological qualities, and frequently fail to relate feelings to other cognitive acts or achievements. In the 1950s, for instance, many psychologists defined the emotion of fear by referring exclusively to its physiological and behavioural correlates. Thus, one writer defined fear as 'one of the primitive, violent, and usually crippling emotions, marked by extensive bodily changes, and by behavior of the flight or concealment character.'[85] Some four decades later, some psychologists added to this definition of fear its relation to reality. Thus, one writer expressed his understanding of 'fear' as an '[u]npleasurable emotional state consisting of psychophysiological changes in response to a realistic threat or danger.'[86] Typically, such writers contrasted fear with anxiety. They defined 'anxiety' as an emotional state in response to an intra-psychic conflict, where the danger or threat is unreal rather than realistic. The first definition expresses an understanding of this feeling of fear as unrelated to the directed, cognitive side of emotions. But even in the revised definition, where there is an effort to relate fear to the reality of a fearful object, there remains a failure to capture the evaluative function of certain emotions. For Lonergan, a key distinction between what one means by fear and anxiety is that fear is an intentional, affective response to some object (i.e., a cognitive act, not merely a state), whereas anxiety is a non-intentional state that has a cause but does not arise out of a cognitive response (i.e., as a response to some known or apparent actual or possible object or event).[87]

4.2 Evaluation

The next term to clarify is 'evaluation,' which is a more general expression than 'value judgment' for Lonergan's fourth level of conscious intentionality. Lonergan distinguishes the 'notion of value' from a 'value judgment.' For him, *value* is a transcendental *notion*: 'It is what is intended in questions for deliberation.'[88] The *notion* of value is intermediate between ignorance and knowledge of values. One moves from ignorance to knowledge of values through, or by means of, a 'value judgment.'[89] Such a judgment states or purports to state what is or is not (would or would not be) truly good or really better. Lonergan further distinguishes the cognitional achievement of a value judgment from consequent decisions to implement, if feasible, this value judgment. Through a value judgment, one achieves cognitional self-transcendence without reaching the fullness of moral self-transcendence. One achieves moral self-transcendence not simply by knowing, but also by deciding to enjoy or act on this knowledge, and proceeding to implement this decision.[90]

Lonergan's views on values and value judgments cast new light on two opinions that originated in the 1890s. Alexius Meinong argued that the source of value was *feeling*, or the expectation or possibility of pleasure in an object. Against him, Christian von Ehrenfels (with Spinoza) countered that the source of value was *desire*. For Ehrenfels, an object possesses value because it is desired.[91] Both of these thinkers argued that some affective elements of consciousness were the source of one's cognitive grasp of values, and that such cognitive achievements grounded real or objective values. In contrast to Ehrenfels's view, Lonergan understands something akin to 'desire' (i.e., the transcendental intention of value) to be the ultimate cognitional criterion of knowing value. But he would reverse Ehrenfels expression by saying that one properly desires an object because it possesses value. Again, in contrast to Meinong's position, Lonergan distinguishes sharply between *feelings* that are intentional responses to satisfactions or pleasures and those that respond to values. Lonergan maintains that the latter feelings play a crucial role in value judgments.

Lonergan's position highlights the distinction between the function of feelings in evaluations and the contents one achieves through or by means of a value judgment. This distinguishes questions about the *epistemic objectivity* of cognitive achievements from the earlier questions about affective, cognitive acts themselves. The term 'epistemic' is an adjective derived from the Greek word *epistēmē*, meaning knowledge. In standard usage, a proposition is said to be epistemic 'if and only if it has some implication for what, in some circumstances, is rationally worthy of belief.'[92] By the term 'epistemic objectivity' I will refer to this characteristic. By contrast, this characteristic is absent if one's knowing is *epistemically subjective*. By this latter term I will refer to those fact or value judgments, and the propositions expressing them, that are cognitionally unsuccessful, false, or invalid.[93]

4.3 Euthanasia

The final term that calls for some preliminary definition is *euthanasia*. The 'euthanasia debate' concerns whether or not to change the received/ traditional legal or moral status of certain deliberate acts of causing death that occur in some medical context of suffering or in the case of a terminal illness. The Canadian Special Senate Committee on Euthanasia and Assisted Suicide set out an understanding of these terms that I will adopt for the purposes of the present discussion.[94] For the committee, *euthanasia* is 'a deliberate act undertaken by one person with the intention of ending the life of another person to relieve that person's suffering where that act is the cause of death.' Assisted suicide is 'the act of intentionally killing oneself with the assistance of another who provides the knowledge, means, or both.' The committee distinguished these activities from a series of others, such as 'palliative care,' 'total sedation,' 'treatment aimed at the alleviation of suffering that may shorten life,' 'withholding of life-sustaining treatment,' and 'withdrawal of life-sustaining treatment.' The debate focuses on the legal status of the most compelling type of case, such as Sue Rodriguez's, in which assisted suicide was performed 'voluntarily' on and by a 'competent' individual. A person is deemed *competent* if he or she is 'capable of understanding the nature and consequences of the decision to be made and capable of communicating this decision.' The act is *voluntary* if it is 'done in accordance with the wishes of a competent individual or a valid advance directive.' At the centre of the public and philosophical controversy are cases of 'voluntary active euthanasia' (VAE), especially those of physician-assisted suicide.[95]

5   Summary

In chapter 2 I suggested that disputants engaging in the euthanasia debate agree that the discussion ought to go forward on 'rational' grounds. Even so, certain apparently 'non-rational' emotions, such as compassion, fear, and despair are part of the experiences of persons with a terminal illness. Such emotions sometimes shape the views and decisions of persons with a terminal illness. They also tend to influence public opinion regarding issues such as euthanasia. For a number of thinkers on both sides of the euthanasia debate, feelings are relevant. Moreover, the proponents' claim that public policy ought to permit euthanasia is based, to some degree, on the methodological stance that the emotions of the person in question who is considering euthanasia are relevant in important ways to their conclusions. In order to explore this contention, I have reviewed the main families of stances on the relation between emotion and reason in the present chapter.

Major thinkers in the history of Western philosophy have conceived of the relation between emotions and reason in diverse and frequently opposed ways. No matter where one stands on the substantive issues of euthanasia, it is surely helpful to be clear on what one thinks 'rational' discourse ought to include and exclude. Moreover, it is also worthwhile to discuss how appeals to such emotions as 'compassion' ought to be interpreted, and just how such notions both (a) do and (b) ought to shape one's evaluations. In this chapter I have attempted to provide an overview of two main families of positions on this issue. It is intended to provide some historical context for the examination in part 3 of Lonergan's account of the role of affect in value judgments.

Summarizing their more extensive historical survey of views on what an emotion is, Calhoun and Solomon conclude: 'Granting that emotions in some way involve cognition, it is an open question and a topic of considerable debate just how cognition is related to emotion.'[96] This chapter has been an effort to locate the tradition out of which Lonergan comes. That tradition advances a position on how cognition is related to emotion that lies somewhere between two extreme historical traditions. On the view I attributed to thinkers such as Hume and Hobbes, feelings are psychologically related to value judgments. Still, at least in Hume's case, the content of the derivative judgments are never epistemically objective. That is, for him *values* refer to nothing other than expressions of emotions. A second family, here exemplified by Kant, rejects the contention made by the first family that all evaluations are merely epistemically subjective. Kant seeks to avoid this conclusion by rejecting the cognitive relevance of feelings in value judgments. That is, Kant argues that emotions have nothing to do with knowing values. I suggested that what is common to both views is the notion that epistemically objective evaluations are quite distinct from emotions.[97]

A second aim of this chapter was to examine the Aristotelian-Thomistic tradition as well as some more contemporary developments that have occurred within it. Beginning with Aristotle, I highlighted several philosophical notions that are important for understanding Lonergan's own position. Aristotle, Aquinas, Scheler, and Stein each holds that feelings are cognitively relevant to value judgments. In fact, they hold that certain feeling responses or 'feeling-functions' are key to grasping values. Moreover, for them the values thus grasped are sometimes epistemically objective.

In this debate regarding the relation of feelings to reason, then, there are two key issues at stake. One issue has to do with the *phenomenal role* that feelings play in evaluations. A further issue is the *epistemic status* of evaluations based, in part, on feelings. In Hume's case, he is adamant that feelings play a phenomenal role in knowing values. The problem, however, lies with the second issue. On the question of the epistemic status of value knowledge Hume seems to reply that all our knowing is never more than epistemically subjective. For him, the contents achieved through one's cognitive processes are at best subjective reports about oneself. In subsequent chapters I will seek to distinguish sharply between the positions of Hume and Lonergan on the question of the epistemic status of evaluations.

I have argued that in contrast to Hume's position Kant affirms at least a practical epistemic objectivity of the moral law. In so doing he rejects the relevance of emotions or 'inclinations' to the cognitive (i.e., formal) processes by which we know values. Not only does Kant affirm what Hume denies, but he also takes the issue of the practical epistemic status of evaluations to be the fundamental one. Despite Kant's apparently negative stance on the role of feelings in the moral life, a notion that plays a fundamental role in his ethics is 'respect.' This notion is arguably a feeling (or at least closely connected to a feeling), which suggests that Kant's position on the first issue might not be as radically opposed to Hume's as it first appears. Indeed, with Scheler, I wonder whether Kant would have grasped the value of the capacity for moral agency without having recourse to his own feeling-functions.

I have also pointed out that Aristotle and Aquinas began their accounts with metaphysics. They articulated their accounts of emotion on the basis of what they believed to be the self-evident relations between real objects encountered in the world and the corresponding feelings. However, even allowing for this world-view, Calhoun and Solomon nevertheless conclude that Aristotle's twenty-five-hundred-year-old theory of emotion stands up to most contemporary criticism.[98] Scheler's account of emotions transposes both Aristotle's and Aquinas's views into the modern context, in which metaphysics is no longer taken to be the usual starting point. With Hume, Scheler agrees that certain emotions or feeling-functions are necessary in order to grasp values. Scheler goes beyond both Hume and Kant by claiming that the knowledge of values thus achieved can be genuine or epistemically objective, and indeed, they are the basis of his ranking of different types of values.

Despite the differences in time and starting points, Aristotle, Aquinas, Scheler, and Stein individually and collectively make some important philo-sophical contributions to understanding the role of emotions in value judgments. I have highlighted several of these: the notion of insight as the act of grasping a form (or intelligible unity) in an image; the metaphysical distinction of potency, form, and act as correlative with the distinctions among cognitive acts of experiencing, understanding, and judging; the doctrine of identity between knower and known in the act of cognition; and the doctrines of connaturality between the lover and the beloved, which is recognized in a moment of complacency. Scheler's thought illustrates the shift from faculty psychology to intentionality analysis, from metaphysics to phenomenology as basic. With contributions from Edith Stein, we already have a detailed analysis of certain emotions, such as empathy, that high-lights both their complexity and their pervasiveness.

A third aim of this chapter was to provide some terminological clarifica-tions of *affect, evaluation,* and *euthanasia.* For Lonergan, the affects that are key in his analysis are those that are intentional responses to objects, by contrast with those that are non-intentional states. The intentional affective responses that are most significant are those that respond to values, by contrast with responses to satisfactions or what is agreeable to me. On this view, affectivity plays a cognitive role in reason when it comes to discerning among values, and between values and mere satisfactions, as will become more evident in chapter 7. By contrast with *affectivity, evaluations,* or more specifically *value judgments,* refer not to elements of one's cognitive activities or operations, but to the content of one's cognitive achievements. I contrasted Lonergan's value theory with subjective and objective alternatives, both of which fail to distinguish clearly between questions about cognitive activities, and those regarding the epistemic status of cognitive achievements.

In addition to defining affect and evaluations, I also outlined the contemporary understanding of *euthanasia*. The form of euthanasia that is at the centre of the debate is 'voluntary active euthanasia' (cf. involuntary or non-voluntary or passive euthanasia). Key moral notions this definition includes are 'voluntariness,' 'competence,' 'intended end,' and 'means.' Voluntary active euthanasia involves a deliberate act by one party, at the request of a second party, that directly causes the second party's death. I will confine the discussion here to voluntary active euthanasia, which many thinkers take to be morally equivalent to physician-assisted suicide. In the latter case, the physician supplies a patient with the means or knowledge to commit suicide. In all cases of euthanasia, the intended end is to relieve suffering. For euthanasia to be voluntary, the individual whose life is to be ended has to make a 'competent' and 'voluntary' request to have it so ended. The issue of the relation between emotion (i.e., affect or wishes) and reason (i.e., competence), therefore, is relevant to the very definition of voluntary active euthanasia.

As Calhoun and Solomon suggest, it remains an open question just how emotions relate to value judgments. If emotions are fundamentally relevant to value judgments, will the resultant knowledge be merely epistemically subjective? On the basis of an affirmative account of the cognitive importance of emotions, could one articulate a systematic moral philosophy? If so, can such an analysis help to meet certain key ethical questions of the day, such as those on which the euthanasia debate hinges?

To begin to answer these questions I now turn to Bernard Lonergan's philosophy. In the next four chapters, I will spell out Lonergan's account not merely of the relevance of certain feelings for value judgments, but also of the precise role that they play in his general cognitional theory.

PART THREE

Lonergan's View of the Role of Affect in Evaluations

4

Lonergan on Cognitional Structure: A Phenomenology of Mind

Existential reflection is at once enlightening and enriching ... But the very wealth of existential reflection can turn out to be a trap. It is indeed the key that opens the doors to a philosophy, not of man in the abstract, but of concrete human living in its historical unfolding. Still, one must not think that such concreteness eliminates the ancient problems of cognitional theory, epistemology, and metaphysics, for if they occur in an abstract context, they recur with all the more force in a concrete context.

Bernard Lonergan, 'The Subject' (*A Second Collection*)

1   An Overview of Lonergan's Account of Human Cognition

As I noted in chapter 1, Bernard Lonergan (1904–1984) was a Canadian-born Jesuit philosopher and theologian, whose best-known writings are *Insight: A Study of Human Understanding* (1957) and *Method in Theology* (1972). As William Fennell points out in the *Canadian Encyclopedia*, Lonergan's principal contribution lay in the area of method, where he demonstrated 'the methodical interrelation of the natural and social sciences, philosophy and theology.'[1] Lonergan's view of the basis for this methodological unity is his critical-realist cognitional theory. Central to Lonergan's realism is his claim, which I will elaborate presently, that *objectivity* (toward which thinkers in various disciplines are striving) is but the fruit of *authentic subjectivity* (grounded in the attentive, intelligent, reasonable, and responsible activities of human knowers and doers). Frederick Crowe, himself a student of Lonergan for more than fifty years, has explained that *Insight* and *Method in Theology* represent distinct periods in the development of Lonergan's interests. *Insight* was written during an earlier period when Lonergan's primary concern was the study of human understanding and knowledge, or 'mind.' *Method in Theology* is the product of a later period when Lonergan turned to address questions about the human capacity for feeling and loving, or 'heart.'[2]

My primary purpose here is to retrieve Lonergan's views on the role of affectivity or *heart* in making evaluations. In order to do this I must begin with his more general views on human understanding or *mind*. Hence, before addressing my focal questions, which are concerned with the evaluations that underpin various decisional responses to suffering and how one makes these evaluations, I will attend to the more basic philosophical questions having to do with knowing. These include the phenomenal question, 'What am I doing when I am knowing anything?' and the epistemic question, 'How does doing this yield genuine knowledge of the real?' Accordingly, I will begin neither with metaphysical questions about which values are, or ought to be, affirmed in cases such as those concerning euthanasia, nor with phenomenal questions about the specific features of one's knowing that form the basis on which one affirms, or ought to affirm, values. Rather, I will begin with an analysis of the phenomenon of knowing that culminates in making fact judgments or, more simply stated, in making judgments as distinct from evaluations.[3] I will address epistemic questions concerning the validity or objectivity of these judgments in chapter 5. And I will address phenomenal and epistemic questions concerning evaluating and deciding in chapters 6 and 7.

I deal with epistemological issues concerning judging and evaluating in separate chapters because I anticipate that for many readers a key difficulty with Lonergan's position on the role affect plays in evaluations will be of an epistemic nature. That is, the question will be 'If our evaluations involve affect, how is this knowledge ever true, genuine or valid?' For Lonergan, such an objection also calls into question the basis of judgments by raising the more general question about the truth or validity of any judgment, and whether a key criterion for the truth of evaluations ought to include a suppression of the knower's own affectivity. By attending to Lonergan's early writings on mind, my strategy is to begin with his account of judgments, and only then respond to the epistemic challenge concerning such judgments. Indeed, for Lonergan, one first knows facts or the real before one evaluates these facts. In addition, questions about the validity of one's knowledge first arise, and are, in many ways, more easily addressed, when one's knowledge concerns factual matters, rather than evaluations. Hence, I will address both of these issues prior to turning to the central questions regarding the role of affect in making evaluations.

2   Cognitional Structure: Bringing to Light My Own Knowing

In Lonergan's original unpublished preface to *Insight*, he sought to orient his readers to his goal of articulating a theory of knowledge based upon the phenomenon of one's own knowing.[4] By attending to his own knowing, Lonergan sought to provide a general theory that accounted for the structured pattern of human cognition. Such a theory would specify and relate the 'internally closed set of partial and complementary functions' of human cognitive activities.[5] Lonergan maintained that such a theory would also serve to make explicit the conditions that are preliminary to effective collaboration between knowers in diverse and specialized fields of human inquiry. Such a collaboration 'supposes at least a central nucleus that somehow could retain its identity yet undergo all the modifications and enrichments that could be poured into its capacious frame from specialized investigations.'[6]

The pivotal act in Lonergan's cognitional structure is the act of insight. He differentiates three distinct apprehensive acts, which I will discuss under the labels 'direct,' 'reflective,' and 'deliberative insights.'[7] Lonergan takes these insights to be the inner focus of his and his readers' own intelligence, reasonableness, and responsibility. His program in *Insight* is to invite his readers to apprehend their own cognitive structure and the pivotal role insights play in that structure. He facilitates this self-knowledge through the use of various exercises that enable his readers to experience themselves engaging in the activities of knowing. On the basis of this heightened self-awareness, Lonergan helps his readers distinguish between the various acts that pertain to the structure of their own cognitive processes, such as 'seeing, hearing, touching, smelling, tasting, inquiring, imagining, understanding, conceiving, formulating, reflecting, marshalling and weighing the evidence, judging, deliberating, evaluating, deciding, speaking, writing.'[8]

By evoking these operations in his readers, Lonergan helps them to discover in their own experience 'the dynamic relationships leading from one operation to the next,'[9] and so to 'know what it is to know one's own intelligence, one's own reasonableness, one's own essential and restricted effective freedom.'[10] The purpose of this arduous process, then, is to promote in his readers an express self-knowledge of their own cognitional performance. And it is not achieved unless the reader is involved in experiencing himself or herself engaging in cognitional activities, in highlighting and distinguishing between different acts, in understanding how each relates to other acts, and finally in affirming the fact that by them he or she is a knower.

The general process of moving from *presence to self*, or consciousness, to *knowledge of self* is the same for anyone who proposes an account of how he or she knows, even if such an account is at odds with Lonergan's. Moreover, the sort of cognitional self-presence that is the basis for articulating one's cognitional structure is rather subtle, and it takes some ingenuity even to evoke the elements of the structure, much less identify and relate those elements.[11] For it is not the sort of self-presence of a woman to her own *physiological* self when, following something like the Creighton Model of Natural Family Planning, she attends to the cyclical patterns of her own fertility by monitoring changes in the quality and quantity of her cervical mucus.[12] Nor is it the sort of self-presence a woman may have to her own *psychological* patterns, which she may acquire through a heightened awareness of her moods, the changes of which she not only notes but also relates to other cyclical physiological changes. Rather, it is a self-presence to her own cognitive acts, through the reflexive acts of understanding and judging, that yields a self-knowledge of her own capacity to *attend to* changes in the physiological data of sense and psychological data of consciousness, and her own capacity to *grasp* some relation between these changes.[13] Indeed, it is this subtle difference that I will be engaging in discussion in part 3. This discussion will involve making a series of distinctions among cognitive acts, such as that between the different kinds of insights to which we have already referred. And it will make sense to readers only if they attempt to invoke in themselves a heightened cognitional self-presence.[14]

Based on his own self-appropriation, Lonergan concludes that knowing is a structured process that involves distinct but related 'levels' of cognitional activities in which the later activities subsume and move beyond the earlier ones. Lonergan uses *level*, in its strict sense, to mean a place in an intelligible pattern of cognitional activities.[15] He summarily refers to these levels as *experiencing, understanding, judging,* and *evaluating,* in accordance with the most prominent characteristic of each set of activities. Lonergan claims that this structure is basic because it underlies all specialized methods in various disciplines. For this reason it also provides common grounds for effective interdisciplinary collaboration. He also claims that this structure is irreducible to any more simple structure because it involves sets of activities that, though interrelated, are nevertheless distinct.[16]

For Lonergan, an accurate account of what one is actually doing when knowing is not only a key type of knowledge but also *the key* to knowledge. Not only in *Insight*, but throughout his studies of mind, and later of heart, Lonergan consistently emphasizes the priority in thinkers of a stance on cognitional theory, even if they never expressly state their stance. He argues that an accurate account of human knowing constitutes a fixed base for philosophy, one that is invulnerable to radical revision. For it would seem that any attempt at revising a valid theory of knowledge would necessarily need to employ the operations distinguished and related in the theory in the very effort of trying to discredit it. Thus, one employs operationally what one tries to reject theoretically. This would involve one in a form of self-contradiction that can be referred to as an act of *operational inconsistency.* Such a self-contradiction would be similar to that which would obtain if one were to argue, 'I am utterly unconscious.' For in the very process of making the argument, one is contradicting the content of the claim.[17]

On the basis of what Lonergan argues is a valid cognitional theory, all of his thought goes forward. He articulates a philosophy that rests on the immanent norms of intelligence and reasonableness, norms Lonergan claims are discoverable no less in his readers than in himself. He presumes that such intelligence and reasonableness reside in his readers. In *Insight* he invites them, with ever more precision and detail, to 'apprehend, to appropriate, to envision in all its consequences' these features of themselves for themselves.[18]

I will be responding to Lonergan's invitation by using a medical example to illustrate some of the key recurring features of human cognition. I will do this with an eye to those distinctions that will be crucial for the subsequent discussion of evaluating and deciding as it pertains to the euthanasia debate. Although this discussion is not meant to provide readers with the sort of detailed self-knowledge that Lonergan sought to promote in *Insight,* it will introduce them to some of Lonergan's distinctive terms and notions regarding what he contends they are actually doing when knowing facts.

Before proceeding with the medical example illustrating the process by which one comes to a judgment, it is worth pointing out that there are at least four advantages of using such an example. First, it provides one with an example of a judgment in an area of knowledge (i.e., cardiology) that is rather *sharply defined.* Lonergan himself engages his readers in problems from other well-defined fields, such as mathematics, geometry, and physics. This is because he maintains that in such areas his readers would more readily recognize and be familiar with just what they have understood. In the case of a life-threatening medical emergency, there is a built-in mechanism that also allows one to recognize readily what one has misunderstood. For the *dynamic* context of a patient's declining medical condition provides an opportunity for prompt feedback on the correctness of one's presumptive diagnoses and treatment decisions, actions or inactions.[19]

Second, such a medical example tends to undermine certain dogmatic philosophical stances. In contrast to some academic philosophers, medical persons of sound common sense proceed on the basis of certain beliefs, such as the belief that their patient actually exists and that the timely diagnosis and implementation of treatment decisions can positively alter the outcome of certain medical problems. Such beliefs constitute elements of concrete human rationality that philosophers, reflecting on the physician's performance as distinct from reflecting in a strictly academic setting, are less likely to neglect or deny.[20]

Third, since our discussion is directed primarily to those with an interest in medical ethics, beginning with the process that led to a fact judgment in a medical context provides a common ground for reflecting on the philosophical features of this process and also prepares the way for reflecting on the philosophical features of value judgments. If one role of medical ethicists is to *mediate* good decision-making in medical matters, then it is no small advantage for them to have an accurate and nuanced grasp of the cognitional processes in which medical persons frequently engage when making medical fact and value judgments and decisions.

Finally, it seems that an important task of a medical ethicist is to invite those making medical diagnoses and decisions also to advert to and make good *ethical* evaluations and decisions. Accordingly, an example of a typical medical judgment concerning the diagnosis and treatment of someone with chest pain will help to highlight the interplay between fact and value judgments in common medical practice. This will prove helpful when later discussing and challenging the sharp contrast between these two types of judgments that characterizes much of modern thought, in both medicine and ethics. A detailed analysis of the diagnosis and treatment of a patient with chest pain will show how dependent one's value judgments are on fact judgments. It will also show how what might be thought to be a strictly 'scientific' fact judgment might actually also involve an evaluation.

3   Cognitional Operations: Acts and Achievements on the First Three Levels

I will begin with an example of the process of diagnosing a patient with an acute myocardial infarction (hereafter AMI). This example is meant to illustrate the first three of Lonergan's four cognitional levels indicated below. I will defer addressing the contents of the fourth level to chapter 6. Throughout this discussion of the four cognitional levels I will maintain, and draw out the implications of, the distinction between the cognitional activities on each level and the resulting cognitional achievements, which table 4.1 summarizes.

3.1 First Level: Experiencing

Lonergan worked out key features of his cognitional theory early in his career, as is well documented in his *Verbum* articles.[21] The context within

Table 4.1 Activities and achievements on the first three cognitional levels

Level	(Activity)	Achievement
1: cognitional	(experiential: sensible-conscious)	awareness of data
2: cognitional	(intellectual)	intelligible unity
3: cognitional	(intellectual)	knowing the unconditioned real
[4: cognitional	(affective)	knowing the unconditioned good
and decisional	(affective)	actualizing or enjoying values]

which the later Lonergan analyses evaluations presupposes an understanding of some of the fundamental categories he articulates in his early work on Aquinas.[22] Despite some terminological differences in Lonergan's *formulation* of his cognitional theory in the early and later periods, he remained consistent throughout his career on the *meaning* of the key cognitional acts to which he refers. In this section, I will highlight and illustrate the meaning of those key cognitional acts on levels one, two, and three, drawing especially upon the early Lonergan writings in works such as *Verbum, Insight,* and *Understanding and Being.*

I will proceed by highlighting both the cognitive *activities* of, and the *achievements* that issue from, each of the first three cognitional levels. Following Michael Vertin's interpretation of Lonergan, there are two key points I will underline regarding the first cognitional level. First, on the first level my cognitive achievement is given *immediately* in the activity of experiencing. This fact makes the first level quite distinct from the subsequent levels in which cognitive activities mediate the achievement of some content. Second, the content I achieve through the immediacy of experience is, nevertheless, one that is discovered rather than one that is merely created by me.[23]

Besides distinguishing cognitive activities and achievements, however, there is also the issue of starting points. Following Aquinas, the Lonergan of the *Verbum* period tended to express the relation between the knower and the known by beginning with the *object* that moves cognition, and then highlighting the apprehensive acts through which the knower gains incremental knowledge of this object. The later Lonergan, more typically, speaks first of the phenomenon of knowing, beginning with the cognitive activities of sensing, and subsequently considers the metaphysics of the known as those contents that result from these activities. Despite these different starting points, Lonergan insists that they are equivalent so long as one completes the cycle, say, from the object to the knower and then back to the object as known. The starting point one chooses, however, ought to be determined by the question one is treating.[24] If my focal question concerns how I come to know actual and concrete existence 'in and through the true judgment,' then I ought to emphasize the subjective processes by which I as a knower make a judgment about being.[25] I will illustrate this process of knowing in the first person, with the example of myself as a medical knower making a judgment about Paul, a medical patient, who presents himself to me complaining about a sensation of pain in his chest.

I first encounter Paul concretely through the activities of sensing him. Still, it is worth pointing out how abstract it is to speak of 'sensation.' Although I am quite familiar with particular activities of seeing, hearing, touching, tasting, and smelling, they never occur in isolation, either from one another or from other events. On the contrary, as Lonergan insists, 'they have a bodily basis; they are functionally related to bodily movements; and they occur in some dynamic context that somehow unifies a manifold of sensed contents and of acts of sensing.'[26]

Along with my sense acts, there is a prior direction and striving that is informed by my medical formation. In light of my knowledge of patterns of symptoms, I am oriented in the stream of successive sensory contents of my experience of Paul. For instance, as a trained physician, I am likely to confront the situation with a number of possible explanations for Paul's symptoms. This background knowledge *directs* my sense experience of Paul to attending to those physical clues that I regard as most likely to be helpful and relevant for diagnosing his pain. Without this medical background, my sense experience of Paul would be much less focused. Still, it is only by sensibly experiencing Paul, through sensory acts, such as listening to his chest with a stethoscope, that I first encounter him concretely. Following Lonergan, I will label the contents of my sense activities, such as his heart sounds, *data of sense*.

I might speak of the *data of sense* as what is *known* through activities of sensing. Even this primitive, preconceptual awareness of data of Paul, as a content of my sensory experience, is *cognitional*. For it is through acts of sensing that I achieve an awareness of sensory contents. Irrespective of how I later interpret them, this awareness of sense data is a cognitional achievement of contents that are distinct from my acts of sensing. Moreover, there is a givenness to these sense data, such that what I apprehend might be surprisingly different from what my medical concepts may have led me to expect.[27]

Strictly speaking, the only experiential activity is sensing. But speaking more broadly, I might say that I also *experience*, or am aware of myself, as engaging in the act of sensing. This experience or awareness is what I mean by *being conscious*. This is not another act but rather it is *an aspect* of the act of sensing, as well as every direct, conscious-intentional act. For instance, concomitant with my awareness of the contents of my hearing is an awareness of myself as currently engaging in the act of hearing. On this basis, I would distinguish between the *intentional* and *conscious* properties of acts of sensing. These acts are intentional in as much as they have the property of being oriented to some sense data and result in an awareness of data that are distinct from the acts themselves. But my sense acts also have the property of being radically self-possessing, so that through sensing I am primitively aware of both my acts of sensing and myself as one who senses.[28] These acts are also conscious in so far as they are primitively self-possessing, such that by them I am present to myself, not as another object, but as an experiencing subject.[29]

By sensing, then, I achieve an *awareness of data*, where by data I would include both *data of sense* and *data of consciousness*. On the first level, such an awareness of data denotes a cognition that falls short of knowing in the strict sense of this word. My empirical awareness is a cognition that is still to be understood and judgmentally affirmed. By including in my experience the awareness of both data of sense and data of consciousness, I refer to the above distinction within the data of experience between my awareness of the contents of sense acts and of the sense acts themselves, and, more basically, of myself as one who senses.[30] On this basis, I distinguish between cognitional processes operating in the *direct* and in the *introspective* or *reflexive mode.*

The *direct mode* of the cognitional process begins with sense data, and advances through the subsequent cognitional levels of understanding, judging, and evaluating, which are data of consciousness. By contrast, the *introspective mode* begins with my data of consciousness, of the self-presence that pertains to me in virtue of my own cognitional acts, such as those of sensing, inquiring, understanding, formulating, reflecting, and judging.[31] As with the direct mode, the introspective or reflexive mode proceeds from an awareness of these cognitional processes (an awareness that is intrinsic to the direct acts themselves), through understanding, judging, and evaluating. Hence, sensing Paul in the direct mode of my cognitional process at the same time provides me with data of consciousness from which I proceed by means of the introspective mode.[32]

I would account for differences among cognitional objects, on this and subsequent cognitional levels, on the basis of distinct *apprehensive acts*. On the level of sensing, then, I would distinguish between apprehensive acts as *receptive* of colours, shapes, odours, etc., and subsequent apprehensive acts as *productive* of images of these data. I distinguish here between receptive and productive apprehensive acts and what results from these acts on the first level. Later, I will emphasize that sense cognition, by contrast to the cognitive acts that occur on the levels of understanding and judging, is predominantly receptive of sensible objects. Moreover, I will show that on the subsequent levels, my knowing is a mediated process that begins in response to wonder occasioned by some sense data.[33]

The point of introducing these distinctions and labels, which figure prominently in the work of the early Lonergan, is to flag a series of issues that are relevant to understanding his later position on affect. First, note that even the act of sensing is *cognitional*, that is, an act of 'sense knowing.' I would distinguish this cognitive act from *non-cognitional* events or processes, such as the physiological process of digestion or the psychological irritability that results from hunger or indigestion. What I achieve through sense knowing is a cognitive awareness of data. By smelling, for example, I am not only physically present to the food, but also the food I smell is cognitionally present to me.

Second, I would characterize the initial apprehensive act on level one as *receptive*. In sensing, I receive cognitionally the sensible form of the object that moves my senses, such as in the case of hearing Paul's heart sounds. The model of this sensory apprehension is that of knowing by confrontation, in which I encounter and passively receive the sensible qualities of an object. This receptive apprehensive act is important because it characterizes the cognitional process on the first level as one that is *unmediated*. This is because there is a direct relationship between the object that moves my senses and the awareness of data I achieve on the first level. Distinct from this first-level cognitive process are those *mediated* processes that occur on the subsequent cognitional levels. This issue will be especially important when I come to distinguish an unmediated awareness of data given in acts of sensing from the mediating function of affects. These mediating affects are aspects of my conscious-intentional response to a possible object of value.[34]

Third, it is important to emphasize not merely the receptivity of the first level of cognition, but also the unmediated character of both receptive and productive first-level apprehensions, that is, that they do not arise as a response to my wonder or to some question. It is this direct or unmediated nature of sense cognition that makes first-level knowing misleading as an analogy for the whole of human cognition.[35] But even on the level of sensation there is the further apprehensive act of imaginatively patterning or representing sense data.[36] Although I label this as a *productive apprehensive act*, it remains an unmediated, first-level act. Nevertheless, Lonergan highlights the significance of this subsequent apprehensive act of imagining by selecting a phrase from Aristotle's *De Anima*, III, 7, 431b 2 for the title page of *Insight*, which one could translate as *the idea stands forth in the phantasm*. On this account, sensing is not merely a matter of producing a photocopy of an object. Rather, there is some imaginative freedom in organizing data of sense. I pattern this data in ways that bear some correspondence to my habitual patterns of experience. These phantasms stimulate and facilitate my second-level drive to grasp some intelligible unity in the multiplicity of sensed data.[37]

Fourth, the distinction between the *data of sense* and the *data of conscious-*

ness is the basis for distinguishing the direct, first-level acts of sense experience and the second, third, and fourth levels of the direct cognitional
process. Data of sense pertain to objects that present themselves to me
through sensation. On the first level, data of consciousness is simply my
awareness of being engaged in acts of sensing. Whether the awareness of
data I achieve on the first level is of data of sense or data of consciousness, it
is on subsequent cognitional levels that I interpret this data, affirm the
contents of my interpretation, and distinguish between contents that are of
self and those that are of the other.

My whole analysis will go forward by considering a medical judgment in
order to bring to light my cognitive processes and, more basically, myself as
constituted as a knower by these cognitive acts. With this background, I will
be in a better position in chapter 6 to attend to affective, rather than strictly
intellectual, cognitive data.[38]

In summary, then, experience for Lonergan is cognitive, primarily receptive, and involves an apprehensive act that is unmediated by my intellect. In
the strict sense, the first level involves direct acts of sense experiencing.
These sense acts are intrinsically conscious, and so consciousness is not a
further act. The *introspective* modes of cognition does not emerge until the
second, third, and fourth levels; it is the folding back of understanding,
judging, and evaluating upon the data of consciousness, which are my
direct acts of understanding, judging, and evaluating. In the present example, the direct mode of cognition refers to the perspective of the patient
or physician seeking to objectify some 'it.' The introspective mode refers to
the point of view of the philosopher analysing distinct cognitional activities
by understanding and judging them, which is what I am primarily concerned with in this chapter. Note that what I achieve at the first level is not
'knowledge' in the strict sense. And because my first-level knowing is
unmediated, Lonergan does not consider it to be a helpful model for
human knowing in the complete sense:

> An act of ocular vision may be perfect as ocular vision; yet if it occurs
> without any accompanying glimmer of understanding, it is mere
> gaping, so far from being the beau ideal of human knowing, is just
> stupidity. As mere seeing is not human knowing, so for the same
> reason merely hearing, merely smelling, merely touching, merely
> tasting, may be parts, potential components, of human knowing, but
> they are not human knowing itself.[39]

3.2 Second Level: Understanding

I have just explained that the first level begins with a sensible thing and
ends with the achievement of my awareness of sense data. The second level

proceeds from this terminal achievement of the first level when I pose the question 'What is it?' The second level reaches its term when I express the intelligible unity I discover in my first-level image in the form of a concept or definition. I will elucidate some features of the second cognitional level by focusing on the pivotal second-level act of a direct insight. It is by means of a direct insight that I grasp an intelligible unity in my first-level sense data. A detailed understanding of how direct insights function on the second level will provide a helpful model for understanding the function of reflective insights in grasping facts on the third level and affective insights that grasp values on the fourth level. I will begin by illustrating the second-level cognitive acts by extending the previously mentioned medical example.

Assume that Paul awakes with a sensation of pressure or squeezing in the region of his chest. For some time he might be primitively aware of this sensation but still fail to wonder about it and ask what it could be. He moves from first-level experiencing to second-level understanding when he begins to wonder about this sensation of pain and asks himself, 'What is it?' As Paul's physician, I am also pressed forward by this question. From his description of the pain, and also from my experience of him during a physical examination, I seek to discover some intelligibility in his experiences.

In time it occurs to me: 'Good Grief! Maybe, Paul, this is an acute myocardial infarction!' This 'Good Grief!' or 'aha' experience signals my apprehension, by means of what I would call a *direct insight*, of a possible correlation between Paul's symptoms and the compromised state of his heart. I experience this insight as an 'aha.' It releases me from some of the intellectual tension connected with my questions regarding the reasons for Paul's pain. It also rewards my striving to understand with the satisfaction of an intellectual discovery of an intelligibility in Paul's experience, which was previously only a bewildering set of symptoms and signs. This 'aha' marks an intellectual shift from my prior state of intending some concrete intelligibility with the question 'What is this?' in relation to Paul's reported experience of pain and the signs and symptoms he exhibits. That is, this 'aha' signals my grasping of a possible intelligible unity in Paul's diverse sense data.[40]

The act of insight well characterizes my achievement of knowledge on this and subsequent levels as involving a process of *discovery*, rather than a matter of positing or creating some content. Although this discovery is shared personally by anyone who has the insight, the conditions for the emergence of my grasp of an intelligibility in Paul's signs and symptoms rests on a long history of similar discoveries first made by others. For instance, the insight that chest pain might manifest an acute myocardial infarction (AMI), and that such an explanation might obtain in Paul's case, is not entirely original to myself. Rather, I come to Paul armed with a whole series of conceptual understandings of common causes of chest pain, and I interpret his signs and symptoms in light of these intelligible patterns with which I am already familiar. This context of accumulated understanding and concepts is the fruit of the labours of my medical predecessors, not simply my own.[41]

It is one thing to grasp a relationship between chest pain and a possible cardiac pathology. It is another to express accurately what an AMI is, or why Paul's pain is cardiac chest pain. So beyond a direct insight, there is a subsequent act of expressing what my 'aha' was all about. I would refer to this further apprehensive act as one of *conceiving* or *formulating* the content of a direct insight. In this case, I express the content of my insight in terms of the concept or definition of an AMI. Such a concept or definition expresses the content of the concrete, intelligible unity I grasp in a direct insight. I express this unity by a *simple mental word*, which is my formulation of the intelligible content of the insight. This concept is the terminal achievement of my level-two cognition.[42]

In my 'aha,' I grasp a *concrete* intelligible relation between diverse elements of Paul's and my own sense experiences. One advantage that I have over Paul is that I bring to this particular encounter with him a knowledge of the abstract concept or definition of an AMI. Not only have I studied this concept, but I have also used this knowledge on other occasions when seeking to understand patients who were having chest pain. At the level of understanding, then, there is some interplay between the concrete data of experience of Paul and my prior knowledge of what an AMI is. This prior knowledge conditions the emergence of my insight into Paul's experience. But I also move from my concrete insight into Paul's experience to formulate and express the contents of this insight by abstracting from all of his particularities only that pattern that is relevant to the concept of an AMI.

The interplay between concrete and abstract intelligibilities, which first arises on the second level, is worth emphasizing now, as it will have a bearing on our later discussion of the relation between concrete value judgments and abstract moral norms. Note that my initial conceptual understanding of an AMI is an abstract one. But in formulating my insight that Paul is suffering from an AMI, I disregard or leave behind a whole range of historical data about Paul that is not relevant to this insight, such as what he happened to be wearing that day. I do this in order to focus solely on the relevant pattern of Paul's experience for this diagnosis.[43] When I subsequently formulate the content of my insight in a conceptual or definitional understanding of Paul as possibly having an AMI, this understanding is not bound to all the particularities of his case. To that extent, it is a form of expression that is universal and general. Hence, all relevant cases can be similarly understood. Conversely, although the meaning of this concept was grasped originally by someone else in some other concrete historical case, I am also able to understand Paul's case in terms of this concept. Indeed, I anticipate that this concept ought to hold for all similarly relevant cases and is not restricted to any particular historical, cultural, or even human context (e.g., dogs also have AMI's). That is, although there are features of Paul's experience that are unique to him, the intelligibility of his pain, expressed in the concept of an AMI, obtains a degree of generality that makes it transcultural and transhistorical.[44]

I can formulate my insight that Paul is having an AMI in two distinct modes, either as a description or as an explanation. For instance, Paul can *describe* his symptoms as consisting of an intelligible constellation of sensations (e.g., pain, sweating, nausea) as these sense experiences relate *to himself*. He might also note that his experience is similar to his sister's description of her experience when she was having her first AMI. Similarly, I can also *describe* Paul's signs as they appear *to me* as an observer.[45] Insights that issue in appropriate descriptions are largely a matter of mastering language, in this case, what is generally meant by 'AMI.' By contrast, I can also *explain* Paul's chest pain in terms of a pattern on his electrocardiogram, one that is characteristic of persons who are suffering from an AMI. Insights that issue in descriptions relate things or intelligible unities to oneself, and insights that issue in explanations relate the same things or intelligible unities *among themselves*.[46] As Lonergan's 'tweezers' metaphor suggests, these two fundamentally different modes of formulating an insight into something such as chest pain are closely related: '[D]escription supplies the tweezers by which we hold things while explanations are being discovered or verified, applied or revised.'[47]

Research, discovering new knowledge, and advancing conceptual clarity are important parts of medicine. Still, as a trained, practising physician, my main concern when investigating a patient such as Paul is typically to 'confirm' or 'rule out' a diagnosis such as AMI. In other words, most of my intellectual effort is not spent on the second level of conceiving and then formulating concepts, such as that of an AMI. This concept is something I have already learned. Rather, my cognitional activity in the clinical setting more typically goes forward according to what I will presently elucidate as a further, third-level process of verification.[48] However, before discussing the third level of cognition, and with the present illustration still in mind, it is worth flagging some further issues arising on the second level that will be relevant to my later discussion of the role affect plays in deliberations.

First, the move from experiencing to understanding is occasioned by my asking the question, with respect to my first-level awareness of sense data, 'What is it?' This particular question expresses my intending some concrete intelligibility in Paul's experience. It is a response to, or is evoked by, both the sense data I encounter in Paul and the radical spontaneity of my 'wonder.' Even prior to my discovering an answer to this question my wonder is made manifest in the question, 'What is it?' But this wonder is a mode of intending different from the intentional responses of acts, such a direct insight, for it intends 'an unknown whole of which our answers reveal only a part.'[49]

This wonder or desire to know, which is the fundamental source of my questions, is similar to what Aristotle referred to in the first line of the *Metaphysics,* when he remarked that 'All men naturally desire knowledge.'[50] It is a desire that motivates, impels, orients, and directs me toward discovery of intelligibility. In general, it moves me from ignorance to knowledge by such mediating acts as direct insights. And on the second level I would label this wonder or desire to know the *transcendental notion of intelligibility.*[51] Here *transcendental* would be in contrast to *categorial* or empirical. It denotes the pre-empirical nature of this desire, which manifests itself in questions intending an intelligibility in some data. It refers to a mode of intending that is qualitatively distinct from categorial intentional responses, such as those direct insights. It is something I bring to anything I experience. It is a structural anticipation of intelligibility, an anticipation that is contained in such questions for intelligence as 'What is it?' and 'Why is it so?'[52] It provides the dynamism of intentional consciousness that heads for answers to the questions for intelligence that arise following some categorial experience.[53] I might formulate the transcendental 'concept' of the intelligible by objectifying the content of this intelligent intending. But even prior to some such conceptual expression, 'there are the transcendental notions that constitute the very dynamism of our conscious intending.'[54]

Second, the apprehensive act of a direct insight is a distinctively *intellectual* cognitional activity, in contrast to sensing. By means of a direct insight I grasp not simply more data but relations within or among data. This cognitional activity might be called *supra-experiential,* for it moves me beyond an awareness of data to grasp an intelligible unity in these data. It is on the basis of a direct insight that I distinguish between, for instance, a heap of stones and a bridge, or a scramble and a play in a football game. Through such insights I grasp or synthesize an intelligible *unity in some diversity* of sense data.[55]

Third, attending to the phenomenon of a direct insight brings to light the *intelligent ground* for the *intelligible content* that I grasp in data. These data, of which I am aware and ask about, first become for me an intelligible content by means of a direct insight. Through this direct insight I grasp a possible connection, say, between Paul's experience and the condition of his heart. That is, my act of insight renders Paul's experience intelligible.

This insight is a second-level, cognitive, intentional response to Paul's experience. It is evoked conjointly by my sense awareness of Paul and my transcendental intending of some intelligibility in his experience. Through my direct insight I grasp a concrete intelligible content *in* Paul's experience.[56]

Fourth, in contrast to the immediacy of my first-level cognitional achievement, this second-level achievement of some understanding is *mediated* by certain cognitive acts, such as direct insights. My sense awareness of Paul is merely receptive. It is evoked by his data as given; and there is an identity between the evoking content and the ultimately known content of these sense data. That is, the received colours, shapes, odours, etc. that move my senses provide the evidence for, and are identical with, the colours, shapes, odours, etc. of which I become aware. That is, these experiences are represented without the *mediation* of intellect since they do not arise as a response to some question.[57]

When I ask, 'What is it?' the second-level, cognitional process is then mediated by distinct and complementary intentional responses to Paul's data. As intentional, my second-level insight is a receptive response to Paul's experience. It also responds by constituting his experience as intelligible. I then complement my direct insight by the productive act of formulating the content that I have grasped. As conscious, my second-level, intentional response is not only self-present, it is also self-constitutive, for in the response I am revealed as one who is actually intelligent.[58]

Fifth, I distinguish between the functions of two second-level intentional responses. A direct insight is *constitutive*; the subsequent act of intending, namely conception, is *productive*. As described above, my insights into Paul's condition constitute the intelligible content of my understanding as well as my own intelligence. I would also speak of my wonder as an original condition for constitutive acts of insight. Just as Aristotle took wonder to be the beginning of all science, so also for Lonergan our state of wonder 'leads to the formation of images that simplify the sensitive data, that throw it [*sic*] into schematic constellations digestible for limited human understanding and [then] there occur acts of insight.'[59]

Wonder also moves me to the productive act of formulating or conceptualizing the intelligibility I grasp through an insight. The product of this apprehensive act is a concept or definition, which I would refer to as a *simple mental word*. My concept expresses an intelligibility that I grasp in my representation or image of Paul. It consists not in an act of grasping an intelligibility, as with an insight, but in an act of meaning or of defining the content of my insight.

Sixth, on the second level there emerges the important distinction between concrete and abstract intelligibilities. I grasp an intelligibility concretely in Paul's data by means of a direct insight. In formulating the content of my direct insight in a concept I produce an *abstract intelligibility*, which could be descriptive or explanatory. Unlike the concrete content of my direct insight, the content of my concept is 'abstract' because it leaves behind those features of Paul that are not essential to my insight into the cause of his pain.[60] Lonergan explains this process this way: 'The intending that is conception puts together both the content of the insight and as much of the image as is essential to the occurrence of the insight; the result is the intending of any concrete being selected by an incompletely determinate (and, in that sense, abstract) content.'[61]

Finally, like experiencing, understanding is not human knowing taken in the strict sense of the word. Neither understanding by itself, nor experiencing and understanding together, yield knowledge of being. In other words, the end I achieve on the level of understanding has merely an indeterminate status as regards knowledge of the real. Without prior sense presentations there is nothing to be understood. Still, the operations of sense and understanding together are insufficient for human knowing, for there must be added judgment.

3.3 Third Level: Judging

> To omit judging is quite literally silly: it is only by judgment that
> there emerges a distinction between fact and fiction, logic and
> sophistry, philosophy and myth, history and legend, astronomy and
> astrology, chemistry and alchemy.[62]

On the third level, I ask of the intelligible unity of Paul's data achieved on the second level, 'Is it so?' or 'Is it true?' In answering 'Yes' or 'No' to this question I achieve knowledge, in the strict sense of the term, that is, knowledge of the real.

I will begin by highlighting the phenomena of making the judgment in the case I have been considering: 'Yes, Paul is having an AMI.' Assume that I have had a number of direct insights into Paul's signs and symptoms. These insights represent alternative, possible interpretations of Paul's condition. I would include these possibilities in my 'differential diagnosis,' which is a series of possible causes for Paul's chest pain. I would also rank these possibilities according to some criteria, such as those causes that are the most serious ones.[63] The third level begins with a global intending of reality, which finds partial expression here in the question 'Is Paul having an AMI?' The third level reaches its term when I make the judgment, 'Yes, Paul is having an AMI.' In the following discussion I will attempt to provide a more expansive account of this third-level process through which I move from a question intending some concrete reality or possible reality to a judgment.

Note that I am not asking questions for intelligibility or understanding, such as 'What is X?' as on the second level, and then conceiving possible interpretations. Rather, I am asking questions that seek to *verify* whether any of my interpretations of Paul's pain is correct. I respond to this question not with a definition (as on the second level) but with a Yes or No answer. Such an answer would make no sense as a response to the second-level question 'What is X?' As a physician, my focal concern is with the correctness of my second-level interpretation of Paul's chest pain, that is, 'Is he really having an AMI?' If he is, then I need to make some important practical treatment decisions. As a philosopher, my focal interest is to highlight and analyse the third-level cognitive process by which I move from a question about the truth of this interpretation of Paul's pain to the answer 'Yes, Paul is, in fact, having an AMI.' Clarity on how I make such a judgment, and how I can be mistaken in this judgment, which I will address in chapter 5, will set the stage for a parallel analysis of value judgments in chapters 5 and 6.

Imagine that I ask myself, 'Is Paul having an AMI?' With this question in mind, I review Paul's data, for instance, from sensing him directly, interpreting the sensations he reports. Knowing *what* an AMI is, or *why* I can say that some patient is having an AMI, I amass data from my encounter with Paul that supports or fulfils the conditions for asserting this diagnosis. For instance, is he someone who is at risk for coronary artery disease?[64] Is his experience of chest pain typical of cardiac pain?[65] Is his physical or laboratory examination consistent with and supportive or confirmatory of this diagnosis and not some other interpretation?[66] What additional data from other investigations do I require to make this diagnosis, such as blood tests, electrocardiogram (ECG), echocardiogram, angiography? For the sake of simplicity, I will assume that a patient with characteristic cardiac chest pain, that is, a retrosternal squeezing or heavy sensation lasting for at least ten minutes, and a positive ECG, is having an AMI.

When finally I conclude, 'Yes, Paul is (or is *probably*) having an AMI,' I purport to know what is, or probably is, the cause of Paul's pain. If such a claim is not merely an arbitrary guess, then somehow I must recognize that the evidence I have is sufficient to infer that Paul is indeed having an AMI. In other words, I somehow grasp that Paul's having an AMI depends upon certain conditions, and I acknowledge that these conditions are fulfilled in Paul's case. Hence, in grasping the truth of the claim that Paul is having an AMI, I have put together diverse elements of knowledge from (a) my sense knowledge of Paul, (b) my understanding of what an AMI is, and (c) my reasoning that (a) and (b) together make my conclusion rationally compelling.[67]

In moving from a state of ignorance to the knowledge that Paul is having an AMI, at some point I grasp the sufficiency of the evidence for this conclusion. This grasp occurs in a pivotal cognitive moment, which is like the 'aha' experience of consciousness that accompanies a direct insight. This might occur moments after I see Paul sweating and clutching his chest, or later on when I examine his electrocardiogram and recognize the pattern that is typical of an AMI. But I could also experience this 'aha' in a less dramatic way when and only after more subtle evidence in favour of this diagnosis becomes sufficient to meet the conditions for this judgment. When I later reflect philosophically upon my performance, I note that I have been involved in a threefold pattern of questioning, having an insight, and producing a judgment. This pattern parallels the pattern of those second-level activities I have already highlighted and, indeed, anticipates a similar pattern for making evaluations.

Thus, on the second level, the source of questions is my desire to know, or what I would call the *transcendental notion of intelligibility*. On the third level, the source of my questions is my desire to know the real, not merely what is apparent, hypothetical, or plausible, a desire I would call the *transcendental notion of reality and truth*. This notion gives rise to my question for reflection concerning Paul, 'Is he really having an AMI?' This third-level question refers not directly to Paul's pain, that is, data of experience, as was the case for my second-level questions for intelligibility. Rather, it is about whether Paul's pain is due to a possible AMI, which regards the data-intelligibility synthesis that I achieved on the second level. That is, this question concerns the *borrowed content* from the second level, and it arises out of my transcendental intention of reality. I intentionally respond to this borrowed content when I raise my question for reflection and in my subsequent cognitive acts of discovering an answer. By raising this question, I move cognitionally from the second to the third level.[68]

I have already described the 'aha' experience of consciousness on the second level that accompanies my grasp of an intelligible unity in some manifold of data. On the third level, this 'aha' accompanies my grasp that Paul is really having an AMI. This 'aha' experience is the conscious dimension of the pivotal third-level, intentional, apprehensive act of 'reflective insight.' It is 'reflective' in the sense that it reflects upon my achievements of knowledge on the first level, such as my awareness of data of Paul, and, on the second level, such as the abstract intelligibility of my concept of an AMI. It is also an act of 'insight' in the sense that, through this act, I grasp some relation among distinct elements of knowledge and the prospective judgment that Paul is having an AMI.

In order to spell this out more clearly in a way that is familiar to philosophers, I will express this pattern using a hypothetical syllogism. My reflective insight grasps a relation among

(a) the prospective conditioned judgment that Paul is having an AMI [**B**];
(b) my understanding of the link between the conditioned judgment that Paul is having an AMI and its conditions (e.g., typical pain and a positive ECG) [If **A** then **B**]; and
(c) my awareness of the sufficiency of evidence, in Paul's case, to fulfil these conditions [**A**].

Hence, in the apprehensive act of reflective insight I grasp intellectually the rational or real relation or unity among these diverse cognitional achievements. This act constitutes the cognitive grounds of, or the intellectual basis for, the 'therefore' that precedes my conclusion, (d) Paul is having an AMI [**B**].[69] Although a reflective insight is far more general than any logical expression I might wish to give it, expressing it in this way simplifies the patterns I wish to highlight. As I have formulated it, (b) is the major premise of syllogism, which expresses an intelligible link between a conditioned **B** and its conditions **A**.

One can formulate this process as follows:

If **A** then **B**.

The minor premise (c) expresses the fulfilling conditions of the major premise:

But **A**.

The conclusion follows these premises:

Therefore **B**.

The conclusion rationally *follows from*, or is *justified by*, the two premises. The term 'therefore' expresses a rational necessity within this pattern. The expressions 'If **A** then **B**' and '**A**' highlight the fact that the evidence for the conclusion is a conjunction of two premises. The conclusion **B** expresses the now virtually unconditioned status of what was the conditioned prospective judgment **B**, which now has its condition 'If **A** then **B**' fulfilled ('But **A**').[70]

Following this apprehensive act of judging, I proceed to express in a fact judgment the content I have grasped in my reflective insight. I *posit* this synthesis, which I previously merely considered, in making the conclusion 'Yes, Paul is having an AMI.' Once I make this judgment I can speak of my 'conditioned' prospective judgment as 'virtually unconditioned.' It is first a 'conditioned' proposition because it is dependent upon certain conditions, that is, Paul is having an AMI **if** he is having typical pain and he has a positive ECG. When the conditions of the antecedent are fulfilled, the consequent stands alone as a 'virtually unconditioned' proposition. That is, Paul **is** having an AMI, no further *ifs*, *ands*, or *buts* about it.[71]

On this analysis, the technical similarities and differences between the second and third levels become more apparent. For instance, the evidence for my judgment that Paul is having an AMI is not given merely in sense data, such as the pattern I note on the electrocardiogram. Rather, it involves conjoining my understanding of an AMI and my experience of Paul. The definition of an AMI, as distinct from the diagnosis or judgment that Paul is having an AMI, is a mere understanding. It is an abstract intelligibility of terms and relations, in particular, the relations between myocardial oxygen supply and demand, which is a second-level achievement. Diagnosing Paul as having an AMI involves more than this second-level process of *grasping* and *conceiving* the potentially intelligible interpretation of Paul's pain as an AMI. It involves the third-level process of *verifying* that Paul does, in fact, fulfil the criteria or conditions of this diagnosis.[72]

Again, on the second level I expressed my direct insight as grasping a *supra-experienceable unity* in data of sense (or consciousness). The cognitive process on the second level involves not only my direct insight as *constitutive* of second-level knowledge, but also my subsequent act of conceiving, which is a *productive* apprehensive act that expresses the contents of this insight. By contrast, on the third level my reflective insight grasps a *supra-intelligible unity* in the data-intelligibility synthesis of the second level. The cognitive process on the third level involves my reflective insight as constitutive of third-level knowledge. It also involves my apprehensive act of judging, which is a productive apprehensive act of expressing the prospective judgment as a virtually unconditioned.

There are four key points of this phenomenological analysis worth highlighting here. First, facts are known only in and through judgments. Even on the second level, knowing an intelligible unity is not merely a matter of having an insight, but of correctly conceiving the contents grasped by means of the insight. Still, this is not yet knowledge in the strict sense. On the third level, I know that Paul is having an AMI not immediately in my reflective insight, but only *in* and *through* a subsequent fact judgment. *In* this productive apprehensive act I express the prospective fact judgment as virtually unconditioned, true, and reasonably justified. *Through* this fact judgment I know the data-intelligibility synthesis as virtually unconditioned, contingently true, a fact. Prior to a judgment, then, there is no knowledge of the real in the strict sense.[73]

Second, like a second-level direct insight, a reflective insight is an intellectual cognition that grasps a relation or unity in some diversity. On the second level my direct insight grasps an intelligible unity in the data of sense or consciousness. On the third level, my reflective insight grasps a relation or unity in the diversity of a prospective judgment, its link to conditions, and the fulfilment of those conditions. On each of these levels, these insights are intentional, intellectual cognitions, which I experience as an 'aha.'

Third, if this unity is said to be grasped *in* either a direct or reflective insight, the force of the preposition *in* is to be taken as equivalent to *by means of*. These insights are my intentional, cognitive responses to an object. On the second level, the object is Paul's sense data; on the third level, it is the prospective judgment that Paul is having an AMI. These insights *partly* constitute my cognitional access to the knowledge I achieve on each level. That is, they are acts of discovery, rather than acts by which I create or posit some knowledge content.

Fourth, by calling this third-level insight 'reflective,' Lonergan avoids any suggestion that the third-level process of knowing is an immediate or intuitive one. Although a reflective insight is itself only a component of knowing facts, this term aptly suggests a reflective basis for a mental word, in and through which knowing goes forward. A fact judgment is a *complex* mental word, by contrast to the *simple* mental word of a concept that issues from a direct insight. Judgment, as a mental word issuing from a reflective insight, can be said to be complex because, beyond intelligibility, it also specifies concrete modes of existence. For instance, I might express my judgment of fact in any of the following modes, as (a) a concrete actual reality (e.g., Paul *is having* an AMI); (b) a concretely possible reality (e.g., Paul *is at risk of having* an AMI); or (c) an abstractly possible reality (e.g., anyone who smokes *is at greater risk* of having an AMI than if they abstained from smoking).

Still, whether I judge that Paul is, or probably is, having an AMI, I am purporting to express my knowledge about what really (or probably) is the case, not what is merely apparent to me. Again, it is through judgment, and not merely experiencing and/or understanding, that I know the real.[74]

To avoid giving the mistaken impression that all of my knowledge is self-generated through mental words constituted by reflective insights, it is important to distinguish between *knowing* and *believing*. *Believing* is knowledge that, though appropriated as my own, is generated by someone else. For instance, Paul seeks medical assistance based upon his judgment that this chest pain might be serious, possibly signifying a life-threatening heart ailment. As his examining physician, I base my judgment that Paul is having an AMI upon the sufficiency of the evidence I gather in examining, listening to, and investigating him. When I relay my conclusion to Paul or his wife, their prima facie acceptance of my fact judgment is predominantly a matter of believing rather than knowing. That is, considering me as a trustworthy authority on these matters, Paul and his wife judge it reasonable to accept my claim that he is having an AMI, and then proceed to decide upon a responsible course of action. In order for Paul or his wife to move beyond accepting this diagnosis on the basis of belief, they would need to share the evidence, insights, and concepts upon which I base my judgment. They would also need to exercise the relevant skills one must have to assess this evidence accurately and make these sorts of judgments.[75]

For Lonergan, it is not until one makes an act of judgment that one achieves knowledge of the real, even if this is a judgment about the reliability of those I would believe. My judgment is my mental word through which I come to know the real – in this case, that 'Paul is having an AMI.'[76] As Lonergan summarizes: '[W]e first reach the unconditioned, secondly we make a true judgment of existence, and only thirdly in and through the true judgment do we come to know actual and concrete existence.'[77]

Although knowledge of the real is achieved through a third-level judgment, such a judgment presupposes that it is based on adequate experiencing and understanding: 'To pass judgment on what one does not understand is, not human knowing, but human arrogance. To pass judgment independently of all experience is to set fact aside.'[78]

Finally, a fact judgment is but a third-level intellectual achievement. The further process of evaluating this fact, and of deciding what I ought to do in light of this evaluation, all are fourth-level cognitional and decisional acts. Although evaluations are distinct in key ways from judgments, they depend upon and sublate these third-level achievements. Without adequate knowledge of facts, my evaluations are apt to be mistaken or irresponsible.[79] I will defer my discussion of the fourth cognitional level to chapter 6 in order first to consolidate this analysis of the first three cognitional levels, and to pause to address some important epistemic issues that have already arisen even prior to those that pertain to values.

4   Re-integrating Lonergan's Theory of Knowledge: From Analysis to Synthesis

Motivation for differentiating the various levels of cognition can be found in Lonergan's crisp advice that the alternative to distinguishing is confusion.[80] Still, the complementary task of emphasizing the integral unity of my cognitional operations returns me once again to the spontaneous pattern already operative in my conscious living and doing before inquiry brings this pattern expressly to light.[81] The motivation for this complementary task of re-integration can also be found in Lonergan's warnings that we risk evacuating the whole spontaneous process by excessively abstract analysis.[82]

But his more frequent warning is against the tendency to puff up a part of the process, such as experiencing or 'the look,' to the status of the whole. For 'just as the pendulum is not a clock so experiencing is not knowing.'[83]

Or again, 'no one of these activities, alone and by itself, may be named human knowing.'[84] With these cautions in mind, I will complement the preceding analysis with a synthesis, in order to emphasize the unity of the cognitional acts and processes I have been distinguishing. [85]

Lonergan expresses the central dynamism of the whole of our knowing in terms of wonder or of our conscious intentionality that we express in our questioning.[86] For Lonergan, the most basic and essential distinction here is between our transcendental (a priori) intending and the categorial (a posteriori) data that our transcendental intending encounters concretely, plus what results from these encounters: 'Sources of meaning are all conscious acts and all intended contents, whether in the dream state or on any of the four levels of waking consciousness. The principal division of sources is into transcendental and categorial.'[87]

Within our transcendental intending, Lonergan distinguishes between intentions of *intelligibility, reality,* and *value.* The categorial determinations of these intentions may be distinguished into *data, intelligibilities, realities,* and *values.* The two are related as question and answer, with our transcendental intending anticipating or prefiguring the answers to questions that arise following empirical encounters:[88]

> A *priori* contents [of intending], by contrast [with abstract contents of conceiving], are HEURISTICALLY 'universal.' They arise through anticipating the components of the thing; they antecede actual knowing, as question antecedes answer, and collectively they prefigure the thing in the totality of its components, intelligible and 'material' as well.[89]

Transcendental intentions, then, unify our cognitive processes by prefiguring categorial determinations. Moreover, the three transcendental intentions are themselves ordered methodologically, and subsequently confer this order on categorial achievements. For the *intending* of reality presupposes the intending of intelligibility, and the intending value presupposes the intending of both intelligibility and reality. Correspondingly, the *achievement* of intelligibility presupposes and sublates an awareness of data, the attaining of reality presupposes and sublates the achievement of intelligibility and an awareness of data, and so, also, the achievement of true value presupposes and sublates the attaining of reality, the achievement of intelligibility, and the awareness of data.[90]

Through the interplay between our transcendental intending and categorial encounters, our questioning relates us directly to being. Nevertheless, Lonergan emphasizes that we come to affirm being through a *mediated* process that builds upon a series of distinct, partial, and complementary cognitional operations. Following a categorial encounter, in my questioning, with some entity, my wonder or transcendental intending of being relates me, in an unmediated way, to being. But I come to affirm being, or know the real, only through an act of judgment. Hence, I am related to being through judgment in a *mediate* way. That is, I am related directly to being through my questions and mediately through my cognitional processes by means of which I discover answers to those questions.[91]

So far I have been exploring the first three levels of Lonergan's cognitional theory by illustrating his answer to the question 'What am I doing when I am knowing?' This question represents, for Lonergan, merely the first of three basic questions that philosophers must consider. The answer to the second basic question, 'Why is doing that knowing?' is an epistemology. The answer to the third basic question, 'What do I know when I do it?' is a metaphysics.[92] In chapter 5 I will take up Lonergan's answer to the second question by exploring his pithy remark that 'objectivity is simply the consequence of authentic subjectivity.'[93] In chapter 6 I will focus on level-four issues. In chapter 7 I will address Lonergan's second and third basic questions about the status of content of my knowledge of values.

5   Summary of the First, Second, and Third Cognitional Levels

I began by reflecting, philosophically, on my own cognitional acts as a physician engaging in diagnosing a patient experiencing chest pain. After becoming aware of relevant data on the first level of cognition, I explained how my subsequent cognitive acts conformed to a pattern of raising questions, having insights, and achieving answers on levels two and three. By way of summary, it would be helpful to reassemble some of the key elements of Lonergan's cognitional theory that I have already discussed in this chapter, for they provide the context for discussing affect as they relate to fourth-level evaluations. This is especially true since Lonergan maintains that fourth-level evaluations are similar in structure, but not content, to third-level judgments of fact.[94] Accordingly, one can anticipate that the fourth level will contain apprehensive acts analogous to reflective insights on the third level.

Thus far I have discussed the following key features of Lonergan's cognitional theory as it pertains to the phenomenon of knowing facts. Knowing involves a series of distinct but related processes of experiencing, understanding, and judging, which I have called levels. On each cognitional level I can distinguish between my cognitive acts and achievements. On the first level, acts of experiencing include those of sense and of consciousness, and on the levels of understanding and judging these acts are intellectual. All my cognitive acts are both intentional and conscious. My cognition goes forward in the direct or introspective modes, but the most fundamental difference in modes of intending is between transcendental and categorial intending. On all levels, knowing is a matter primarily of discovering and not of creating or positing. My knowing is a mediated process that begins with both an object and a question on all but the first level, which is unmediated. The pivotal cognitive acts on all but the first level are insights; by means of an insight I grasp a unity in some diversity. Second-level direct insights are intellectual cognitions that grasp an intelligible unity in experience and issue in a concept or definition. Third-level reflective insights are also intellectual cognitions that grasp a relation among elements of a prospective fact judgment and issue in knowledge of the virtually unconditioned real or a fact. By means of a fact judgment I gain cognitional access to the virtually unconditioned real, thereby achieving knowledge in the strict sense.

Beyond knowing that Paul is having an AMI, I have still to pose the evaluative question of whether or not this AMI is good or bad, whether it would be worthwhile for me to do something about it, and how I should carry out my decision responsibly. My focal concern will then be to highlight the role, if any, that my affectivity would play in such evaluations and decisions. In order to provide some clues for the relevance of the preceding discussion of knowing facts for the later discussion of knowing values, I will close by making explicit some of these connections.

First, one can anticipate that the structural similarity between the fourth and prior levels ought to include the cognitive events of transcendental intending, categorial questioning, having insights, and the production of a mental word. On this basis alone, I have some clues for where affect fits into the deliberative process. The transcendental intending of value, as was the case for the prior levels, is the source for my categorial value questions about the realities known through third-level fact judgments. It also provides the ultimate measure of the adequacy of my answers. Hence, if affect plays an important role in my categorial achievements of value, I might also anticipate a correspondingly key role for affect in my transcendental intending of value.

Second, I might also expect my fourth-level acts to sublate the achievements of the prior three levels. Hence, I anticipate that my fourth-level question 'Is it good?' will seek to evaluate the 'borrowed object' of my third-level judgment. In the case of Paul's chest pain, the question is whether having an AMI is good or whether some alternative possibility is better. In this way, the achievement of the prior levels, which culminates in a judgment, becomes the object of my question of value.

Finally, Lonergan locates the role of affect in my responses to third-level achievements or facts. He contends that I apprehend the value of such facts *in feelings.* From my discussion of apprehensive acts on the second and third levels, I am already familiar with the distinction between the *activity* of an insight and the *content* I grasp by means of that insight. I anticipate locating the fourth-level role of affect in acts of apprehending values. But I also think that if I understand Lonergan's analysis of knowing facts, it should not be too difficult to extend this analysis and understand how affect might play a role in my grasp of values.[95]

In order to make my account of Lonergan's position more plausible and convincing, I need to pause in this analysis of cognitional structure to address some questions that I anticipate are becoming of increasing concern to readers, namely, how can I be sure that my knowing is genuine or true. To address this question, I will devote chapter 5 to discussing Lonergan's account of an epistemology of knowing as regards the first three levels. This will involve bringing expressly to light a self-awareness of myself as a knower who is able to sense not automatically but attentively, to understand not mechanically but intelligently, to judge not unwittingly but critically, and to decide not arbitrarily but responsibly.[96]

5

Lonergan on Cognitional Objectivity: An Epistemology and Metaphysics of Mind

Once those ambiguities [underlying naive realism, naive idealism, empiricism, critical idealism, absolute idealism] are removed, once an adequate self-appropriation is effected, once one distinguishes between object and objectivity in the world of immediacy and, on the other hand, object and objectivity in the world mediated by meaning and motivated by value, objectivity is simply the consequence of authentic subjectivity, of genuine attention, genuine intelligence, genuine reasonableness, genuine responsibility. Mathematics, science, philosophy, ethics, theology, differ in many manners; but they have the common feature that their objectivity is the fruit of attentiveness, intelligence, reasonableness, and responsibility.

Bernard Lonergan, *Method in Theology*

1 Lonergan and the Issue of Cognitional Objectivity

In the previous chapter I gave an exposition of Lonergan's answer to what he takes to be the first of three basic questions for philosophy, namely, the phenomenological question, 'What am I doing when I am knowing facts?' His answer was that when I am knowing facts I engage in a series of complementary cognitional acts of experiencing, understanding, and judging. In the present chapter I will continue to focus on judging and address Lonergan's second basic question, which is the epistemological question, 'How does engaging in the phenomenon of judging result in epistemically valid knowing?' That is, how does this cognitive process result in my achieving knowledge that is more than epistemically just subjective?[1]

My purpose in this chapter is threefold. In a later chapter I will highlight the importance of Lonergan's distinction between the phenomenological and epistemological questions for his position on the role of affect in evaluations. I anticipate that a key difficulty that readers will have with the claim that certain affects play a cognitive role in evaluations is an epistemological one. That is, there is the fear that if one grants affect or any kind of feeling a role in evaluations then one cannot avoid the conclusion that all such evaluations are merely epistemically subjective. The initial aim of this chapter is to begin to undercut some of these concerns by an exposition of Lonergan's various senses of 'objectivity,' and by addressing the problem of the bridge between subject and object as it arises at the level of judgments, even prior to dealing expressly with evaluations.[2]

Second, I hope to emphasize how Lonergan's answer to the epistemological question follows from his answer to the phenomenological question. For Lonergan understands epistemic objectivity to be the consequence of 'authentic subjectivity.'[3] The present discussion will address the 'performative' aspect of my cognitional structure with the aim of highlighting those features that are characteristic of 'authentic' cognitive performances. At the level of judgment, Lonergan summarizes these features as matters of experiencing *attentively* rather than *inattentively*, understanding *intelligently* rather than *unintelligently*, and judging *reasonably* rather than *unreasonably*. By this approach, I hope to illustrate how the quality of my cognitive performance is reflected in my cognitive achievements.

Third, I hope to provide a nuanced and persuasive account of what Lonergan means by objectivity, and to contrast his view with a series of other, more typical stances on objectivity. I will illustrate various senses of objectivity by extending the medical example of diagnosing an AMI in order to reflect on ways in which I as a physician might fail to achieve the correct diagnosis. My own concrete, mistaken performance when making this medical judgment provides me with data on my own conscious, cognitive acts, and this will serve as a starting point for philosophically reflecting on the issue of epistemic objectivity. On the basis of such data I can then go on to assess the accuracy of Lonergan's account. To the extent that I am able to grasp accurately the distinct qualities that characterize my own successful cognitive performance, then, I shall have an express knowledge of the basis for my confidence, or anyone else's, in making judgments.[4] Furthermore, by contrasting this account of epistemic objectivity with some rival views, I will highlight the fact that objections that arise from these views bear as much upon insights and judgments as they do upon affects and evaluations.

2   A Peer Review of a Medical Misjudgment

I will begin, then, by taking as an example for examination my failure to make the diagnosis that Paul was having an AMI. I will consider the various ways that I might fail to arrive correctly at this diagnosis from the point of view of my medical peers reviewing my performance. For the sake of simplicity, I will assume that I have followed Lonergan's purportedly normative cognitional structure of experiencing, understanding, and judging in order to show that even if I follow this pattern, errors can arise at each level. By examining the patterns of my own faulty performance in making this judgment, correctly, I hope to highlight distinct, positive features that characterize my authentic cognitive performance. These characteristics are also the distinguishing features of consistently excellent diagnosticians, such as William Osler.[5]

Assume that my peers have in mind some notion of a competent diagnostician as a realistic standard of care, and this notion includes the exemplary performance of the cognitive acts of experiencing, understanding, and judging. On the first level, what are the standards for experiencing adequately that my peers might presuppose when assessing my competence? They would hardly excuse me, for instance, for failing to attend to significant findings, such as Paul's low blood pressure or changes on his cardiogram characteristic of an AMI. Nor would it be enough for me to claim that I did a complete physical examination if, when listening to Paul's lung and heart sounds, I missed the signs of congestive heart failure. For even if I understand that among persons experiencing an AMI I ought to anticipate impaired cardiac function, when examining Paul I might not have attended to the relevant data that manifest the physical signs of heart failure. To miss these signs, however, is to err on the cognitional level of experiencing, by what might be called *inattentively* experiencing.[6]

On the second level of understanding, even if Paul's symptoms were less than characteristic of cardiac disease, my peers might insist that in the course of deciding upon the cause of Paul's complaints I should have at least considered the possibility that he was having an AMI. If I failed to conceive of this possibility, I would most likely have overlooked the tell-tale signs and symptoms of an AMI. The contrast here is between an 'empty head' approach and the questioning 'full head' approach. Being mindful of a full range of probable causes for a symptom such as chest pain and systematically probing them is a distinguishing feature of an *intelligent* diagnostician. Conceiving of the possibility of an AMI is an achievement of second-level understanding. One way of my failing to meet some minimal standard of *intelligent* understanding that my peers might presuppose would be my neglect even to wonder whether Paul might be having an AMI, especially if Paul had already been wondering about this possibility himself.

Assuming that I had thought of the possibility of an AMI and had attended to the typical manifestations of this condition during my examination of Paul, I still might fail to understand Paul's data according to my peers' standards of intelligent performance. For instance, assume that Paul told me that his chest pain began soon after falling from a ladder and injuring his chest, and that his pain felt sharp, which is unlike the typical 'squeezing' or 'heavy' sensation of an AMI. Assume also that the only significant finding upon examining him was a tender bruise in the region of his chest and that all his other cardiac tests were normal. On the basis of this evidence, I might misinterpret Paul's chest pain as simply the result of his fall, and assume that this interpretation excludes the possibility that he might be having an AMI. That is, I might not seriously consider the possibility that he was having two causes for his chest pain, one from a chest-wall contusion and the other from cardiac ischemia. My peers might point out, however, that such an understanding of the matter is not an intelligent one. For although the prior probability of two types of chest pain occurring simultaneously might have been low, these two events are not mutually exclusive. Moreover, with the advantage of hindsight, they are able to confirm that not only was there a possibility of a double diagnosis, but that this was, in fact, the correct diagnosis.[7]

A similar difficulty at the second level of understanding could arise in the effort to distinguish between a diagnosis of an AMI and one of gastritis. If Paul's chest pain improved after he drank an antacid medication, I would be mistaken to interpret this outcome as *incompatible* with a cardiac cause for his chest pain. As with the case of a chest-wall contusion and an AMI, my peers might point out that his improvement following treatment with an antacid did not exclude the possibility that his pain was from an AMI. This would be especially relevant when the other non-excluded diagnosis involved a condition such as an AMI for which my peers would consider early recognition and treatment to be the standard of care. My efforts to distinguish intelligently between, and even logically to exclude, various possible causes of Paul's chest pain, such as chest-wall contusion, gastritis, or AMI, involved me in a process of constructing *arguments* for and against the conclusion that Paul is having an AMI. Consequently, my misdiagnosis might have resulted simply from a logically flawed argument.[8]

On the third level of judgment, I can again consider how my misdiagnosis could be related to some fault in my performance. On the one hand, assume that my peers would have withheld their judgment as to whether Paul was having an AMI, and decided instead simply to observe him longer. Taking this as their standard, they might conclude that my judgment 'Paul is *not* having an AMI' and my subsequent decision to send him home were *rash* or insufficiently critical. Indeed, it would have been rash if I lacked sufficient evidence to support this negative conclusion. They might insist that to make a reasonable diagnosis of a non-life-threatening cause of chest pain, such as a muscular or gastrointestinal cause, I should have ordered further tests, or perhaps observed Paul for a longer period of time. Given Paul's description, which was suggestive of cardiac pain, my peers might argue that the probability of the cause being an AMI was too high to be dismissed by the story of the injury to his chest, by relief of the pain using an antacid, or by the negative initial investigations. The probability that Paul was having an AMI would diminish, however, if no further evidence emerged to support this diagnosis, as he continued to be monitored and have repeat investigations.

On the other hand, if, according to my peers, I took too long observing Paul as he was having a heart attack (i.e., infarcting his cardiac muscle) by doing further tests on him, they might fault me for being overly *hesitant* in making the diagnosis and proceeding with definitive treatment. This hesitancy would be most obvious if all my peers agreed that, given the high probability of an AMI on the basis of the evidence I had already collected, these tests were superfluous to deciding whether I should treat Paul for an AMI. My peers might argue that I should have proceeded to treat Paul based on the presumed diagnosis of an AMI. For according to the relevant standard of care, a person who is having or is likely to be having an AMI should receive certain drugs, such as ASA and streptokinase, within the first hour following his arrival in an emergency department. Decisions concerning treatment were urgent in this case because there was a window of opportunity within which I could have prevented further damage to Paul's heart muscle.[9]

Hence, when judging whether Paul was, or was not, having an AMI, I can err by being either rash or overly hesitant. I would err by being rash if I made a judgment without sufficient evidence. On the other extreme, I would err by being overly hesitant if I failed to make the appropriate judgment even though I already had sufficient evidence. All my experiencing and understanding is presupposed in, and directed toward, my act of judging. Still, even if I intelligently understood Paul's reported experience and attentively experienced his signs and symptoms associated with his condition, my peers could justly criticize my judgment that he was not having an AMI because it failed to meet their standard of reasonableness.[10]

3   Elements of Epistemic Objectivity

I have illustrated different kinds of errors my peers could point to if they were to criticize my cognitive performance that led to my missing the diagnosis that Paul was having an AMI. The sorts of problems that I have been illustrating do not arise simply as a result of failing to follow Lonergan's purportedly normative cognitional operations of experiencing, understanding, and judging. Rather, they have to do with some deficiency in the quality of my concrete performance of these cognitive acts when making fact judgments. The judgment that my performance was deficient in any of the ways indicated presupposes that my peers have some performative norms that serve as criteria for knowing reality. My effort here will be directed to highlighting these presupposed norms in an express theory of objectivity.

Relating cognitional theory to objectivity, Lonergan points out:

> This complexity of our knowing involves a parallel complexity in our notion of objectivity. Principally the notion of objectivity is contained within a patterned context of judgments which serve as implicit definitions of terms 'object,' 'subject.' But besides this principal and complete notion, there also are partial aspects or components emergent within cognitional process.[11]

The meaning that Lonergan assigns to *objectivity* corresponds to the meaning of the term 'object' (i.e., being, thing, entity) as understood in the context of the world mediated by meaning, rather than the world of immediacy. Just as objects are for him what I come to know through experiencing, understanding, and judging, so also objectivity has three partial aspects or components:

> There is experiential objectivity constituted by the givenness of the data of sense and the data of consciousness. There is the normative objectivity constituted by the exigencies of intelligence and reasonableness. There is the absolute objectivity that results from combining the results of experiential and normative objectivity so that through experiential objectivity conditions are fulfilled while through normative objectivity conditions are linked to what they condition. The combination, then, yields a conditioned with its conditions fulfilled and that, in knowledge, is a fact and, in reality, it is a contingent being or event.[12]

I will begin by discussing these three components of epistemic objectivity before turning my attention to what Lonergan calls 'the principal notion of objectivity.' In the example of my peers assessing my performance, I might press them on the criteria for knowing the real that they are presupposing in their critique of my performance. That is, what do they take to be the distinguishing features of one's conscious acts, features that correspond to one's successful cognitional achievements, that make them genuinely cognitional, epistemically valid, or cognitionally true? How do they think these features were lacking in my performance, such that my cognitional achieve-

Table 5.1 Meanings of *objectivity* for Lonergan

A. Phenomenal objectivity: the subject-object distinction as experienced

B. Epistemic objectivity – genuine knowing

Cognitional activity	*Cognitional activity as genuine*	*Objectivity achieved*
1. experiencing	attentive experiencing	Experiential objectivity
2. understanding	intelligent understanding	Normative objectivity
3. judging	reasonable judging	Absolute objectivity (real)
[4. evaluating	responsible evaluating	Absolute objectivity (good)]

5. Principal notion of objectivity – the subject-object distinction as known

C. Metaphysical objectivity

---

ment was mistaken, epistemically invalid, untrue? Answering this question for them in Lonergan's terms will entail spelling out a series of different meanings of the term 'epistemic objectivity,' as outlined in table 5.1.

I will begin with *epistemic objectivity* by distinguishing what Lonergan labels *experiential, normative,* and *absolute* epistemic objectivity. Following this, I will distinguish these senses of objectivity from what Lonergan calls the *principal notion of objectivity,* and finish by distinguishing these types of epistemic objectivity from what Lonergan takes to be *phenomenal* and *metaphysical* objectivity.[13] He maintains that together these distinct notions of objectivity provide an accurate articulation of the criteria of knowing genuine facts that my peers are operatively presupposing in their criticism of my performance.[14]

3.1 Experiential Objectivity

Experiential objectivity is the consequence of experiencing *attentively.* That is, experiencing attentively, as distinct from experiencing inattentively, characterizes those acts of experiencing that are genuinely cognitional. In Paul's case, he might sense chest pain and other symptoms of his cardiac crisis, and I might also sense some of the manifestations of his AMI during my examination of him. But the question that a peer review would insist upon answering is whether I erred in this case because I was, in some sense, inattentive to, and consequently unaware of, important physical manifestations of his condition.

In reviewing my cognitive performance that resulted in my mistaken diagnosis, my peers might ask themselves how my experience of Paul was deficient or substandard. The criterion of genuine experience that Lonergan would suggest is being presupposed in their criticism of my performance is that one ought to experience attentively. The distinction between my experiencing attentively or inattentively corresponds to the distinction between my achieving and failing to achieve an adequate awareness of sense data. My peers' criticism of my failure to achieve an adequate sense awareness of Paul follows from their judgment that I failed to experience him attentively.

The precise meaning and nuance of such a general criterion as experiencing *attentively* is only brought to light by reflecting on concrete failures to attain such experiencing. I have already alluded to this process in the discussion of the self-correcting process of learning. Such a review reveals myriad ways in which acts of experiencing can be cut short or undermined by various fears or desires. But there is also the basic problem of selecting, from among the manifold data of experience, those that are relevant, and then attending to these data in a careful, orderly, and deliberate manner.

In the act of sensing I achieve an awareness of sense data. Still, if sensing attentively is a property of my first-level performance, distinguishing between relevant and irrelevant data is something that would seem to be guided by higher-level concerns, such as my intending intelligibility in these data. Data given to me in first-level sense experience are preconceptual and unstructured contents, which I unify or integrate, to some extent, at the first level of perceptual experience. I grasp further unities in my sense experience as I move to understanding and judgment. Since sense data are initially unstructured, discovering and affirming a structure is what my subsequent questions for understanding and judgment are about. I can wonder about the possible structures that can be revealed in the data through understanding, and so I raise questions about what I have become aware of through sense experience. Subsequent cognitive acts add structure to the preconceptual contents of sense experience and, in the process, further promote my attentive unpacking of these data. These further acts give my experiencing, as it were, not only an ulterior motive for attentiveness, but also an orientation to selecting relevant data.[15]

In the previous chapter I spoke of the formation of images as a cognitive act on the first level of experiencing. Images facilitate the demand to simplify the manifold of data and to promote insights into these data. But images can also lead one astray. For instance, by simplifying the data in an image I might be omitting relevant data. This immanently generated image, then, would impede the emergence of correct insights into the data. Alternatively, images might even be produced by some psychological aberration (e.g., hallucinations) that results in a perfect counterfeit of sense data. If I attend attentively to the experience of a hallucination, I might meet the criterion for experiential objectivity. But interpretations of the data and judgments regarding the correctness of the interpretations are still to occur. In the case of a hallucination, these interpretations and judgments are within the province of the study of aberrant psychology.

Hence, not only is sense experiencing the fundamental cognitive act, but experiential objectivity also captures the fundamental (though partial) notion of objectivity. All subsequent acts go forward from contents of experience; they add structure to those contents and return me once again to experience, where I test my hypotheses through further attention to data. By experiential objectivity, then, I refer to the genuineness of first-level acts of sensing that ground my achievements of awareness of data. In summary, I can say that experiential objectivity obtains in as much as my experiencing is 'attentive.'[16]

3.2 Normative Objectivity

For Lonergan, *normative objectivity* is a consequence of understanding 'intelligently.' That is, I progress successfully from an objective awareness of data to an objective understanding of these data according to the second-level, cognitive norm of *intelligence*. Like the presupposed criterion of genuine experiencing, Lonergan considers these norms to be operative in intelligent persons even prior to their expression in rules of logic, such as the algorithms for medical decision-making. As table 5.1 highlights, the normative objectivity of my second-level achievements follow from the genuine quality of cognitional acts of understanding, which Lonergan characterizes as understanding intelligently.[17]

To understand intelligently is to be faithful to my transcendental intending of intelligibility in any concrete or categorial encounter. The alternative is not merely to fail to yield to my desire to know; it is to be oriented by other norms, such as my own satisfactions and dissatisfactions: 'There is a normative aspect that is contained in the contrast between the detached and unrestricted desire to know and, on the other hand, merely subjective desires and fears.'[18]

To understand intelligently at least means that my understanding is internally consistent. I illustrated possible ways I might violate the norms of rationality or logic in interpreting Paul's reported experience and his signs and symptoms, even though I had considered the diagnosis of an AMI. If I thought that Paul could not have both an AMI *and* a chest-wall injury, or that I need not verify that he was *not* having an AMI on the basis of the prior statistical improbability of him having both diagnoses, then such illogical arguments could be responsible for my misdiagnosis. Here, normative objectivity reveals itself as one of my peers' presupposed criteria of genuine knowing, namely, that acts of understanding ought to be intelligent. So when it came to the question of my understanding the logic of a double diagnosis, they might have judged that I did not attain the norm of under-standing intelligently.

3.3 Absolute Objectivity

By *absolute objectivity* I refer to that property of judgments whereby I move into the absolute realm of being through a true judgment about reality. The normative, genuinely cognitive activity here is that I judge *reasonably*, on the basis of a reflective understanding. I illustrated how my peers might judge that my performance in diagnosing Paul failed to meet this criterion of *reasonableness* in two ways. First, they might judge my misdiagnosis that Paul's chest pain was from a chest-wall injury to be *rash* because I failed to gather sufficient evidence to exclude safely the possibility that he might also be having an AMI. They might also criticize my delay in offering Paul standard drug therapy to be overly *hesitant* because I already had enough evidence to support the diagnosis of a probable AMI. On the basis of the likelihood that he was having an AMI, they might judge that I ought to have decided to treat him. For my peers to agree that in this case my judgment was unreasonable, they also need to have some operative notion regarding what distinguishes a reasonable judgment on this matter from the extremes of overly *rash* or *hesitant* judgments.[19]

For Lonergan, then, genuine knowledge of facts involves the conjunc-tion of experiential, normative, and absolute components of objectivity. The resultant criteria of epistemically objective judging is that I experience *attentively*, understand *intelligently*, and judge *reasonably*. Moreover, he main-tains that the requisite experiencing, understanding, and judging do, at least sometimes, occur. In each of these acts, a distinct but related meaning of epistemic objectivity arises. As my illustration highlights, they are distinct because experiencing *attentively* (experiential objectivity) is quite different from understanding *intelligently* (normative objectivity). Each of these is different from judging *reasonably* (absolute objectivity). But each of these distinct meanings of objectivity is related to the others in a manner similar to that in which the underlying cognitive acts are related to one another, as I have already indicated.

Hence, I understand *intelligently* data that I have experienced *attentively*. I judge *reasonably* what I have intelligently understood in the data I have attentively experienced. *Absolute* objectivity sublates objectivity in the prior meanings in a judgment in which I affirm a proposition as virtually uncon-ditioned. This is a conditioned proposition whose conditions are, in fact, fulfilled. Through this judgment I reach the absolute realm of being: 'The process of knowing, when you grasp the unconditioned and affirm it, moves beyond subjectivity by the mere fact that you reach an unconditioned. You step in, through the judgment, into the absolute realm. There is nothing outside being that can take a look at it and have being as its object. If it is outside being, it is nothing.'[20]

In the previous chapter I discussed three of Lonergan's cognitional levels and how each is related to the next. As Frederick Crowe expresses Lonergan's position, the discovery of these levels gives us 'a rule for life and work: be attentive, be intelligent, be reasonable, be responsible.'[21] These rules or precepts point to what Lonergan means by 'authenticity.' What I am calling 'epistemic objectivity' refers to a property of my acts of knowing and, derivatively, to the validity of my claims about the purported real, known in and through true judgments. For Lonergan, such objectivity is nothing other than the consequence of authentic subjectivity, that is, of following my own internal cognitive norms, which, I will later argue, are the same ultimate norms to which my peers are striving.

In the previous chapter I also distinguished between the transcendental intentions and categorial determinations that follow encounters of these transcendental intentions with data. These transcendental intentions can be understood as differentiations of the notion of wonder, such as the distinction between wonder that intends intelligibility and wonder that intends reality. These differentiations are not only the radical motivators of my concrete cognitive acts of discovery; they also provide the ultimate criteria for the success of my apparent cognitive achievements. Hence, for Lonergan, epistemic objectivity is found not merely in my fidelity to wonder, spelled out in terms of transcendental striving for intelligibility and reality, but most importantly in meeting the criteria set by these intentions. This occurs when I live up to the norms of the transcendental precepts: Be attentive, Be intelligent, Be reasonable. A sign of my successful fidelity to these precepts is given when I have satisfied myself that I have met all relevant questions. By contrast, the hallmark of my infidelity to these precepts is given in my agitation or restlessness, which might result from my resistance to raising or addressing further, relevant questions. From these experiential, normative, and absolute components of objectivity, I will now turn to what Lonergan calls the 'principal notion of objectivity.' This will involve the crucial discussion of the subject-object distinction, and the problem of the bridge.

4   The Principal Notion of Objectivity

So far in this analysis of the possible factors contributing to my misdiagnosing Paul as not having an AMI when in fact he was, I have been speaking of myself, a 'subject,' intending to achieve real or genuine knowledge about the cause of Paul's chest pain. Paul's experience of pain is the 'object' of my inquiry. In the previous chapter I spoke of the distinct and related cognitive acts in which I engage in diagnosing his chest pain. As a physician, my focus is on Paul who is the 'object' of my inquiry. At the same time, as a conscious subject I am also present to myself as engaging in this inquiry. But as a physician, the contents of my cognitive subjectivity are, for the most part, merely *experienced, lived,* and *implicit* in my performance. As a philosopher, however, I bring to light my cognitive subjectivity by attending to and reflecting on the features of my medical judging. From this perspective, I come to *judge, know,* and make *explicit* these features of my subjectivity, and to account for the difference between my subjectivity as 'authentic' or 'inauthentic.' In so doing, I argued that questions about the genuineness of my knowledge follow from questions about the authenticity of my cognitional subjectivity.

In order to understand better what Lonergan takes to be the 'principal notion of objectivity,' I will need to address the *subject-object* distinction. I begin by defining what Lonergan means by 'object' and 'objectivity' and, on the other hand, by 'subject' and 'subjectivity.' Part of the terminological difficulty here regarding the meaning of 'objectivity' arises from the fact that *Insight* was written from a moving viewpoint. In it, the meaning of the term 'knowing,' for instance, expands when one moves from the context of a phenomenology of knowing to an epistemology of knowing. In chapter 4, knowing merely denoted an 'apparently epistemic conscious process,' one that 'purportedly grasps being.' In the present context, it may be defined as 'a genuinely epistemic conscious process,' one that 'actually grasps being.'[22]

Michael Vertin offers the following clarification of Lonergan's position:

> '[B]eing' means 'the goal of intelligent inquiry and understanding and of reasonable reflection and affirmation.' 'Objectivity' means 'the distinctive property of that knowing which grasps some being other than the knower *as* being other than the knower and, correlatively, the knower *as* knower.' On the [i.e., Lonergan's] positional stance, 'reality' means nothing other than 'being'[23]

The principal notion of epistemic objectivity emerges in the context of discussing judgments that are instances of absolute objectivity. In this setting, I can make the further distinction between knowing non-self *as* non-self, and, correlatively, knowing self *as* self.[24] In discussing absolute objectivity, I spoke of moving into an absolute realm where I discover not only objects, but also myself as a subject.[25] Lonergan defines the principal meaning of 'objectivity' as emerging from a pattern that I grasp within a series of judgments, and this brings to light the difference between those series of facts that pertain to the non-self and others that pertain to the self.

The principal notion of objectivity arises when the true judgment, 'some object A is,' is complemented by at least two other judgments, 'I am a knower' and 'I am not A.' Put more amply, the judgment 'I am a knower' can be expressed as the judgment 'I am a unity-identity-whole that senses, perceives, imagines, inquires, understands, conceives, reflects, grasps the virtually unconditioned, and judges.'[26] As a knower, I know some real being or beings (represented by A). But the key judgment that gives rise to the principal notion of objectivity is, 'I am not this A.' This is the account of the subject-object distinction, not as experienced, lived, and implicit, but as judged, known, and made explicit, as arising within a pattern of judgments that mark off those contents that refer to self from those referring to non-self. This distinction becomes judged, known, and explicit only as a result of some philosophical reflection and introspection. Moreover, it is referred to as the principal notion of objectivity because it highlights the concern to account not merely for genuine knowledge (i.e., absolute objectivity) but, more specifically, for genuine knowledge of objects (i.e., non-self).

In the background of this principal notion of objectivity is the 'problem of the bridge,' that is, how it is that self can come to a genuine knowledge of non-self. Lonergan maintains that the subject-object distinction is *known* only at the third level of judgment. And although the subject-object distinction underpins what Lonergan refers to as the principal notion of objectivity, for him this distinction does not provide a fundamental category within which all experience falls. What is fundamental for Lonergan is the distinction between the transcendental and the categorial. The transcendental notions or intentions, such as those of intelligibility and reality, can be objectified as transcendental concepts. Conscious acts work out categorial determinations of these intended contents. From among my knowledge achieved through categorial acts of judgment there emerges the subject-object distinction between the being whose unity-identity-whole I affirm as 'self' (as lived and objectified) and other beings I judge to be 'non-self.' On this account, once I reach the third level of making these judgments in the sense of knowing I have already arrived in the objective world; and there is no problem of bridging a gap between my activities of knowing and the content I achieve through those activities. If I reach the judgment, I am there:

> An object means no more than that A is. If I am A, and A is, and B is, and A is not B, then we have a subject: I am a knower (established in [*Insight*] chapter 11); and we have an object: something that A knows, that I know, that is not myself, that is not the subject. Through true propositions, you can arrive at an objective world. That is the principal notion of objectivity.[27]

The principal notion of objectivity, then, combines the notion of absolute objectivity in achieving knowledge of the real and the notion of personal responsibility for this knowledge. That is, my knowing is 'objective' not only in the absolute sense of a genuine cognitional achievement, but also I expressly affirm this achievement as the result of my own authentic cognitive performance. The principal notion of objectivity grounds all of my knowledge about being in my cognitional subjectivity, or my world of interiority, so that as originator of that knowledge I know both objects distinct from myself and myself. Hence, 'objective,' epistemic knowledge of objects, in its principal meaning, is knowledge of them 'both as beings and *as* beings other than the knower.'[28]

In summary, knowledge of self *as* self is epistemically 'objective' in at least two senses. First, I can have genuine knowledge of 'self-as-objectified,' which is an instance of absolute objectivity. Second, I can also judge this 'self-as-objectified' to be myself, and so distinct from other objects who are knowers and thus other selves. This is an instance of the principal sense of objectivity as regards my own subjectivity.[29]

5   Correlative Basic Senses of Objectivity for Lonergan

Thus far I have distinguished four meanings of epistemic objectivity: experiential, normative, absolute, and the principal notion of epistemic objectivity. Lonergan did not always restrict *objectivity* to the epistemic sense as he did in his later writing. In his earlier writings, for instance, he also used the term 'objective' to speak about the emergence of the subject-object distinction in the phenomenal sense and in the metaphysical sense. In the phenomenal sense, the subject-object distinction is an aspect of every intentional act insofar as it is also a conscious act, such as with an act of sensing I am aware of myself as engaged in this act. In the metaphysical sense, the subject-object distinction contrasts objects that have the capacity for subjectivity, such as persons, from those that do not, such as chairs. Although I have just discussed the difference between the subject-object distinction as experienced and as explicitly affirmed, this distinction is not merely between *self* and *non-self* at the level of experience. It will be helpful to underline two other ways that the term 'objectivity' can be used in order to link this discussion with the discussion of cognitional phenomenology in chapter 4 and the metaphysical discussion to come in chapter 7.

In the phenomenal sense of the subject-object distinction, Lonergan pins down the meanings of 'subject' and 'object' in terms of my psychological activities. For instance, in the sentence 'I examine Paul,' I am the subject doing the examining; examining is the activity I perform; and Paul is the object of this activity. On one side of the activity there is the subject (myself) engaging in acts of knowing. On the other side there are contents, or the object of my cognitive acts (Paul).[30]

A distinction that emerges in every conscious-intentional act is that between my cognitional acts and their contents or achievements. What might be called 'phenomenal objectivity' has to do with the contents of these cognitive acts (e.g., red-as-seen), which are distinct from the acts themselves. 'Phenomenal subjectivity,' on the other hand, refers to the cognitive acts themselves (e.g., seeing red), which are given as acts that are mine; they are acts that I perform. This sense of the subject-object distinction, which first emerges in living, is subsequently known through judgment; and it is made explicit when I distinguish between my 'subjective' intentional acts (e.g., sensing) and the 'objective' contents or achievements of those acts (e.g., awareness of data).

By contrast, the sense of the subject-object distinction that the principal notion of objectivity makes explicit is the distinction between self and non-self. This is a subsequent distinction made within phenomenally objective contents, and it involves at least three epistemically valid judgments, as I previously explained. From this perspective, the problem is not one beginning with knowledge of self, from which I proceed to knowledge of some object that is non-self. Rather, both self and non-self are, in the first instance, phenomenally objective contents of my cognitive acts. They subsequently become known in the absolute meaning of epistemic objectivity through authentic judgments. Finally, by means of the principal notion of objectivity, I distinguish between those facts that pertain to self and those pertaining to non-self.[31]

Finally, the very possibility of a subject-object distinction rests on the fact that there are subjects. In the metaphysical meaning of objectivity, I can distinguish between those beings who have some capacity for self-presence and those beings who do not have this capacity. What may be called 'metaphysical objectivity' is the hallmark of those real beings, such as stones, that are totally lacking in consciousness, and so are in no way present to themselves. By contrast, what may be labelled 'metaphysical subjectivity' denotes a capacity of certain types of beings, such as humans, for self-presence. Metaphysical subjectivity, then, is a condition for the emergence of the phenomenal subject-object distinction. By contrast to both phenomenal and metaphysical objectivity, 'epistemic objectivity' has to do with the genuineness or truth of my cognitive achievements. Once again, the validity of my knowledge claims is intimately connected to the quality of my cognitive activities that undergird these achievements. The principal notion of objectivity, therefore, denotes a property of my knowing that grasps some being other than self *as* a being other than self (i.e., a non-self) and, correlatively, self *as* self.

6   Contrasting Lonergan's Notion of Objectivity with Common Medical Uses

In common medical parlance the term 'objectivity' has several meanings that can helpfully be contrasted with Lonergan's meanings. The purpose of this contrast is twofold. First, it will enable us to clarify further Lonergan's views on objectivity. Second, it will enable us to begin to understand better the main outlines of some stances on objectivity that are dialectically opposed to Lonergan's and that figure prominently in the euthanasia debate. Thus, I will have a basis for criticizing these stances later from Lonergan's perspective. Here, I will confine myself mainly to pointing out differences between certain common medical uses of 'objectivity' (cf. table 5.2) and Lonergan's use of the term in the context of judgments.[32]

6.1 Objectively to Know As: Attentively to Sense

Corresponding to Lonergan's experiential objectivity, there is some currency to the notion that 'genuinely to know is nothing other than attentively to sense.' That is, being or the really real is what is given in unmediated sense experience and, moreover, such sense experience can actually occur. In this context, various forms of the term 'objectivity' seem to function as indicators of emphatic qualifiers for acts of sensing. Accordingly, I might say, 'I examined Paul's cardiogram objectively.' What this usage of the term 'objective' presupposes is a notion of elementary knowing that is given in an unmediated manner at the level of sense experience. This usage implies that genuine knowledge not only begins with concrete sensible data, but is also restricted to the sensibly given. Although Lonergan acknowledges a sense in which I may speak of the objectivity of sensing, for him knowing is not merely sensing, nor is genuine knowing reducible to some property of acts of sensing.[33]

6.2 Objectively to Know As: To Understand from the Second- or Third-Person Perspective

Although medical practitioners often presuppose the primacy of sense experience in genuine knowing, they are also ready to move beyond the 'subjective' experience of patients to what they take to be the more 'objective' medical perspective. This difference in perspectives is highlighted in the way that clinical records are organized. Standard medical procedure organizes clinical findings according to the categories 'Subjective,' 'Objective,' 'Assessment,' and 'Plan.'[34] According to this scheme, I would list under 'subjective' *Paul's* descriptive account of his chest pain. Under 'ob-

Table 5.2 Meanings of *objectively to know* in common medical usage

1. Attentively to sense.
2. To understand from the perspective of the second or third person.
3. To understand in the explanatory (and person-neutral) mode.
4. To abide by the procedural norms and definitions of my profession as a group.

jective' I would include findings from *my* physical examination of Paul, such as his temperature, blood pressure, and cardiac and respiratory findings. This objective category would also include the results of laboratory measurements, such as his cardiac enzymes, cardiogram, and X-ray results. Following this, I would then write my assessment and plan, such as 'Chest pain: probable AMI or chest-wall contusion' and, under 'plan,' 'advise that he be admitted to the Intensive Care Unit for cardiac monitoring, medications, and further investigations and consultations.'

Note that on this usage, the distinction between what is subjective and what is objective seems to correspond, in part, to some difference between Paul's perspective, as the one who is experiencing the chest pain, and my perspective, as the physician examining him. The advantage of my perspective as Paul's physician over Paul's perspective on his own problem, which this use of the term 'objective' seems to underline, is that I enjoy a certain detachment from the immediacy of Paul's painful sense experience of himself, as well as other complicating and possibly biasing experiences, such as his associated fears and compensatory psychological responses. Moreover, as a trained and experienced physician, presumably I also have the advantage of understanding certain patterns of physical experiences, having learned from many cases involving apparently similar experiences of chest pain. Nevertheless, labelling Paul's account 'subjective' because it is his account of himself, and my account 'objective,' suggests that there is something inherently epistemically deficient about a perspective on something in which one is personally involved. This seems to be a sort of ad hominem argument against any judgment about one's own experience simply because the content regards oneself.[35]

6.3 Objectively to Know As: To Understand in the Explanatory Mode

In terms of Lonergan's categories, another interpretation of the subject-object distinction underpinning common medical usage is that objectively to know is to understand in the explanatory mode. This use of objectivity draws on the difference between two forms of understanding: description and explanation. For instance, Paul is thought to express his 'subjective' experience in describing his chest pain as it relates to himself. By contrast, I express my understanding of Paul's experience by noting those findings that best allow me to compare his chest pain to other instances. By performing tests and making measurements, such as quantifying the rise in his cardiac enzymes, I move toward the explanatory perspective of relating findings on Paul's condition to findings on others who have had AMI's. I locate these findings under the 'objective' category. In other words, the contents that fall under the 'objective' category are objective not merely because they are from my perspective as a trained physician rather than from Paul's perspective. These contents are also unified by the fact that I am able to relate these data to the data from other patients who have had an AMI. In the move from subjective to objective, then, there is a shift from Paul's sense experience of himself to my sense experience of him, which is oriented by the ulterior motive of relating his experience to those of others who have had chest pain from various causes. I make this relation by expressing it in the explanatory mode, rather than being restricted to the descriptive mode.[36]

There are a number of ramifications that follow from these last two notions of objectivity that involve differences from Lonergan's account. For instance, if the subject-object distinction has to do with perspective, then any first-person description or explanation is inherently 'subjective.' This gives rise to the biased view that any judgment by oneself about oneself is inevitably epistemically just 'subjective.' On the other hand, if the subject-object distinction is primarily linked to the difference between descriptive and explanatory modes of understanding, then this gives rise to a bias against any descriptive account, expressed either from a first- or second-person perspective, again as epistemically just 'subjective.'[37]

By contrast to these medical uses, Lonergan's absolute epistemic objectivity emerges at the levels of neither experiencing nor understanding, but with third-level judging, which in medical terms is 'assessment.' It is at the level of judging that one achieves knowledge of the real. For Lonergan, explanations, even from the perspective of the second or third person, are never epistemically objective in their absolute meaning simply because they are not judgments. On the other hand, the purported 'subjectivity' of knowledge claims that are first person in perspective or descriptive in content is not to be discounted as epistemically just 'subjective' simply because the subject is implicated in the knowledge claims. The issue of whether the contents of one's cognitive achievements regard oneself or not is related to what Lonergan calls the principal meaning of epistemic objectivity. For him, this determination merely involves further judgments, and the distinction between self and other is not a fundamental category phenomenologically, epistemically, or metaphysically.

6.4 Objectively to Know As: To Abide by the Procedural Norms of One's Group

A further commonly presupposed meaning of objectivity in medical circles corresponds to Lonergan's normative objectivity, but it conceives of the relevant norm as sociological. For instance, if cardiologists agree on the criteria that must be met in order to make the diagnosis that a patient such as Paul is having an AMI, then they might find fault with my judgment not primarily because I came to a different conclusion, but because I failed to follow these standard criteria of good medical decision-making. Accordingly, my diagnosis that he was having an AMI would be 'non-objective' if I based it on different criteria than those followed by my peers, or established this diagnosis following a methodologically novel approach to the one agreed upon by my group or profession. That is, my peers need not also complain that my diagnosis was, in fact, wrong. Nor need they insist that the presence of standard criteria necessarily means that the patient is having an AMI. All that is presupposed by this use of 'objectivity' is that genuinely to know is nothing more than abiding by the procedural norms and definitional criteria of my group.

In other words, what might be presupposed here is some notion that genuinely to know is exhaustively to understand and thereby to transcend the limitations of my historical situatedness. But there is also the admission that such knowing never occurs. So on this presupposition there never is absolute objectivity in Lonergan's sense of a knowing that reaches the unconditioned through judgment. Rather, I must be content with normative objectivity where all I can do is make contingent judgments that are inescapably historically conditioned.

In contrast to Lonergan's sense of absolute objectivity, this medical view seems to be willing to acknowledge peer standards for correct understanding and judging, but still resists the notion that absolute, epistemic objectivity can sometimes be attained by reaching a virtually unconditioned judgment. That is, this view presupposes that genuine knowing is achieved by transcending all historical perspectivism, but then concludes that such knowing never occurs. From Lonergan's perspective, such a stance might itself be an instance of 'group bias.' To be sure, there are some advantages of a group's perspective over that of an individual.[38] But individuals might also be negatively influenced by group biases. For instance, it is probable that a widely held belief that genuine knowledge does or does not occur is bound to influence what people think about some matter, and how they interpret their own experience. Similarly, as regards feelings, a group consensus against the cognitive relevance of feelings might also influence how a person interprets his or her own experience. If the norm is biased, it will promote a similar bias in individuals. Indeed, for Lonergan, the issue of bias is connected to that of objectivity, and he expresses the crux of the difficulty of objectivity in terms of the difficulty of rooting out not merely individual bias, but group bias as well: 'No problem is at once more delicate and more profound, more practical and perhaps more pressing. How, indeed, is a mind to become conscious of its own bias when that bias springs from a communal flight from understanding and is supported by the whole texture of a civilization?'[39]

7   Summary

Lonergan treats the question of objectivity as the second basic question of philosophy. The first basic question of philosophy is the question of phenomenology, 'What am I doing when I am knowing?' One's answer to the second basic question follows from one's answer to the first. In this chapter I addressed Lonergan's answer to the second basic question, in which he argues that epistemic objectivity results from our performing cognitional activities *authentically*. For him judging objectively is the consequence of our fidelity to the precepts of life and work: be attentive, be intelligent, be reasonable. In so far as our cognitional performance exemplifies these precepts, we are operating as authentic subjects, and this is the key basis for our confidence in our cognitional achievements.

Lonergan's answer to the second basic question expresses theoretically what he claims people performatively presuppose genuine knowing to be. For him, genuinely to know facts is nothing other than *attentively* to experience, *intelligently* to understand, and *reasonably* to judge. In addition, he affirms that the requisite experiencing, understanding, and judging sometimes do occur.

I distinguished four meanings of Lonergan's notion of 'epistemic objectivity.' These were further distinguished as two partial meanings of objectivity, experiential and normative objectivity, which are combined in acts of judgment to yield absolute objectivity. Lonergan's principal sense of objectivity involves the further judgment of oneself as a subject who is capable of self-presence, and who is a unity who consciously performs certain cognitional operations as distinct from objects which may or may not also be subjects. All these meanings of objectivity can be understood as differentiations of the notion of 'epistemic' objectivity, as distinct from 'phenomenal' and 'metaphysical' objectivity.

Finally, I sought to clarify further Lonergan's stance on objectivity by contrasting his distinct but related notions of objectivity with other views that are common in medical parlance. By contrast to Lonergan's account of knowing in his answer to the first basic question of philosophy, these other views presuppose different accounts of knowing – that to know, for instance, is simply a matter of experiencing, or that objectivity is achieved simply in virtue of compliance with some group norm. Corresponding to their underlying notions of knowing, these opposed views also presuppose different accounts of what genuine knowing is. From Lonergan's perspective, each of these views is deficient because they inflate what he takes to be an element of knowing to the status of the whole. Consequently, they mistakenly promote a partial meaning of objectivity to the status of a criterion for 'absolute' objectivity. Finally, I suggested that these different accounts of how judgments are genuine will have important implications for my focal question regarding the role one believes feelings play in evaluations and their objectivity.

6

Lonergan on the Role of Affect in Evaluations: A Phenomenology of Heart

Intermediate between judgments of fact and judgments of value lie apprehensions of value. Such apprehensions are given in feelings.

Bernard Lonergan, *Method in Theology*

1   Lonergan's Account of the Role of Affect in Human Cognition

From the account of the phenomenology and epistemology of *mind* I now move to a phenomenology and epistemology of *heart*. In this chapter I seek to highlight Lonergan's view regarding where, as a matter of phenomenal fact, feelings enter into our cognitive processes in general and, more particularly, where they enter into our apparent knowledge of actual or possible values.[1]

Although I will distinguish between the knowing mind and heart, I want to begin by emphasizing the fact that feelings and evaluations first emerge in concrete living. The distinctions I will be making between knowing facts and knowing values, and correlatively between the activities of judging and evaluating, are philosophical differentiations of what is given as a single whole in ordinary human living.[2] I emphasize the prior unity of human knowing because any discussion of where feelings enter into moral judgments risks becoming an overly abstract way of talking about something that is utterly concrete and common. In the subsequent analysis I hope to minimize this risk by basing the discussion on examples of medical evaluations that arise in the context of treating patients, such as the one discussed earlier involving my patient Paul who was having chest pain.

Despite my best efforts to pin down Lonergan's views on these issues by recourse to my own concrete evaluations, the issues themselves remain subtle and difficult to articulate accurately. Moreover, my task of interpreting Lonergan's views is made even more difficult because of his rather cryptic remarks on the relation between feeling responses and evaluations. Both of these factors have given rise to diverse interpretations of his position by various Lonergan scholars.[3] Despite the ongoing discussions among Lonergan scholars regarding the role of feelings in evaluations, all agree that for the later Lonergan certain feelings play a crucial role in evaluations. Lonergan made this clear in his often repeated remark that those feelings that are intentional responses give intentional consciousness 'its mass, momentum, drive and power,'[4] and the further remark that '[i]f you have not got feelings, you are a psychopath.'[5]

A precise understanding of Lonergan's view of feelings as 'the mass and momentum of intentional consciousness,' and as a necessary prerequisite for psychological health, is the main goal of the present chapter. However, before launching into a detailed interpretation of Lonergan's views, it will be helpful to recall how Lonergan's general position on the role of feelings in evaluations relates to other prominent views on this issue in the history of philosophy.

Lonergan's position is clearly at odds with a rationalist or intellectualist denigration of feelings. On the rationalist account, knowing and ideas are quite distinct from feeling; although feelings can be psychologically important, they typically have no properly philosophical or cognitive import.[6] Still, if Lonergan disagrees with this rationalist position, it does not follow that he is in agreement with all of those positions that endorse the cognitive role of feelings, such as the emotivist, voluntarist, or sentimentalist positions. For although thinkers who express these positions emphasize the importance of feelings, they frequently view these feelings, as well as the values such feelings grasp, as strictly private matters.[7]

For Lonergan, the genuine good, which he equates with value, is what I intend in questions for deliberation, and what I know in and through evaluations. But my knowing apparent values is based on feelings that are intentional responses to values. On his account, it is a radical mistake to oppose both knowing and feeling. Although the ultimate evidential basis for Lonergan's stance is his own cognitive processes of making evaluations, other evidence can also be cited to support it. Thus, Antonio Damasio has recently expressed a view that is similar but based instead upon the evidence of neurology:

When reason is conceptualized as free of biological antecedents,
it is easier to overlook the role emotions play in its operation, easier
not to notice that our purported rational decisions can be subtly

manipulated by the emotions we want to keep at bay, easier not to worry about the negative consequences of the vicarious emotional experiences of violence as entertainment, easier to overlook the positive effect that well-tuned emotions can have in the management of human affairs.[8]

Not only does Lonergan think it a radical mistake to oppose knowing and feeling, he is also critical of the consequent opposition between discoveries of fact and value knowledge.[9] In this chapter I will aim to address both of these issues by expressing and grounding in a detailed manner Lonergan's view of where feelings enter into the process of evaluating and deciding. As in prior chapters, my procedure will be to highlight these cognitive and decisional moves by using the medical example of my response to Paul's chest pain. By attending to the types of evaluations that are commonly made in medicine, I hope to illuminate a number of easily overlooked distinctions. These include distinguishing between third-level judgments and fourth-level evaluations, as well as the correlative distinction between feelings that arise in the context of knowing facts and feelings that enter into the process of knowing and acting on values. In all of this, my focal concern will be to explicate Lonergan's view that 'values are apprehended in feelings.'

2   Affective Cognitional Structure: Bringing to Light My Own Medical Evaluating

Assume that I have correctly diagnosed Paul's chest pain as being due to an AMI. As a physician my usual procedure would be to inform Paul of this diagnosis, and discuss with him what is actually happening and what will probably happen either with or without treatment. I would help Paul to decide what to do by summarizing for him the forms of treatment that are available, what each involves, and how successful they tend to be in minimizing the risks of this AMI to his life and future health. The goal of this discussion is not merely to understand, but also to enable Paul to arrive at a decision about how he wants to proceed.

An initial consideration is whether or not Paul would accept my recommendation that I admit him to hospital. If he questioned this recommendation, I might let him know that the norm of the medical profession is to admit patients who are having, or are probably having, an AMI to a coronary care or intensive care unit. This would allow his cardiac function to be monitored using special equipment, and skilled staff be available to respond effectively to any problems that might arise due to his AMI. Paul's AMI puts him at risk of having a cardiac rhythm disturbance, that is, a change in the normally sequential electrical conduction to, and stimulation of, his cardiac muscle. This might result in an overly rapid heart rate, called a tachycardia, and possibly disorganized and ineffective contractions, such as in the case of ventricular fibrillation. So if Paul chose to stay in the coronary care unit, this would give hospital staff members an opportunity to respond more rapidly and effectively to any life-threatening cardiac rhythm problems that might develop.

Even if Paul is willing to stay in hospital and be treated, there are still further decisions to be made about what this treatment should be. One such decision has to do with whether, besides symptomatic treatment, he would also allow some form of definitive treatment that will halt the progression of his AMI. If he opts for some definitive treatment, he will need to decide whether this should be a medical or surgical approach. Since the degree of ischemic damage to the cardiac muscle supplied by the obstructed coronary artery increases with time, the sooner one intervenes the better. Hence, Paul needs to decide about some form of definitive treatment as soon as possible.[10]

Unless Paul makes these decisions arbitrarily, that is in a groundless way, he will need some basis upon which to choose a treatment plan from among the available alternatives. As his physician, I am morally and legally obliged to ensure that he understands the relevant facts concerning the proposed treatments. This information includes what the proposed treatments involve, their probable short-term and long-term benefits, the accompanying risks, the skill and experience of those who will provide the treatment, the availability and costs of each option, and so forth. If Paul has had a stroke in the last six months, for instance, or recently bled from a stomach ulcer, the risks of causing further harm by giving him a thrombolytic drug would be sufficiently high that choosing this form of treatment would be much less worthy.[11] In such a case, Paul might judge that, even though the greatest possibility of benefit would derive from a medical treatment to dissolve the clot in his coronary artery, the accompanying risks of this treatment are too high in his case. On this basis, he might decide against this form of treatment.

Assume that Paul understands the different options available to him and the risks and benefits of each. Assume also that in his case, in contrast to symptomatic treatment, both forms of definitive treatment substantially lower his risk of sudden death and long-term cardiac disability. Assume, lastly, that he is also aware that, in contrast to symptomatic treatment, both forms of definitive treatment carry with them a slightly increased risk of causing a stroke. If Paul is more concerned about living with a stroke than with living with compromised cardiac function or of dying from his AMI, he might choose only symptomatic treatment. That is, he might value his intact cognitive function over his intact cardiac function or even the risk of death. Having expressed these concerns, assume that he then turns to me and asks, 'What do you think would be best?'

Paul's question seeks an answer that goes beyond the medical facts I have just explained to him. In order to provide an adequate answer to his question I need to know, at least in general terms, not only what Paul means by *best*, but also what I mean by *best*, how I would go about deciding which option is *best*, and what in his case I think is *his best* option. I might judge that thrombolysis would be the best option because it offers him the greatest reduction in the risk of mortality and morbidity, in comparison to other available treatments. In addition, the risk of a stroke with this treatment is not substantially greater than with other options. Hence, I might be inclined to recommend a more aggressive form of treatment than Paul would be inclined to choose.[12]

If physicians are to help patients to make these sorts of complex decisions, they not only need to be able to make good decisions themselves, but also be able to facilitate this process in their patients. As a philosopher, I might best help caregivers in this facilitating role by bringing to light for them how their own value judgments differ from fact judgments, and what the distinctive cognitional processes are that underpin their evaluations and decisions. In the physician's role as a mediator helping patients make wise choices, I would argue that the cognitive function of feelings needs to be taken seriously. Although feelings are fundamentally personal and spontaneous, I would also maintain that they are not simply private.[13]

3   A Phenomenology of Fourth-Level Feelings

The medical world provides ample illustrations of the lived phenomenon of making an evaluation. Patients with an illness feel threatened, and they enter the medical world hoping to understand their experience better and find some remedy for their distress. If the illness is an AMI, I can often easily identify and distinguish a variety of feelings that are part of their experience: feelings of physical pain in the chest area, of anxiety when the significance of the pain is uncertain, and of fear concerning the genuine threat to one's life that the diagnosis of an AMI signifies. There can also be feelings of hope that might arise when a possible cure is offered, of gratitude when the pain is relieved or the hoped-for cure is effected, and of despair if the condition cannot be remedied.[14]

Of primary concern in the present discussion are feelings that arise in response to a physical illness such as an AMI, and how such feelings relate to evaluations. These feelings need to be distinguished from feelings that are themselves the primary illness. Two examples of the latter are the set of feelings that characterize a major *depression*, and what is commonly referred to as *stress*. A major depression can negatively influence a patient's cognitive processes, causing such things as a lack of concentration, loss of interest, feelings of worthlessness, thoughts of death, and suicidal plans. It also influences many non-cognitive processes, such as one's level of energy, appetite, mood, capacity for pleasure, and ability to sleep.[15]

Although stress is a less dramatic condition characterized primarily by negative feelings that influence cognitive and non-cognitive functions, it is even more common than depression. Some experts consider stress to be the single most common underlying cause of ill health in North America, accounting for as many as 70 per cent of all visits to family physicians.[16] Although feelings of depression are frequently considered to have a primary biological basis, and hence tend to be treated with antidepressant medications, feelings of stress or anxiety are more commonly considered to arise as dysfunctional responses to life events. In both cases, these feelings frequently underpin certain evaluative conclusions, such as about one's own self-worth. Hence, health-care providers recognize the importance of feelings for well-being, and have devoted considerable energy toward understanding and treating feelings that are detrimental for well-being. What I will focus on, however, are not those pathological feelings that are the subject of study in psychiatry, but rather those feelings that arise in every physician–patient interchange, beginning with a problem and concluding with a plan to address the problem. This process involves the weighing of options, and feelings inevitably enter into such weighing in important ways. The present chapter is aimed at better understanding these fourth-level feelings from Lonergan's perspective.[17]

I begin by assembling some of Lonergan's reflections on the feelings that emerge on all cognitive levels in ordinary living. On the first level of experiencing, for instance, Lonergan identifies affect-laden images as *symbols*:

> The symbol for me is the 'affect-laden image.' It's evoked by an affect, or the image evokes the affect. They're linked. It's the means of internal communication between psyche and mind and heart. Where mind is experience, understanding, judgment; and heart is what's beyond this on the level of feeling and 'is this worthwhile?' – judgment of value, decision. Without feelings this experience, understanding, judgment is paper-thin. The whole mass and momentum of living is feeling.[18]

Lonergan also speaks of the purely experiential dimension of art, which evokes affective experiences: '[Art] is of the seen as seen, of the heard as heard, of the felt as felt. It is accompanied by a retinue of associations, affects, emotions, incipient tendencies that are part of one, that arise spontaneously and naturally from the person.'[19]

Not only does artistic imagination evoke feelings, Lonergan also considers certain forms of art to be especially suitable for expressing and objectifying feelings. For him, music is the most apt artistic expression of the life of feeling:

> Measured time is unidimensional, but the time that is the 'now' of the subject is a time in which many things are going forward at once. The music expresses this by taking one theme, and then another, and blending them. There are oppositions, tensions, resolutions. The life of feeling that is in that 'now,' in its rhythms and turmoil and peace, is expressed in music. The time of the music is a non-spatial movement and has a nonspatial shape. And this nonspatial shape corresponds to the way in which feelings multiply and change.[20]

To these experiences and expressions of feelings can be added the further refinements of judgment and decision in such universal symbolic expressions as poetry and rhetoric:

> The universal style is symbolic. Its language is instinct with feeling. At its liveliest it is poetry. At its profoundest it is rhetoric. It lacks neither attention to detail nor keen insight nor balanced judgment nor responsible decision. But it has all these, not stripped of feeling, but permeated with feeling. The calm, the detachment, the clarity, the coherence, the rigor of the logician, the mathematician, the scientist – these are just beyond its horizon.[21]

As I outlined in chapter 3, a key distinction for Lonergan is between intentional and non-intentional feelings. *Non-intentional* feelings are neither evoked by nor oriented to what I know through judgments. Such feelings can be evoked by biological or psychological needs, such as hunger or insecurity, and oriented to whatever will meet those needs, such as food or shelter. Although these feelings are conscious, they are states or trends rather than cognitive responses to some object. However, besides these feelings, Lonergan also identifies *intentional* feelings as those that respond to what is known. Intentional feelings presuppose knowledge, in the strict sense, and constitute an important part of my cognitive response to this knowledge. They are part of the phenomena of living, and are particularly prominent in personal relations:

Such feeling gives intentional consciousness its mass, momentum, drive, power. Without these feelings our knowing and deciding would be paper thin. Because of our feelings, our desires and our fears, our hope or despair, our joys and sorrows, our enthusiasm and indignation, our esteem and contempt, our trust and distrust, our love and hatred, our tenderness and wrath, our admiration, veneration, reverence, our dread, horror, terror, we are oriented massively and dynamically in a world mediated by meaning. We have feelings about our respective situations, about the past, about the future, about evils to be lamented or remedied, about the good that can, might, must be accomplished.[22]

Intentional feelings, then, are evoked by what we know. They respond to, and orient us in, a world of meaning and values. But although some objects of knowledge are simply good or bad, and evoke unequivocally positive or negative responses, other objects of knowledge are complex mixtures of good and bad and evoke mixed affective responses.

Even on the basis of these few selections from Lonergan on the phenomena of feelings, one can appreciate not only the range of the life of feeling, but also the importance of feelings for the process of knowing, and especially for evaluating. For the sake of clarity, I will focus on simple affective responses to objects of knowledge in order to highlight the central issue regarding where fourth-level feelings enter into the cognitional process.

4   Locating Fourth-Level Affective Cognitive Operations

In chapter 4 I provided a schematic outline of cognitive activities and achievements on the first three cognitional levels. I will now return to that outline to extend the analysis to include the activities and achievements of the fourth cognitional level. The four levels, with the appropriate activity and achievement on each level, are represented in table 6.1.

The fourth level of intentionality is the level of evaluating or deliberating in Lonergan's scheme. The role that feeling or affect plays on the fourth level is central to my consideration of Lonergan's analysis. In particular, I aim to explicate Lonergan's contention that '[i]ntermediate between judgments of fact and judgments of value lie apprehensions of value. Such apprehensions are given in feelings.'[23]

I will argue that by 'apprehensions of values' Lonergan means that there is some cognitive act that occurs on the fourth level that results in the discovery of values. This act is similar to direct and reflective insights insofar as it is a proximate, constitutive apprehensive act in which I grasp a unity in some diversity. But these fourth-level apprehensions differ from direct and

Table 6.1 Activities and achievements on the four cognitional levels

Level	(Activity)	Achievement
1. cognitional	(experiential: sensible-conscious)	awareness of data
2. cognitional	(intellectual)	intelligible unity
3. cognitional	(intellectual)	knowing the unconditioned real
4. cognitional	(affective: moral/religious)	knowing actual or possible values
and decisional	(affective: moral/religious)	*enjoying* actual values or *actualizing* possible values

reflective insights because they 'are given in feelings.' On the interpretation I will argue for, the *in* of 'in feelings' means that the value I discover is given to me in a fourth-level apprehension that is an affective cognition. *In* or *by means of* this affective apprehension, I grasp some fact as a good or a value.

In order to draw out and clarify this interpretation of Lonergan's remark that 'apprehensions of values are given in feelings,' I will select some key similarities and differences between the fourth-level process as a whole in comparison to the processes on the prior levels. Following this global comparison of levels, I will contrast particular fourth-level cognitive acts with the corresponding acts on the prior levels. The schematic outline in table 6.2 of the sequence of operations on each of the four cognitional levels will facilitate this comparison.

4.1 Fourth Level versus the First, Second, and Third Levels

Let us begin by highlighting some global similarities and differences between the fourth and prior cognitional levels.

There are at least four similarities between acts on the fourth and prior levels that are worth noting. First, as our schematic outline illustrates, on the fourth level, as on the prior levels, one can distinguish between cognitional activities and achievements. The cognitional achievements on each subsequent level add an increment of knowledge to what was achieved on the prior level. Each of these incremental cognitional achievements is a discovery I make on the basis of the cognitional activities of that level. Moreover, as on each prior level, so on the fourth level one can distinguish between at least two sequential cognitional acts of discovery – a proximate constitutive act and a subsequent productive act.

Secondly, the second, third, and fourth levels all begin by my posing a question directed at the knowledge achieved on each prior level. That is, each successive level sublates the earlier levels. In Lonergan's language of

Table 6.2 Cognitional operations on the first to fourth levels

---

First level: Experiencing
  1.1 Data as given, and potentially sensible.
  1.2 *Sensing.* Receiving data of sense (e.g., Paul feels chest pain).
  1.3 *Imagining.* Forming an image of data of sense (e.g., Paul imagines a band around, or a weight on, his chest).

Second level: Understanding
  2.1 *Question for understanding.* 'What is this?' (e.g., Paul asks himself, 'What is this pain I sense?').
  2.2 *Direct insight.* Grasping a possible intelligible unity in data (e.g., Paul grasps a possible relationship between his pain and his heart).
  2.3 *Conception:* Formulating the intelligible unity grasped as a definition or concept (e.g., Paul expresses a possible cause of his chest pain in terms of an AMI).

Third level: Judging
  3.1 *Question for reflection:* 'Is this conceived, possible intelligible unity real (or really possible)?' (e.g., 'Is Paul's chest pain an AMI'? 'If so, is it possible to limit Paul's AMI with thrombolytic therapy?').
  3.2 *Reflective insight.* Grasping the evidence for positing this conceived, possible intelligible unity as real (or really possible) (e.g., grasping the evidence for positing that Paul is having an AMI or that it is possible to limit this with thrombolytic therapy).
  3.3 *Fact judgment.* This understood and conceived intelligible unity is real (or really possible) (e.g., 'Paul is having an AMI,' or 'It is really possible to limit Paul's AMI with thrombolytic therapy').

Fourth level: *Evaluating, deciding, and doing/enjoying*
  4.1 *Question for deliberation:* 'Is this understood and conceived intelligible unity that is judged as real (or as really possible) worthwhile?' (e.g., 'Is Paul's real AMI good?' 'Are the really possible benefits of treating Paul with thrombolytic therapy really worthwhile, and/or better than the alternatives?').
  4.2 *Apprehension-of-value.* Grasping the evidence for positing the worthwhileness of the understood and conceived intelligible unity that is judged as real (or really possible) (e.g., 'The really possible benefits of treating Paul with thrombolytic therapy are good and/or better than the alternatives').
  4.3 *Value judgment.* This understood and conceived intelligible unity that is judged as real (or really possible) is worthwhile (e.g., 'Paul's concretely possible improvement with thrombolysis is worthwhile').
  4.4 *Decision:* a choice to enjoy this understood, conceived intelligible unity that is judged as real, a worthwhile (or to actualize this possible, really worthwhile understood and conceived intelligible unity) (e.g., 'Paul chooses to proceed with thrombolytic therapy').
  4.5 *Execution,* if pertinent: Actualizing this worthwhile, really possible, understood and conceived intelligible unity, if I have the requisite skill and there is no impediment (e.g., 'I treat Paul with thrombolytic therapy, since I am able to do this and have access to the necessary medications').[24]

---

intentionality analysis, these achievements are of data, data-intelligibility synthesis, and being or quality, actual or possible, as asked about.

Third, the source of each of these questions is the corresponding transcendental intention. Moreover, the move from raising a categorial question to achieving an answer is not an immediate one, but rather is a process that is mediated by a series of cognitive activities. As the transcendental intentions are the sources of my questions, so also they serve as the ultimate criteria for the adequacy of my answers.

Fourth, the third and fourth levels result in knowledge of the real, or knowledge in the strict sense of the word. That is, on the third and fourth levels insights grasp (a) a prospective judgment as conditioned; (b) conditions for the prospective judgment that, if fulfilled, justify my asserting the judgment; and (c) the fulfilment of those sufficient conditions. Although reflective insights, in the case of judging, and deliberative insights, in the case of evaluating, are distinct cognitive activities, each grasps how the above diverse elements 'all hang together'; that unity is what in turn justifies my positing the prospective judgment and evaluation as virtually unconditioned. *In* and *through* asserting a judgment or evaluation as true I come to knowledge of the real or really good. These third- and fourth-level insights combine normative and experiential cognitive achievements into a single unity. By means of them I grasp cognitive unities in these diversities. Still, the real is only known in and through an act of judgment.[25]

Besides these global similarities between the fourth and prior levels, there are also some important differences. First, by contrast with the first level, the fourth-level achievement of knowledge is a mediated process. On the first level, sense data are simultaneously given and received sensibly in the act of sensing. That is, the cognitive process is immediate or intuitive because there is an identity between the sense data as given and as received. In the categories of metaphysical psychology, the agent object and the terminal object are the same; hence, no mediation is required. By contrast, the fourth-level process is mediated by cognitive acts that respond to the conditioned real as asked about. By means of these acts, I achieve knowledge of the really good, which is distinct from my potential knowledge of the conditioned real. Again, on the first level, the agent object and terminal object are identical; on each of the subsequent levels they are distinct. Hence, I know values not immediately, for instance, simply by feeling, in a way analogous with sensing, but rather through, or by means of, the mediation of cognitional, fourth-level operations that follow a question for deliberation.

Second, in contrast to the second and third levels, the key move in the mediated process on the fourth level is affective rather than intellectual. Although my questions, insights, and productive apprehensive acts on the second and third levels have an affective dimension, this affectivity only enters into the cognitive process in a crucial way on the fourth level. Moreover, this fourth-level affectivity has a specifically moral/religious quality that does not characterize the affectivity on prior levels. Hence, discovering values on the fourth level, unlike discoveries of the prior levels, depends on my capacity to respond affectively to concrete values. This is the central claim of this work, and I will expand on it further in the subsequent discussion.

Third, by contrast with the third level, the cognitional achievement on the fourth level is knowledge of an actual or possible value, rather than an actual or possible fact. In addition, beyond this cognitional achievement, the fourth level reaches completion through the further acts of deciding and executing a decision. Only on the fourth level is there a distinction between cognitional and decisional activities. Hence, to my third-level achievement of knowledge of some concrete actual or possible reality is added the further achievement of whether these realities are or would be good. Finally, the fourth-level process culminates not just in knowing, but in doing something to achieve some future good, or in enjoying some present good.

The notion of value motivates the fourth level. The distinctiveness of this notion is worth highlighting. Lonergan recognized explicitly the distinction between the notion of the real and the notion of value sometime between the writing of *Insight* and the writing of *Method*. In *Method*, the notion of value includes and goes beyond the second-level notion of intelligibility and the third-level notion of reality:

> In *Insight* the good was the intelligent and reasonable. In *Method* the good is a distinct notion. It is intended in questions for deliberation: Is this worthwhile? Is it truly or only apparently good? It is aspired to in the intentional response of feeling to values. It is known in judgments of value made by a virtuous or authentic person with a good conscience. It is brought about by deciding and living up to one's decisions.[26]

This shift is correlative to Lonergan's increasing interest in affectivity or feeling responses as cognitive activities by means of which one grasps values. *Insight* focuses primarily on understanding and the intellectual side, or mind:

> There is in *Insight* a footnote to the effect that we're not attempting to solve anything about such a thing as personal relations. I was dealing in *Insight* fundamentally with the intellectual side – a study of human understanding – in which I did my study of human understanding and got human intelligence in there, not just a sausage

machine turning out abstract concepts. That was my fundamental thrust.[27]

In *Method* Lonergan came to focus more attention on the feeling side, or heart: 'What I did in *Insight* mainly was intentionality analysis of experiencing, understanding, judging. Add on to that ... the different types of feeling.'[28]

The clarification of how precisely feelings enter into the cognitive operations on the fourth level is the central philosophical contribution of this work. It is to this issue that I shall now direct my attention.

5   Evaluating: Fourth-Level Activities and Achievements

5.1   Question for Deliberation, 'Is it worthwhile?'

The fourth level arises when I ask of my third-level achievement of knowledge of some real, or really possible X, 'Is this real X, or really possible X, worthwhile?' There are at least four similarities between this fourth-level act and the corresponding acts on the two prior levels. First, posing a question is the first act of the second, third, and fourth levels. On each level, the raising of a question is my initial response to some content given as the cognitive achievement of the prior level, that is, a diversity of data, abstract intelligibilities, or actual or possible realities. The raising of a question also expresses my desire to discover some unity in the diversities of the object I am asking about, and it thereby advances my knowledge. Second, these questions are evoked conjointly by this content that is given and my transcendental intending.[29] Third, the transcendental intentions and the concrete questions that express them all have an affective dimension insofar as they express something about my present lack of knowledge and my desire to correct this state of affairs by discovering answers. My question arises out of a sense of wonder or a restlessness that seeks fulfilment or satisfaction in adequate answers. Finally, the transcendental intentions, which my questions express, provide the criteria that any answer I might discover must satisfy.[30]

How, then, do questions for deliberation differ from those on the prior levels? Key differences between these questions stem from differences in the categorial cognitional content that is given and the transcendental intentions, which conjointly evoke them. This fundamental distinction between the transcendental and the categorial underpins Lonergan's whole discussion of feelings:

The principal division of sources [of meaning] is into transcendental and categorial. The transcendental are the very dynamism of intentional consciousness, a capacity that consciously and unceasingly both heads for and recognizes data, intelligibility, truth, reality and value. The categorial are the determinations reached through experiencing, understanding, judging, deciding. The transcendental notions ground questioning. Answers develop categorial determinations.[31]

According to this division of sources of meaning, that is, all conscious acts and all intended contents, Lonergan distinguishes transcendental intending into intentions of intelligibility, reality, and value. These ground the second, third, and fourth cognitional levels. The answers to the questions raised on successive levels develop my knowledge of data, intelligibilities, realities, and values.

Hence, a first set of differences between my question for deliberation, 'Ought it be so?' and those of the prior levels can be derived from differences between the categorial cognitional content and transcendental intentions. Together, these evoke questions for understanding, reflection, and deliberation, and thereby give rise to the corresponding levels. Accordingly, on the second level, a question for understanding, 'What is it?' is evoked by the data of sense or consciousness I encounter with my transcendental intention of intelligibility. On the third level, a questions for reflection, 'Is it so?' is evoked by a possible intelligible unity I encounter with my transcendental intention of reality. Finally, on the fourth level, a question for deliberation, 'Is it good or worthwhile?' is evoked by an actual or possible reality I encounter with my transcendental intention of value.

A second difference has to do with the type of answer my fourth-level question prefigures or anticipates, by contrast with my third-level question. My third-level question, 'Is it so?' seeks knowledge of some actual or possible fact. My fourth-level question seeks to know the good and perhaps to do something on the basis of this knowledge. That is, in my fourth-level question I express my desire, first, to know whether this actual fact is good or that possible fact would be worthwhile, and, second, to decide whether I should act on this knowledge. Hence, the force of my fourth-level question goes beyond the cognitional query of 'Ought it be so?' to raise the decisional issue, 'Ought I enjoy this actual good or actualize this possible good?'[32]

This difference between *fact* and *value* questions expresses in terms of intentionality analysis what is traditionally expressed in the terminology of faculty psychology as the distinction between *intellect* and *will.* In intentionality analysis, knowing the real is a third-level achievement that corresponds to the faculty of intellect. Deciding and doing what I judge I ought to do are fourth-level activities that correspond to the faculty of the will. The nuance introduced by intentionality analysis is the distinction between the capacities and acts of knowing the good (which are not merely intellectual) and the further capacity to decide to do the good (which is captured by the notion of the will). That is, the advance of intentionality analysis is in affirming a capacity to know the good that is not merely an intellectual knowing.

A third difference between fourth-level questions for deliberation and second- or third-level questions has to do with the relative importance of the affective dimension pertaining to the transcendental intentions these questions express. I noted above that transcendental intending is already thoroughly affective. In *Insight*, Lonergan speaks of the *eros of the mind*, and the *desire to know*. In *Method*, this dynamic orientation, renamed the transcendental intending of intelligibility and reality, is sublated and complemented by the transcendental intending of value.[33] All three intentions of intelligibility, reality, and value, and not just the third, are thoroughly affective. Even so, only on the fourth level does the affective dimension of my 'transcendental intention' of value, or my 'intending' of transcendental value, serve as a criterion for the adequacy of categorial answers I develop in response to a categorial question of value. That is, there is an importantly affective dimension of my transcendental intention of value; in discovering some purported value I experience an affective fulfilment of this prior anticipation.[34]

In summary, categorial questions for deliberation are evoked, in part, by the transcendental intention of the good. The affective dimension of my transcendental intention of the good first enters into the fourth-level process in these questions for deliberation. This affectivity orients me to certain answers and provides an affective criterion for any answer I might propose.

5.2 Apprehensions of Value in Feelings or Deliberative Insights

Distinct from the affectivity of my transcendental intentions, as previously described, there is also an affectivity that enters into all my conscious-intentional acts of discovery. Thus, there are feelings correlative with sensing, feelings correlative with direct insight and conceiving, feelings correlative with reflective insight and judging, and feelings correlative with the apprehension of value, evaluating and deciding. Moreover, just as direct insight and conceiving, reflective insight and judging, apprehension of value and evaluating presuppose but are distinct from the transcendental intentions of intelligibility, reality, and value, so also these feelings presuppose but are distinct from the feelings that are correlative with each of the transcendental intentions.

Lonergan maintains that feelings enter into fourth-level evaluations in a key way in the cognitive act of apprehending values. By 'apprehension of value,' Lonergan refers to the pivotal fourth-level act by means of which I move from a question for deliberation, 'Is this actual or possible X truly worthwhile?' to a value judgment, 'Yes, this X is truly worthwhile.' This pivotal fourth-level act is similar to the already discussed second-level act of direct insight, and is even more closely analogous to the third-level act of reflective insight. An apprehension of value is similar to a direct or reflective insight insofar as each of these acts involves grasping a unity in a concrete diversity.

In order to highlight the continuity between these acts of grasping a unity in a diversity, I will follow Vertin's suggestion and refer to what Lonergan calls *apprehensions of value* as insights that follow a process of deliberation, that is, as *deliberative insights*. This term neatly suggests the continuity between cognitional processes on every level beyond the first. That is, in a manner analogous to the second and third levels, an act of deliberative insight is a mediate activity that involves the grasp of some unity in a diversity, and is part of the fourth-level discursive process of deliberation about values or the worthwhileness of some actual or possible reality.[35]

By the term *deliberative insight*, then, I will henceforth be referring to those fourth-level intentional responses that are apt to follow a question for deliberation in a responsible person intending value and provide the basis for an evaluation by that person. These fourth-level deliberative insights are analogous to direct and reflective insights in at least three ways. First, in terms of the sequence of cognitive acts on each level, these insights are the first element of my response to some object asked about. Second, these insights are constitutive acts that grasp a unity in some diversity. By means of such a response, I grasp some novel unity in the diversity of some content asked about. Although the precise nature of this unity differs in each case, as I will indicate presently, grasping this unity is a constitutive act in as much as it represents a pivotal cognitive advance from the state of questioning. And on the basis of this pivotal cognitive advance I am moved in each case to produce a mental word (i.e., the act of conceiving or of judging).[36] Third, as I suggested above, there are feelings that are a dimension of, or correlative with, each of these insights. These feelings are given in the *aha* experiences that accompany my grasp of unities, where the *aha* signifies an affective fulfilment of my desire to know. That is, like all my conscious-intentional acts, these cognitive acts of insight all have an affective dimension.

To these similarities that deliberative insights share with direct and reflective insights, I will now add four key differences. First, although a deliberative insight, like a direct or reflective insight, is the first element of my response to some object asked about, a response in which I grasp a unity in a diversity, and a response on the basis of which I am moved to a subsequent act of producing a mental word, that is, a conception or a judgment, the response of deliberative insight is specifically different from a direct or reflective insight in that it is an *affective cognition*. Although direct and reflective insights have feelings that are a dimension of these responses, they are both instances of *intellectual cognition*. But, in the proximate response to the question of deliberation, I *affectively* grasp the virtually unconditioned worthwhileness of some option.

Although there is some disagreement among Lonergan scholars about the precise manner in which Lonergan thinks that one 'apprehends values in feelings,' most agree that Lonergan considers certain feelings to have cognitive significance when it comes to knowing values. Vertin amplifies the uniqueness of Lonergan's stance on how one comes to know values by contrasting acts of apprehending values, which he identifies as instances of 'affective cognition,' with those acts of direct and reflective insight, which he calls instances of 'intellectual cognition.' On this point, Vertin acknowledges that he is at odds with Patrick Byrne's interpretation of Lonergan. For Byrne, Lonergan characterizes value as 'concretely realized intelligibility – intelligibility which there is good reason to bring about.' This manner of expression, for Vertin, does insufficient justice to the uniqueness of value apprehensions for the later Lonergan, which sublate intelligibility's 'good-reason base.' In support of Vertin's interpretation is Bernard Tyrrell, who contrasts Lonergan and von Hildebrand on this issue. Tyrrell suggests that von Hildebrand considered the type of cognitional activity that perceives value to be located within the sphere of the intellect (similar to the Lonergan of *Insight*). Although Lonergan largely accepts von Hildebrand's phenomenal analysis of value judgments, by the time of *Method*, Tyrrell suggests, Lonergan 'had cleanly broken free from the restrictive classifications of faculty psychology.' Accordingly, on Tyrrell's reading, Lonergan does not insist on sharp distinctions between 'the intellect, the will, and the heart.' Instead, Lonergan speaks, in the language of intentionality analysis, of the intentional response of feelings, which he expressly locates in the realm of Pascal's 'reasons of the heart, ... which reason does not know.' Here, 'the heart's reasons' are what Lonergan calls 'feelings that are intentional responses to values.'[37]

Second, although each insight grasps a unity in a diversity, the unities, and the diversities in which I grasp the unities, are different on each level. My direct insight, as I have already described, is an *intelligent* grasp of a unity in the diversity of data of sense or consciousness; and that is what in turn enables me to produce a conception of these now understood data, that is, a simple word. My reflective insight is a *rational* grasp of a unity in the diversity of contents on which I reflect. These contents include (a) a prospective fact judgment and (b) the link of that judgment to conditions sufficient to justify its reasonable affirmation. In that reflective insight I grasp how these 'all hang together'; and that is what in turn justifies my positing the prospective fact judgment as virtually unconditioned, that is, a complex word.[38] In contrast to both of these, my deliberative insight is a 'positive affective response' with cognitional value, a positive affective cognition of how (a) the prospective value judgment and (b) the link of that judgment to conditions sufficient to justify its responsible affirmation 'all hang together.' My apprehension of value is a *responsible* grasp of a unity in this diversity upon which I deliberate. Affectively grasping how these diverse elements all hang together is what I am calling a deliberative insight; and this insight is what in turn justifies my positing the prospective value judgment as virtually unconditioned, that is, a complex mental word.[39]

Let us now consider the difference between an intelligent and a rational grasp of a unity in a diversity, on the one hand, and the grasp of a responsible unity in a diversity, on the other. This difference can be illustrated more concretely by using the example of my decision to go hiking with friends and, in a more detailed way, by using the example of my medical decision to treat Paul in a certain way.

In the first case, I might, following some deliberation, decide to go for a hike with some friends. In this judgment, I am positing the value or worthwhileness of going for a hike. The proximate basis that justifies this evaluation is an affective cognition, which, at best, is a responsible grasp of how the elements that underpin my conclusion all hang together. Note that I might not be able, at least initially, to articulate the elements upon which I have deliberated, and affectively grasped, and thanks to which, on the basis of that affective grasp, I concluded that I should go on this hike. With some prompting and encouragement, I might eventually identify something of the complexity behind this decision, including those factors that swayed me in opposite directions.[40] In contending that 'values are apprehended in feelings,' Lonergan is highlighting the fact that, even in such common evaluations, there is an affective cognition that is specifically distinct from the feelings that correspond to the earlier described intentional responses of direct and reflective insight. In this case of apprehending values, the relevant feelings are prior to everything else.[41]

In the case of my medical decision about treating Paul's AMI, one can further highlight the diverse elements in which I responsibly grasp a unity, and contrast this diversity to that in which I rationally grasp a unity. Earlier I represented this diversity in the form of a syllogism, emphasizing that, for Lonergan, the actual context in which I rationally grasp a unity is far more diverse than the general form represented by a syllogism suggests.[42] Letting A and B each stand for one or more propositions, one can illustrate the diversity of elements that may be rationally grasped in the form of a deductive inference: 'If A, then B; but A; therefore B.' In the example of deciding whether Paul is having an AMI, I might formulate the diversity of contents among which reflective insight grasps a unity as follows:

(a) the prospective fact judgment ('Paul is having an AMI');
(b) the link of that judgment to conditions sufficient to justify its reasonable affirmation ('If Paul is having typical symptoms and signs of an AMI as well as a positive ECG, then he is having an AMI');
(c) the fulfilment of those sufficient conditions ('But Paul is having typical symptoms and signs of an AMI as well as a positive ECG').

For Lonergan, 'the function of the form of deductive inference is to exhibit a conclusion as virtually unconditioned. Reflective insight grasps the pattern, and by rational compulsion there follows the judgment.'[43] Lonergan also contends that '[j]udgments of value differ in content but not in form from judgments of fact.'[44] Hence, in deciding that treating Paul with thrombolytic therapy would be worthwhile, one might formulate the diverse elements my deliberative insight grasps as all hanging together according to the above form of a deductive inference. Thus I have:

(a) the prospective value judgment ('Paul's possible improvement with thrombolysis is worthwhile');
(b) the link of that judgment to conditions sufficient to justify its responsible affirmation ('If the extent of damage to Paul's heart from his AMI can be reduced with thrombolysis, then Paul's possible treatment with thrombolysis is worthwhile'); and
(c) the fulfilment of those sufficient conditions ('But the extent of damage to Paul's heart from his AMI can be reduced with thrombolysis').

For Lonergan, the act of grasping how the diverse elements represented in this deductive inference 'all hang together' is what he calls an apprehension of value, or what I am calling a deliberative insight. Moreover, he insists that this apprehension of value is given in feelings; or on this interpretation, it is an affective cognition. It is this affective grasp of a unity in the above diversity that in turn justifies my positing the prospective value judgment as virtually unconditioned. Hence, it is by a *responsible* (and not merely a *rational*) compulsion that there follows a judgment of value.

The key difference I wish to highlight here is between the feelings that are associated with second- and third-level insights, and the fourth-level feelings in which I apprehend values. On the second level, there is surely an affective dimension that is manifest not only in the *aha* of my direct insight that Paul's pain might be due to an AMI, but also in my prior transcendental intending of some intelligibility in his data. But what is crucial about both my intending of intelligibility and my direct insight is not the affective dimension of my striving to understand his data nor my response to it, but rather their intellectual dimensions. The direct insight that moves me to conceive of Paul's data in terms of an AMI grasps an intelligible unity among his signs and symptoms and brings to light how these data might hang together intelligibly. The affectivity of my intending of intelligibility and the subsequent *aha* experience that accompanies my discovery of an intelligible connection among Paul's data are not crucial to either act. More to the point, the feelings associated with my direct insight do not provide me with cognitive access to the intelligibility I discover.

Similarly, on the third level there is surely an affective dimension to both my transcendental intending of the real and the *aha* of my reflective insight. But, again, what is crucial about both my intending of reality and my reflective insight that grasps how (a), (b), and (c) all hang together is the intellectual dimension of these acts. The affectivity of these acts, though surely present, is not crucial to the discovery of the real. The *aha* associated with my reflective insight accompanies my discovery but does not play a crucial role in providing me with cognitional access to this content.[45]

By contrast, my fourth-level intending of value and my deliberative insight are thoroughly affective in a way that is importantly different from the affectivity of the corresponding acts on the second and third levels. In the case of my transcendental intending of value, this difference seems to involve a restlessness of heart, rather than of mind. Although I might know that going on a hike or treating Paul with streptokinase are concrete possibilities, what I now seek to know is whether realizing these possibilities would be truly good or worthwhile. The *aha* is my deliberative insight that affectively grasps how the prospective value asked about, its link to conditions, and the fulfilment of those conditions all hang together. This response can be objectified as the affective fulfilment of a certain restlessness of my heart, as expressed in my question for deliberation. This affective response is, at the same time, my grasping a unity among this diversity.[46] This *aha* experience provides the cognitional access to the values asked about, rather than the content of these values.[47] That is, the *aha* experience that is apt to follow a question for deliberation and precedes a judgment of value is the manner in which feelings enter into my fourth-level cognitive process. These fourth-level feelings are not merely associated with my deliberative insight, as is the case with feelings associated with direct or reflective insights. Rather, they are centrally constitutive of my cognitive access to particular values.

Although deliberative insights are thoroughly affective, one ought not infer from this that they are not also thoroughly cognitive. Rather, the affectivity of my deliberative insight provides the total cognitional grounds, justification, basis, foundation for my subsequent value judgment. Knowing values brings about a synthesis of mind and heart, or of the intellectual and the affective sides. On this account, it is, in general, a radical flaw to disjoin knowing and feeling, to disjoin cognition and affectivity on any level, but especially on the fourth level.[48]

Besides the difference in the way affectivity enters into the process of discovering values by comparison with the feelings associated with my acts of discovering intelligibilities or realities, one can also contrast differences between the content of the unities grasped by deliberative insights and reflective insights. The unity grasped by a deliberative insight goes beyond, but not against, the strictly rational unity grasped by a reflective insight and known in and through a fact judgment. I presuppose the content of my fact judgment when I move to the fourth level and raise a question for deliberation. The content of the unity I grasp in my fourth-level insight sublates my fact knowledge. It includes, as the objects on which I deliberate, those really actual or possible facts I know through the rational acts of fact judging. But it also goes beyond these contents by grasping a unity that justifies my positing the prospective value judgment as virtually unconditioned.[49] Hence, my deliberative insight goes beyond my fact judgment by grasping that I am *responsibly,* not merely rationally, compelled to affirm the disvalue of Paul's AMI and/or to affirm the possible value of Paul's improvement with thrombolytic treatment. Grasping this value is an addition that moves one beyond mere fact knowledge.[50]

Unlike a direct or reflective insight, a deliberative insight has a specifically moral/religious dimension. The unity I grasp in deliberative insight occurs in the context of my whole life and horizon that is oriented to, and motivated by, values. These apprehensions of value are given in my affinities and repulsions to facts. In and through judgments of value they result not only in constituting my knowledge of values, but these responses are also expressions of myself as constituted morally. A deliberative insight then is the *aha* experience (in a responsible person) that is apt to follow a question for deliberation concerning some concrete or concretely possible fact. As with second- and third-level insights, this fourth-level insight is a pivotal, conscious-intentional response to an entity asked about. By contrast with the *intellectual* character of direct or reflective insights, fourth-level deliberative insights are crucially *affective,* and this affectivity has a moral/

religious quality. Finally, the affectivity of my categorial deliberative insight is distinct from, but related to, the affective dimension of my transcendental intention of value.

To summarize, then, on the second and third levels, affectivity enters as the context and by-product of an insight. The affective context of an insight is set by the transcendental intention of intelligibility or reality. The affective by-product of an insight results when I achieve the knowledge sought in my prior questioning. Similarly, affectivity enters in both these ways on the fourth level. But in addition, it also enters in a central and distinctive manner in my deliberative insight. Here it is by means of my intentional affective response to a value that I come to a judgment of value, through which I know what is good or worthwhile.

Before proceeding to discuss value judgments that follow deliberative insights, I can further clarify what Lonergan means by feelings that are 'intentional responses' to 'values' by situating these fourth-level feelings within his division of feelings. Lonergan begins his discussion of feelings in *Method* by distinguishing those feelings that are non-intentional states and trends from these fourth-level intentional responses. He then proceeds to subdivide intentional responses according to two main classes of objects: satisfactions and values. Following von Hildebrand's phenomenological analysis of feelings, Lonergan relates non-intentional states, such as fatigue, irritability, bad humour, or anxiety, to causes; and trends or urges, such as hunger, thirst, or sexual discomfort, to goals:

> [T]he relation of the feeling to the cause or goal is simply that of effect to cause, of trend to goal. The feeling itself does not presuppose and arise out of perceiving, imagining, representing the cause or goal. Rather one first feels tired and, perhaps belatedly, one discovers that what one needs is rest. Or first one feels hungry and then one diagnoses the trouble as a lack of food.[51]

Non-intentional states and trends, then, 'are feelings whose causes or goals are not, at least initially, also intentional objects.'[52] Non-intentional feelings are evoked by such factors as biological needs and are oriented to whatever will meet those needs. By attending to these data, that is, as an intended content of my cognitive acts, they become sources of meaning. Meaning is achieved, for instance, when I come to understand and judge my experienced state of fatigue to be caused by a lack of rest, or my experienced urge of hunger to be directed to the goal of food.[53] But there might not be any properly biological or human meaning. Rather, they might be adequately explained in strictly physiological terms. For instance, an experience of anxiety or elation could simply be due to deficiencies or excesses of certain neuro-substrates, such as lithium or thyroxine.

By contrast with these non-intentional states and trends, intentional responses answer to what is intended, apprehended, and represented. They are evoked by, or oriented to, what I know. That is, they presuppose knowledge and are responses to it. Such feelings relate me, not just to a cause or end, but to an object. Moreover, a conflict could arise between a non-intentional feeling, such as fatigue and, say, my intentional response to the value of staying awake to complete some task. Without opposing feelings that are intentional responses, I might simply be inclined to follow my non-intentional feelings of fatigue. For Lonergan, the feelings that go beyond, and might even oppose, non-intentional urges and trends are what give 'intentional consciousness its mass, momentum, drive, power. Without these feelings our knowing and deciding would be paper thin.'[54]

By means of my affective responses, I distinguish between classes of objects, and in each class I respond either positively or negatively by orienting myself toward some and away from others.[55] Lonergan distinguishes between two main classes of objects to which my intentional, affective responses can orient me, namely, *satisfactions* and *values*: 'Feelings that are intentional responses regard two main classes of objects: on the one hand, the agreeable or disagreeable, the satisfying or dissatisfying; on the other hand, values, whether the ontic value of persons or the qualitative value of beauty, understanding, truth, virtuous deeds, noble acts.'[56]

As Vertin elaborates,

> ... Some intentional objects evoke feelings of pleasure, gratification, and fulfilment that are not necessarily more than self-oriented, self-centred, self-immanent. Lonergan denominates such objects 'satisfactions.' Other intentional objects evoke feelings of delight, joy, and fulfilment that derive from one's encounter – via such objects – with what stands beyond the objects themselves, feelings that are totality oriented, universe-centred, self-transcendent. Lonergan denominates such objects 'values'; and the self-transcending feelings they evoke, 'apprehensions of value.'[57]

The first key distinction, then, is between non-intentional and intentional feelings. Non-intentional feelings are not necessarily anything more than some affective data or contents of consciousness, rather than part of my cognitive activities (e.g., feelings of hunger, which are related to some physiological cause). By contrast, intentional feelings are part of my activities of knowing and arise on the fourth level of cognition. The further distinction between intentional, affective responses to satisfactions or values is a distinction between fourth-level affective responses that are not necessarily more than self-oriented and those that are totality-oriented. Affective responses that are totality-oriented are in harmony with my transcendental intending of value. By this distinction Lonergan contrasts those intentional feelings that are evoked by, or by means of which I apprehend, satisfactions and those feelings that are evoked by, or by means of which I apprehend, values. From the perspective of intentionality analysis, it is crucial to highlight the type of intentional, affective response that underpins my claims about purported values.

If I claim truly to love another person, for instance, on what basis would I be justified in making this claim? From Lonergan's perspective of intentionality analysis, my claim of love would not be justified if I regarded this person as a mere source of satisfactions, rather than as a value. That is, I would not be justified in making this claim if this person were for me merely an object of lust. This would be the case if my intentional, affective response to him or her was not necessarily anything more than self-oriented, or self-immanent. By contrast, if I truly loved this person, my intentional, affective response to him or her would have the self-transcending orientation and the quality of a response to value. In other words, I must justify any claim I might make about an object of value by attending to my affective response to this object.

But even if I am able to distinguish between satisfactions and values reliably and consistently in my own living, when philosophically justifying these judgments I could subscribe to a philosophy that directs me to avoid attending to my own intentional, affective responses because this philosophy deems them to be 'merely subjective.' This philosophical bias against subjectivity can be especially strong if the intentional activities in question are affective. For they not only seem more intimate to the subject, but they also seem more inherently ambiguous as regards values. For Lonergan, however, all my knowing, and not just my valuing, is intentional. Still, this does not necessarily entail that all knowledge is merely subjective. Moreover, when I am knowing values, my intentional activities necessarily involve my own affectivity, such that 'the eye of love reveals values in their splendor, while the strength of this love brings about their realization.'[58]

5.3 Value Judgment

I indicated above that one way in which categorial feelings enter into the evaluative process on the fourth level is in acts of deliberative insight. I will now consider the subsequent act of value judging to show how categorial feelings also enter into these acts.

Just as I distinguished between apprehensive acts as constitutive and as productive on the first three levels, so also a similar distinction obtains on the fourth cognitional level. I will begin to clarify the act of value judging by describing it and then pointing out similarities and differences between this act and corresponding acts on the prior levels.

According to Lonergan: 'In a judgment of value three components unite. First, there is knowledge of reality and especially of human reality. Second, there are intentional responses to values. Thirdly, there is the initial thrust towards moral self-transcendence constituted by the judgment of value itself.'[59] Knowledge of actual or possible reality is achieved on the third level through fact judgments. To this knowledge is added moral feeling in deliberative insights that respond affectively to these actual or possible facts and reveal their absolute and/or relative value. The content that I grasp in my deliberative insight is subsequently expressed in an asserted value judgment. In this judgment, I express the virtually unconditioned status of a value, its contingent truth, or my preference among actual or possible values (e.g., 'It is a true statement that it would be good to treat Paul with streptokinase'). Through this asserted value judgment, I know a concrete actual or possible value, or the better option (i.e., 'It really would be good to treat Paul with streptokinase'). Prior to my value judgment, I do not know this value, in the strict or absolute sense. That is, it is only through this value judgment that I know a particular value.

The value judgment described above is a productive apprehensive act that is similar, in at least three ways, to the corresponding acts on the two prior levels. First, on the second and third levels I distinguished between those proximate constitutive apprehensive acts of grasping a unity-in-a-diversity and the subsequent productive apprehensive acts of expressing the content of this unity. Still, in the case of the second level, subsequent to a direct insight there is an act expressing the unity I grasp, but it is not a judgment. In my reflective and deliberative insights, however, there is a further factor that is not present in the case of a direct insight, namely, that it is in and through the expression of the unity-in-diversity that I come to know reality, in the case of reflective insight, and real value, in the case of deliberative insight. That is, reality is not grasped initially in reflective insight, and real value is not grasped initially in deliberative insight, hence leaving the act of judgment in both instances as some *rubber stamp* on what I have already come to know in the insights. Rather, it is in and through fact judgments and value judgments that something else emerges, which is knowledge of reality, in the case of fact judgments, and real value, in the case of value judgments.

Second, like my third-level fact judgment, my value judgment either affirms or denies some reality in a complex judgment. That is, the answer to both questions of fact and questions of value is either 'Yes' or 'No,' and each answer can concern either an actual, or a possible, fact or value.

Third, a criterion for the adequacy of the contents I express in my productive apprehensive acts is some experienced satisfaction with what I have discovered. This 'satisfaction' is a sign of the harmony between my categorial deliberative insight and my transcendental intending of value, about which I will have more to say later.

There are, however, three salient differences between the fourth-level productive apprehensive act of value judging and the corresponding acts on the prior levels. First, on the first level, the terminal object, which I represent in my act of imagining, is a content (i.e., data) that is identical to the agent object. By contrast, the content expressed and affirmed in the fourth-level productive apprehensive act of value judging (i.e., the unconditioned good) is distinct in important ways from the fourth-level agent object (i.e., the unconditioned real). That is, the mere fact that Paul could be treated with streptokinase is now known, through a value judgment, as something that ought to be done. Moreover, this 'ought' is not entirely determined by the facts concerning the safety or efficacy of this particular option, although these considerations will factor into this evaluation.

Second, my value judgments differ from fact judgments because in addition to absolute judgments, which determine whether an actual or possible fact is a value, there are also relative judgments that compare these instances to one another in determining which is better, more pressing or urgent. Such a comparison or weighing is what the term *deliberation* suggests. This is a process that is analogous to comparing things according to their weight. It is part of the complex process of reaching an evaluative conclusion.[60]

Third, feelings are a dimension of the productive apprehensive acts on each level, and they serve as a criterion for the adequacy of the contents I express in these acts. In the case of the second-level apprehensive act of conceiving, my intellectual being is affectively satisfied only when there are no further, relevant questions for understanding. In the case of a third-level judgment, my rational being is affectively satisfied only when there are no further, relevant questions for reflection. But in the case of a fourth-level evaluation, my moral being is affectively satisfied only when there are no further, relevant questions for deliberation. I will refer to this affective satisfaction of my moral sensibilities that comes with a discovery of some value as an experience of *complacency*.[61]

On the basis of this account of fourth-level affective cognition, Lonergan interprets Pascal's remarks about the reasons of the heart:

> First, then, there is a knowledge born of love. Of it Pascal spoke
> when he remarked that the heart has reasons which reason does not

know. Here by reason I would understand the compound of the activities on the first three levels of cognitional activity, namely, of experiencing, of understanding, and of judging. By the heart's reasons I would understand feelings that are intentional responses to values; and I would recall the two aspects of such responses, the absolute aspect that is a recognition of value, and the relative aspect that is a preference of one value over another. Finally, by heart I understand the subject on the fourth, existential level of intentional consciousness and in the dynamic state of being in love. The meaning, then, of Pascal's remark would be that, besides the factual knowledge reached by experiencing, understanding, and verifying, there is another kind of knowledge reached through the discernment of value and the judgments of value of a person in love.[62]

For the sake of simplicity of expression, I have spoken of value judgments in positive terms, as referring to either actual or possible values. But a more exhaustive categorization would also include negative judgments referring to actual or possible disvalues, of evils to be lamented and/or remedied, and possible evils to be avoided. In Paul's example, I judged his AMI to be a disvalue not only because he declined physically from his prior state of robust health, but also because this condition put him at a much higher risk of sudden death in the near future. Four comments about this form of expression are worth registering at this point.

First, even though the content of my evaluation regarding Paul as having an AMI is negative, that is, that this is a disvalue, this evaluation is still a cognitive achievement. In this sense, even the discovery that some X is a disvalue is a positive cognitive advance.

Second, even if I affirm that Paul's AMI is a disvalue, I need not generalize this judgment to conclude that Paul's AMI is an unmitigated evil, that is, without any possible redeeming features. To take another example, I need not conclude from the fact that humans undergo physical disintegration, like all material things in the universe, that this process is radically at odds with human dignity. Indeed, this knowledge of a decline in Paul's physical status also provides him with an opportunity to discover and actualize certain other values that he might bring about as a result of this event. For instance, he might decide to remedy his poor health by making lifestyle changes. Also, this event might enable him to face certain existential questions that he had never before considered seriously, such as the value of his own being. Paul's AMI, then, might ultimately prove to be a valuable personal experience that heightens his sense of responsibility toward himself and others. This event might also provide members of Paul's community with the opportunity to concretely manifest their care and concern for him through their decisions and actions in response to his AMI.

Third, for Lonergan, what I judge to be good or a value is what I intend in my questions for deliberation and know through my value judgments. What I judge to be a disvalue is what I judge ought not to be. The good that I affirm, then, is always some concrete actual or possible reality, especially a human reality. On the one hand, I might be prone to judge concrete reality negatively if much of what I discover falls short of my transcendental notion of the good, serving as a criterion for my judgments. Not only is there a limitation in concrete reality, and in attempts to achieve the good, there is also, most proximately, the moral limitations I recognize in myself, the stain or 'inner bentness' that reveals itself in my own history. As Lonergan suggests:

> [T]he transcendental notion of the good heads for a goodness that is beyond criticism. For that notion is our raising questions for deliberation. It is our being stopped with the disenchantment that asks whether what we are doing is worthwhile. That disenchantment brings to light the limitation in every finite achievement, the stain in every perfection, the irony of soaring ambition and faltering performance. It plunges us into the height and depth of love, but also keeps us aware of how much our loving falls short of its aim.[63]

On the other hand, for every negative value judgment I make there also seems to be a positive correlative judgment. For instance, judging Paul's actual AMI to be a disvalue is linked to my positive judgment that some treatment would be good. Conversely, the positive judgment that some future possible good is worth achieving is linked to the negative judgment about something that is actually lacking in present reality. So even the emphasis on positive values to be achieved also implies a corresponding negative evaluation of the present. In an effort to become more, I might be overly negative in my judgment of what I am, or ungrateful for what I have been given.

Fourth, moral idealism can also play a role in negative value judgments. Moral idealism results when knowledge is deficient. For value judgments 'presuppose knowledge of human life, and human possibilities proximate and remote, of the probable consequences of projected courses of action. When knowledge is deficient, then fine feelings are apt to be expressed in what is called moral idealism, i.e., lovely proposals that don't work out and often do more harm than good.'[64]

It would seem that moral idealism can lead not only to moral ineptitude, but to moral impotence, as when one decides that there is no point trying to do what one judges one ought to do.

Finally, consider the range of meanings that my evaluation that Paul's

AMI is an actual disvalue might open up. First, this might be a negative, absolute value judgment about the actual fact that Paul is suffering from this particular form of physical evil which entails the risk he could die or be physically restricted in the future. Second, it could also be a relative negative value judgment, namely, that Paul's current chest pain is worse than the transient angina he experienced the day before. Third, for each of the above cases, this negative value judgment could be a negative evaluation of some moral, rather than merely physical, reality. For instance, Paul's AMI could have resulted from a deliberate attempt, by himself or another person, to harm his health or end his life. Or, again, the possibility that Paul will die as a result of this AMI might be deliberately increased by certain courses of action or inaction taken by himself or others. In these cases, my negative evaluation would be of a moral evil versus a physical one, where I would distinguish between the agent who chooses the evil by doing something or by failing to do something, and the patient who suffers the evil.[65]

5.4 Decision: Choosing to Enjoy Actual Values or to Actualize Possible Values

Distinct from making a value judgment or evaluating is deciding, if pertinent, to enjoy an actual value or actualize a possible value. The move from judging to deciding involves a fourth-level shift from cognitional issues regarding how I discover values to decisional issues regarding how I voluntarily, that is, willingly, come to make a personal choice and commitment to some course of action on the basis of this knowledge. Strictly speaking, these decisional acts go beyond our focal concern to analyse where feelings enter into evaluations. Even so, the good that is intended in my question for deliberation is not merely a cognitional good of knowing what ought to be, but also includes choosing that which I know I ought to enjoy or do. Since affectivity also enters into such decisions and actions, a brief discussion of how this occurs will complete our account of where feelings enter into the fourth level.

As I quoted from Lonergan above, a judgment of value constitutes 'the initial thrust towards moral self-transcendence.'[66] In addition, I offer the following:

> True judgments of value go beyond merely intentional self-transcendence without reaching the fulness of moral self-transcendence. That fulness is not merely knowing but also doing, and man can know what is right without doing it. Still, if he knows and does not perform, either he must be humble enough to acknowledge himself to be a sinner, or else he will start destroying his moral being by

rationalizing, by making out that what truly is good really is not good at all.[67]

I have discussed how feelings enter into the fourth-level process of value judging. Transcendental affectivity is expressed in the searching, sometimes wrenching question 'Is it worthwhile?' Categorial feelings reveal values to us in deliberative insights and dispose us to commitment. But, of themselves, the feelings that respond to values 'do not bring commitment about. For commitment is a personal act, a free and responsible act, a very open-eyed act in which we would settle what we are to become.'[68]

By the act of decision one not only settles ends and objects, but also one's own habitual ways of feeling and acting:

> [Choosing] gives rise to dispositions and habits. It makes me what I am to be. It makes it possible to estimate what probably I would do in a given situation. It gives me a second nature, and that second nature is what existentialists frequently refer to as the essence of man ... It is the essence you get insofar as you develop habits and dispositions by your choices.[69]

Decisions are choices I make regarding the contents of value judgments. These decisions also have an affective dimension, which can be given either in a pattern of complacency or of concern. Recall that whether a value judgment manifests an actual or possible value, the truth of that judgment is given in the satisfaction of my moral being, what I called a sense of complacency. Decisions can be either about an actual good, in which case I can choose to enjoy this value; or they can be about a possible future good, in which case I might choose to act in a way that will bring about this good. The decision to enjoy some actual good might be said to be given to me in the mode or pattern of complacency. This is a *decisional complacency*, which is distinct from the *cognitive satisfaction* I referred to previously, which arises when I make a true value judgment. The decision to do something or actualize some possibility follows from the deliberative process of weighing alternative options, and my choice might be said to be given to me in the pattern of concern. In treating Paul, then, there is an affective progression from the mode of complacency, when I arrive at the conclusion about what I ought to do in a value judgment, to the mode of concern, which motivates me to decide to live up to what I know I ought to do (i.e., to achieve some future good).[70]

If I affirm, as in Paul's case, that some possible good is truly worthwhile and ought to be actualized, I might decide (a) Yes, I will (help to) actualize this possible good, (b) No, I will not actualize this possible good, or (c) not to decide, that is, decide to postpone or simply refuse to make a decision. In deciding to do what I discern I ought to do, that is, in opting for (a), there is a synthesis or integration of my intellectual and affective cognition with my decision, or will, such that my knowing and doing are of a single piece. In this case, the initial thrust toward moral self-transcendence, constituted by the judgment of value, is extended into my decision without reaching its fulfilment in action. If I decide not to do what I judge I ought to do, or to do what I judge I ought not do, that is, if I opt for (b), there arises a rift between my knowing and doing. Although I am morally constrained to decide in accord with the good I grasp through my value judgment, I am still free, in fact, to decide not to respond to this knowledge, that is, to act in an irresponsible way. In that case, the initial thrust toward moral self-transcendence, constituted by my value judgment, is aborted by this negative decision. This inconsistency between my knowing and doing could be interpreted as a 'lack of integrity.' Finally, if I decide not to decide, that is, if I opt for (c), then I have chosen to drift, refusing to face the decisional issue. Such a refusal is a failure to be affectively moved by my concern to make a decision following a value judgment; and this could become habitual over a whole range of decisions.

This analysis is in congenial continuity with the traditional moral recommendation, for instance, as articulated by Aquinas, that one ought never do something that goes against one's conscience. In the terms of intentionality analysis, a guilty conscience arises when there is an incongruity between what I know to be good and what I decide to do or not do, and actually carry out. In this context, rationalization would seem to be an effort on my part to avoid a value judgment that, in the first instance, I grasp affectively in a deliberative insight. The fact that I can be aware of my own pangs of conscience when I decide to follow some irresponsible value judgment and decision, and can recognize my own abortive attempts to sooth my affective unrest by rationalizations, is evidence for the cognitive interplay between mind and heart. Even mistaken evaluative performance, then, highlights the affective base for value judgments and decisions.

Lonergan's analysis of decision-making is also in continuity with some aspects of the traditional emphasis on doing one's duty. For instance, it could be that in good conscience I know I ought to treat Paul with streptokinase. But I might also know that actually to carry out the proposed treatment would be fraught with difficulties, not the least of which might be that I would need to postpone desires for such things as food, rest, or entertainment. Traditional recommendations always to do one's duty come into play precisely at the level of deciding to do what one knows one ought to do. On this analysis, my duty can be understood not as some abstract rule, but rather as concrete, in this case, the concrete exigence to decide to treat Paul in accordance with my, or his, value judgment, that is, to treat him with streptokinase. Doing my duty suggests that I resolve to do what I know to be good, even if I also know this will be, in some ways, unpleasant. For, as Lonergan suggests, 'What is agreeable may very well be what also is a true good. But it also happens that what is a true good may be disagreeable. Most good men have to accept unpleasant work, privations, pain, and their virtue is a matter of doing so without excessive self-centred lamentation.'[71]

The traditional emphasis on the importance of doing one's duty, then, could be understood as an effort to instruct persons to conform to their decisions to do the good, irrespective of whether the good happens to be agreeable or pleasant to oneself.[72]

5.5 Execution of One's Decision, if Appropriate

I might effect my decision not only by actualizing some possible value, or remedying some actual disvalue, but also by enjoying some actual value. So I might decide that Paul ought to be treated with streptokinase in order to actualize the value of limiting the extent of his AMI, or to remedy, as much as possible, the disvalue of his AMI. I could also decide that I am the one who should carry out this treatment, that is, rather than another physician to whom I might refer Paul.

But my decision could also be a decision simply to enjoy some actual value. For instance, I could decide to spend some time with Paul, following his treatment, to enjoy the value of his company. Alternatively, if Paul's condition turns out to be a terminal one for which no treatment would be effective, I (and/or his loved ones) might decide to do those things that would bring him comfort, and simply to enjoy being with him during his remaining time. Hence, decisions are not merely to actualize some possible good. The inattention to and oversight of decisions made to enjoy the good promote the false dichotomy that one either actualizes some possible good or one does nothing. On this view, the implication of doing nothing is that one is useless. I would urge that when there is nothing more that one can do medically to treat a patient's or family member's medical problem, it is still possible to decide to enjoy being with them and remain in solidarity with them, rather than to abandon them. Indeed, the possibility of hope being present throughout this process would seem to rest upon the patient's or caregiver's discovery of some positive actual or possible value(s). As future possible goods to be achieved diminish, there is a greater need to affirm actual values and to decide to enjoy these values (e.g., loved ones) in the mode of complacency.[73]

The affective modes of complacency and concern, as previously described, also set the pattern in which I execute decisions. My enjoying some actual value occurs in the mode of complacency. By complacency, I refer to the affective unity that encompasses my whole evaluative process; from my question of value, through activities of deliberative insight, value judging, deciding, executing a possible good, and/or enjoying an actual good. If the good is a possible future good that is to be actualized, my affectivity shifts keys during the evaluative process from the mode of complacency, which corresponds to achieving a value judgment, to the mode of concern, which corresponds to my decision to commit myself to bringing about this good. For example, I affirm the value of treating Paul with streptokinase in the mode of complacency. Subsequently, I respond to this judgment in the mode of concern, when I resolve to treat Paul as I know I ought. I then begin actually to implement this treatment plan in the mode of concern, which eventually gives way to complacency as I realize my goal.[74]

As I act on my decisions, they become effective and/or constitutive. The execution of a decision is effective in the sense that, in actually bringing about some state or end, I effect some change in the world. In Paul's case, this change is most obviously a material or external one brought about predominantly through some physical means and activity, for instance, treating Paul's AMI. But I can also effect changes by executing a decision to enjoy some actual value. Much of friendship involves the execution of a decision simply to enjoy the other.

The execution of decisions, whether they involve actualizing a possible good or enjoying an actual good, are also constitutive in the sense that these acts determine not only what I do, but who I am. For instance, if I carry out Paul's treatment in a responsible manner, then, in the process, I also constitute myself as a responsible physician. On the contrary, if I fail to effect Paul's improvement, and I am culpable for this failure, for example, due to my lack of skill and my resistance to acknowledge this deficiency and so refer Paul to a cardiologist, then my deeds have not only failed to make my decision effective in action, but also, in the process, I have constituted myself as an irresponsible, or at least an inept, physician. Beyond constituting myself through particular acts, executing decisions also develops my habits or dispositions to act in certain ways. The term of this development is my character.

On the fourth level, then, one comes to know and do the good. On this level one moves from the cognitional issues of evaluating to the decisional issues of *praxis*. Executing decisions can be a matter of actualizing possible values that are given in the pattern of concern, or enjoying actual values that are given in the pattern of complacency. Through my actions, I am concomitantly engaged in effecting changes in the world and constituting my moral character.

Lonergan on the Objectivity of Evaluations: An Epistemology and Metaphysics of Heart

For your judgment of values, for the objectivity of a judgment of value, the criterion is the good conscience of the virtuous man. It's very Aristotelian, incidentally. Aristotle made ethics empirical by postulating the existence of virtuous men.

Bernard Lonergan, 'Milltown Park Lectures on *Method in Theology*'

1 Lonergan's Account of the Objectivity of Evaluations

In chapter 4 I examined Lonergan's answer to the phenomenological question, 'What am I doing when I am knowing *facts*.' In chapter 5 I considered Lonergan's second basic question for philosophy, which is the epistemological question, 'How does this process of experiencing, under-standing, and judging yield genuine knowledge of facts?' In chapter 6 I extended the phenomenological analysis of knowing facts or judging to include those cognitive activities of evaluating, by means of which one comes to know *values*. In this chapter I will provide an account of how, according to Lonergan, this purported knowledge is sometimes genuine. Lonergan's answer to the question of the possibility of knowing values objectively parallels his answer to the prior, and more basic, question of the possibility of knowing anything.[1] For him, objectivity, whether in matters of fact or value, is 'simply the consequence of authentic subjectivity.'[2]

Lonergan's position concerning what constitutes a genuine evaluation follows from his conclusions regarding what one is doing when knowing apparent values. As discussed in the previous chapter, the cognitional reason for every evaluation is some apprehension of value or deliberative insight. At a minimum, in order for an evaluation to be correct, my deliberative insight must be authentic. Since my deliberative insight is an affective cognition, the objectivity of this insight is best expressed in terms of its affective dimension. On the interpretation of Lonergan I will be proposing, the key issue is whether a particular deliberative insight is made in affective fidelity to the *self-transcending*, transcendental notion of value. I will attempt to illustrate the meaning of this claim by means of the medical example previously mentioned of diagnosing and treating a patient with chest pain.[3] In addressing briefly Lonergan's third basic question for philosophy, 'What are the general features of the truly good that I come to know?' I will outline his notion of the scale of preferences among values.

2   A Critical Peer Review of a Medical Treatment Decision

I will proceed, as in chapter 5, by illustrating an instance of an evaluation made by a physician that contravenes the normative view of the profession. Once again, the main point of this illustration is to highlight concretely an evaluative dispute centring on differing apprehensions of the apparent values at stake. By beginning with a concrete example, I hope to focus the discussion on the objectivity of evaluations, and on the difference in meaning of the labels 'inauthentic,' or 'irresponsible,' and 'authentic' or 'responsible,' phenomenal subjectivity.[4]

Resuming the discussion of my encounter, as a physician, with a patient, Paul, who is having chest pain, assume that I have correctly diagnosed his chest pain as an acute myocardial infarction (AMI). Assume also that I discover that Paul's chest pain began soon after he ingested some crack cocaine, since I know that an AMI can be caused by coronary vasospasm resulting from using cocaine. In order to minimize the damage to his heart and the risk of a life-threatening cardiac rhythm disturbance, I recommend to Paul that he remain in hospital and receive the usual treatment for this condition, namely, monitoring of his blood pressure, cardiac rhythm, and blood chemistry, and treatment with oxygen, nitroglycerine, aspirin, and other drugs, as indicated by his condition.

Assume further that, to my surprise, Paul rejects these recommendations and, with full knowledge of the risks of non-treatment, decides to go home and treat the pain himself. Paul refuses to stay in hospital because that would restrict his access to, and use of, cocaine. Paul also rejects my suggestion that he receive counselling for his addictive behaviour, since he sees nothing wrong with the life he is leading, so long as he is able to continue to obtain cocaine.

As Paul is about to leave the emergency room, I inform him that he may die from a heart attack if he continues to use cocaine. To this he responds, 'Then give me another drug *like* cocaine that will give me a high but won't affect my heart.' In fact, morphine is an example of an opioid that produces euphoric effects but does not cause the cardiac problems associated with cocaine, and is commonly used to treat the pain of an AMI. Eventually, I agree to Paul's request and provide him with a prescription for morphine, and I arrange to examine him again soon. Following several repeat prescriptions for morphine, I am charged by a medical review body for prescribing narcotics inappropriately.

It is likely that my decision to continue to prescribe morphine to Paul would be criticized by the medico-legal body that oversees such prescriptions, that is, the Bureau of Drug Surveillance. My medical peers might object to treating Paul with regular prescriptions for morphine, and this view would likely hold even if he had significant pain, so long as it was non-malignant pain.[5] One reason for their objections is a rejection of the value of pharmaceutically induced euphoria and the subsequent addictive behaviour that results from a physical and psychological dependence on these drugs. Indeed, the addictive power of cocaine is already evident in Paul's continuing use of this drug despite its harmful effects on his health. My peers may interpret the decision to substitute one narcotic for another, which happens to have fewer harmful physical side-effects, to mean that I condone the use of drugs for recreational purposes, or a life oriented to the pursuit of chemically induced euphoric feelings. Moreover, they might be concerned about the social consequences of members of the medical establishment colluding with, or somehow promoting, chemical dependencies among persons in their care.[6]

This brief illustration highlights a dispute over different notions of the good and how one comes to know it in particular contexts. The dispute between Paul and myself highlights fundamentally different operative orientations to the good, and this is the basis of our disagreement. The disagreements between Paul and myself, as well as that between myself and my medical peers, prompt one to wonder who is correct, whose judgments are more genuine or 'objective.' Moreover, if Paul is content with receiving a regular supply of morphine, on what basis might I or my medical peers both understand and sympathize with him, and yet still be critical of the content of his evaluation? That is, what other values are at stake in this case and how might they be compared?[7]

Note that my encounter with Paul as a patient in the emergency department occurs within the context of an already existing and accepted field of values and practical skills associated with these values. All of this is part of a rich human and medical heritage. Some of these values might only become evident when they are challenged or contravened, such as the values Paul, his family, the hospital staff, and members of the public hold and express through their attitudes, decisions, and actions.[8] More remotely, this field of values may or may not be supported by institutional, societal, and political values, often expressed in cultural stories and religious traditions. Hence, even prior to Paul's encounter with me and other health-care workers, there are more widely held sets of mores that are part of the tapestry of our encounter. These values condition Paul's interaction with the health-care system and shape, for me and my peers, what will count as an acceptable outcome.[9]

3   Intentional Affective Responses to Satisfactions or to Values

In chapter 6 I distinguished between non-intentional and intentional feelings and then went on to assert that feelings that are intentional responses are the cognitional grounds, or reason, for evaluations. The above medical example illustrates how different evaluations might stem from distinct intentional, affective orientations. For Lonergan: 'Feelings that are intentional responses regard two main classes of objects: on the one hand, the agreeable or disagreeable, the satisfying or dissatisfying; on the other hand, values, whether the ontic value of persons or the qualitative value of beauty, understanding, truth, virtuous acts, noble deeds.'[10]

In an apprehension that grasps a value (versus what is merely a satisfaction), the relevant feeling is a *self-transcending*, affective response. For Lonergan, *value* and *true good* are synonymous. A response to value 'both carries us towards self-transcendence and selects an object for the sake of whom or of which we transcend ourselves.'[11] By contrast with *value* or *true good*, Lonergan maintains that those feelings that respond to what is agreeable or disagreeable are ambiguous guides to knowledge of what is genuinely good. That is, the agreeability of an object is insufficient to ground an authentic evaluation. Evaluations made on the basis of agreeability at best coincide with authentic evaluations accidentally: 'What is agreeable may very well be what is also a true good. But it also happens that what is a true good may be disagreeable.'[12]

I have explained that, for Lonergan, one achieves *rational* self-transcendence on the third level of conscious intentionality when reflection reaches a virtually unconditioned judgment. Through or by means of such a judgment, 'we acknowledge what really is so, what is independent of us and our thinking.'[13] Similarly, one achieves *moral* self-transcendence on the fourth level of conscious intentionality when, through the operations of deliberation, decision and action, 'we know and do, not just what pleases us, but what truly is good, worthwhile ... It is, finally, only by reaching the sustained self-transcendence of the virtuous man that one becomes a good judge, not on this or that human act, but on the whole range of human goodness.'[14]

What does Lonergan mean by these two main classes of objects? He seems to be flagging what he later refers to as a dialectical difference between subjects making fourth-level evaluations, some of whom are oriented to, and motivated by, satisfactions in a world of *immediacy*, and other subjects who are oriented to, and motivated by, values in a world he refers to as *mediated by meaning*, rather than immediacy. I used the example of Paul to illustrate an orientation primarily to objects that are satisfying or agreeable, even when this pleasure-seeking activity has an obvious detrimental effect on one's own health or causes sorrow for one's family or loved ones.[15]

Satisfactions and dissatisfactions need not be confined to sensible experiences. For instance, addictive behaviour typically involves the pursuit of the psychological euphoric effects of drugs, such as cocaine, even when this is accompanied by, or results in, significant physical dissatisfactions, such as hunger and painful injections. Indeed, one might prefer the satisfaction of experiencing this euphoria even if this is accompanied by, or results in, significant psychological or mental anguish, for instance, the harm that one's behaviour causes one's family. Alternatively, in order to avoid the risk of experiencing certain psychologically disagreeable experiences, such as terrifying hallucinations that might accompany the use of narcotic analgesics, one might prefer to accept significant physical pain rather than use certain analgesics. Although there seem to be certain acts that would never be satisfying or agreeable to a virtuous person, such as rape or murder, for Lonergan, such a person might decide to proceed with an action they believe is good, even though he or she finds it to be disagreeable on some level, for instance, accepting Paul as a patient even though one knows that this may lead to legal difficulties. Lonergan's main point is that affective responses to the agreeable or the disagreeable are too ambiguous to be useful criteria on which to base ethical evaluations.[16] The corollary of this is that, if at least sometimes one is unable to discern the difference between one's responses to satisfactions and responses to values, then all of one's affective life will remain a confused and ambiguous guide to knowledge of values. As Walter Conn puts it, 'Sometimes the valuable and the satisfying coincide, and self-transcendence comes easily. But often enough, as we all know too well, the valuable is dissatisfying, disagreeable, and then self-transcendence means overcoming the disagreeable for the sake of doing the good. Not having that second or third drink so that one can drive home safely is choosing value over satisfaction.'[17]

Paul's decision to use narcotics is, in some sense, a personal one. He makes this decision using his own mind, and this decision primarily concerns his own life and his own fulfilment or loss. Assume that Paul had sufficient knowledge and effective freedom, at least originally, to assent to using narcotics. This discussion will focus on the criterion on which he bases his decision. In so doing, I will set aside for now the further issue of how others who challenge the grounds for Paul's decision ought to proceed in helping him to reconsider the matter.

The most basic challenge of Paul's behaviour, I suggest, would be to question his conclusion that using cocaine actually is a good one. More generally, the kinds of mistaken evaluations that patients such as Paul tend to make seem to imply other actions that, from my vantage point as his physician, are also mistaken. This might involve pursuing a proposed action based upon a desire for something agreeable, such as a narcotic. Or it might involve pursuing a plan that affirms what seems to me to be a less pressing value, such as the need to return home over the urgency to attend to a life-threatening illness.

On Lonergan's account, what is at stake in my difference of opinion with Paul on whether cocaine is a value is fundamentally a divergence in orientations between Paul and myself. His decision is deficient, I would argue, primarily because it is not properly based on his self-transcending affectivity that responds to values. Like Aristotle's claim that all humans desire to know, Lonergan adds that they also desire the good. The fact that Paul is mistaken in this instance about the value of cocaine does not contradict this claim. Even if Paul does not yet have any critical feelings toward the effects of cocaine on his life, he could have them, and at some future point he actually might have them.[18] Lonergan allows for the possibility that someone such as Paul can radically shift his orientation in the world from satisfactions to values. He calls such a shift in orientation a *moral conversion*. This consists in 'opting for the truly good, even for value against satisfaction when value and satisfaction conflict.'[19] Since this shift in orientation is something like falling in love, intellectual arguments are insufficient to effect such change in core values.

Lonergan conceives of values or goods as that content I grasp in and through self-transcending affective responses to things or persons – past, present, or future. Even more basically, he conceives of value or the good (singular) as that which I transcendentally intend, even before I actually grasp it affectively. That is, it is my transcendental intention, rather than any categorial object, that provides the basic content of what Lonergan means by *value*. It is possible to distinguish between Paul's transcendental intending of value and his grasp of particular categorial values and disvalues. The key questions are whether Paul is oriented to values, and if so, whether the affective grounds of his value judgment are in accord with the affectivity of the self-transcending orientation to value. Perhaps one sign of the self-transcending orientation of one's affective responses is the presence of self-disinterestedness or the absence of self-concern as regards the contents one grasps. Although this might be difficult to determine concretely, the general point is that one is a person of integrity if one has resolved to live on the level of moral seriousness. A further sign of a genuine orientation to values is one's openness to further questions and considerations about the values on which one is deliberating.[20]

This view of values can be contrasted with other, historically prominent views. On the one hand, there is the view of goods commonly associated with *puritanism* or *altruism*. This view tends to conceive of values as being in some essential conflict with what is experientially satisfying-to-self, with things that are agreeable to me; that is, if it feels good, it cannot be truly good.[21] On the other hand, Lonergan's view of the good is also in stark contrast to what has come to be labelled as *Epicureanism*, which is a way of life based on the view that values are whatever is pleasurable; that is, if it feels good, it is good.[22] Values, for Lonergan, are not necessarily in conflict with what is satisfying. Feelings that respond primarily to that which is satisfying, either to self or even the sum total of self and others, as some utilitarians might insist, are not what Lonergan takes to be the proper affective *criterion* for evaluations. For him, as I have pointed out, if it feels good, it may or may not also be truly good.

When speaking of the role of affect in evaluations, Lonergan is referring to intentional, affective responses to values or true goods. His distinction between an orientation to satisfaction and an orientation to value is key to his positive stance on the philosophical import of feelings. It is also a fundamental distinction for discussing the epistemic objectivity of evaluations. For him, in order for evaluations to be epistemically objective they must be based on authentic deliberative insights, which are given in and through feelings that are self-transcending. These are feelings that orient me not merely to the good for me, to what is agreeable or disagreeable to myself. Rather, they are oriented to the good of the whole; they are *totality oriented*. The most obvious example of such an orientation is self-sacrificing love.

Although there are many other ways that my evaluations might fail to be epistemically objective, some of which I will discuss shortly, those who reject the distinction between satisfactions and values are apt to deny that feelings have any genuinely cognitive import in evaluations. John Finnis, for instance, is one prominent contemporary thinker who, despite his many points of agreement with Lonergan, nevertheless has written that all feelings are of merely psychological interest with no properly cognitional relevance. For Finnis, all human affectivity would seem to fall into Lonergan's categories of non-intentional states or trends, for instance, hunger or free-floating anxiety. If he allows that some affective responses are intentional, then it seems that he would still have trouble accepting that they are anything more than responses to objects merely as satisfying or dissatisfying.[23]

Admittedly, on Finnis's phenomenal account of the affective life, feelings are surely ambiguous guides to knowledge of values. However, if the reader suspects, or has a *gut feeling*, that there is something problematic about Paul's choice to continue using narcotics, or about my response to Paul, or my profession's critical response to me, then at least operationally he has become engaged in what Lonergan contends is the crucially affective cognitive process of making an evaluation. Another disagreement between Finnis and Lonergan concerns the commensurability of distinct values, such as vital, social, cultural, and religious values. Against Finnis's position, Lonergan maintains that the moral life frequently involves making *relative* evaluations, which is a process of weighing and choosing among competing values when, for practical reasons, both cannot be promoted.[24]

4 Affective Responses to Values according to Some Scale of Preference

For Lonergan, there are grounds to help us relate these different kinds of values to one another. He argues that feelings respond to the ontic value of persons or to the qualitative value of beauty, understanding, truth, virtuous acts, noble deeds. Moreover, he observes that they do so according to some scale of preference:

> [W]e may distinguish vital, social, cultural, personal, and religious values in an ascending order. Vital values, such as health and strength, grace and vigor, normally are preferred to avoiding the work, privations, pains involved in acquiring, maintaining, restoring them. Social values, such as the good of order which conditions the vital values of the whole community, have to be preferred to the vital values of individual members of the community. Cultural values do not exist without the underpinning of vital and social values, but none the less they rank higher. Not on bread alone doth man live. Over and above mere living and operating, men have to find a meaning and value in their living and operating. It is the function of culture to discover, express, validate, criticize, correct, develop, improve such meaning and value. Personal value is the person in his self-transcendence, as loving and being loved, as originator of values in himself and in his milieu, as an inspiration and invitation to others to do likewise. Religious values, finally, are at the heart of the meaning and value of man's living and man's world.[25]

What Lonergan highlights here are some relations among distinct types of values. The achievement of certain values is a *sine qua non* for realizing subsequent ones. One needs to achieve certain vital values, such as freedom from pain or disease, in order to pursue other values, such as the social value of an improved system of care for the dying. Conversely, certain social values, such as systematic improvements in the environment, can condition the vital values of the whole community. Hence, these two values can be related reciprocally, in a mutually conditioning manner. Although subsequent values, such as the social value of a ministry of the environment, may depend on earlier vital values, in some sense they also go beyond them. Even when there is a greater urgency to secure the earlier ones, one can still affirm that the later ones are more excellent. As Walter Conn explains, 'Cultural values such as education and art, though dependent on vital and social values, go beyond them, just as the meaning and value we search for in our living go beyond that living.'[26]

It is also evident that there are what Scheler calls 'strata of values,' and these exist even within the level of vital values. In treating someone who is in cardiogenic shock, for instance, one gives priority to certain organ systems in the resuscitation process. This order is captured in the *ABC*'s, which are taught in basic cardiac life-support courses. These letters serve to remind caregivers of three words: 'airway,' 'breathing,' and 'circulation.' This order indicates the priorities of a resuscitation. One begins with efforts to (1) establish an airway, (2) support breathing, and (3) enhance the circulation of blood. These activities are ordered according to the end or goal of the resuscitation procedure. This end is to support or restore an individual's vital functions. But the goal of resuscitation is also to prevent the harm of irreversible brain injury. Although this is called *cardiac* resuscitation, it is evident that the efforts are directed toward the heart because the circulation of oxygenated blood through the heart is the means for rescuing an individual's brain from irreversible damage and subsequent cognitive impairment. Therefore, even in the midst of a procedure that focuses on vital values, one distinguishes among a series of vital values, which are ordered as means to certain ends, such as the capacity for higher cognitive functioning.

On this account, a key source of different views on questions regarding values, such as those involved in the euthanasia debate, concerns differing scales of preferences. Lonergan notes, as a matter of fact, that these differences occur in communities: 'There are common or opposed feelings about qualitative values and scales of preference. There are mutual feelings in which one responds to another as an ontic value or as just a source of satisfactions.'[27]

Lonergan maintains that the manner in which members of a community rank values can either bind it together or tear it apart. But on what basis does one decide between opposed rankings of values? If fundamentally this is an issue of feelings, how is this whole account not irredeemably subjective? In an effort to answer these important questions I will provide some account of the criteria on the basis of which Lonergan would reflect on opposed scales of value preferences.

5   Epistemically Objective Evaluations as the Fruit of Authentic Subjectivity

Central to Lonergan's account of the objectivity of evaluations is the fact that, on some level, everyone desires the good. That is, prior to any determination of categorial values, everyone has a transcendental notion of value. Given this prior orientation to the good, my affective response to particular objects conditions my apprehension of them as values. Lonergan's account of the relation between this prior orientation and my activities of apprehending a particular object as a true value involves not only a number of philosophical distinctions but, most importantly, a familiarity with one's own activities as an evaluator. Moreover, these philosophical distinctions ultimately flow from one's personal attention to, understanding of, and affirmation of these cognitional and decisional activities. I will highlight, in this section, some of the noteworthy features of Lonergan's account of how these activities yield epistemically objective evaluations.

As I have pointed out in chapter 6, on Vertin's interpretation of Lonergan, all of my intentional, cognitional acts are conscious. The principal division of these conscious-intentional acts (as well as all intended contents) is into the *transcendental* and the *categorial*. Again, on Vertin's reading of Lonergan, one may distinguish further between *categorial feelings* that constitute my intentional responses to particular objects and *transcendental feelings* that are a dimension of the transcendental notion of value.[28] Following any categorial encounter of data, the transcendental notion of value is what gives rise to questions of value that underpin, penetrate, and go beyond any particular area of questioning. This intending of value is transcendental because it applies to all areas, whether in biology, psychology, world affairs, or one's daily life.[29]

When I raise the question 'Is it really good?' I am intending value insofar as I already have some notion of what would count as an adequate answer. It is in light of this transcendental notion of value that I affectively grasp some particular object as genuinely valuable, good, or worthwhile. Thus, 'when I ask whether this is truly and not merely apparently good, whether that is or is not worth while, I do not yet know value but I am intending value.'[30]

Lonergan distinguishes between the *meaning* and *criterion* for the good or value. I have suggested that, for him, the meaning of the good is fundamentally that which I intend in answer to the question 'Is it good?' This intending is the transcendental notion of value, which is a dynamic intending rather than a static concept of the good. The criterion for the good is the standard I use when I judge that I have achieved knowledge of particular values through some categorial value judgment. As was the case with the pattern on the two prior levels, so also on the fourth level the transcendental notion of value provides the criterion that reveals whether I have achieved genuine or epistemically valid knowledge, in this case, of the good. I apprehend a value proximately through, or by means of, those categorial feelings that are self-transcending, intentional responses to some thing or person. As Vertin interprets Lonergan, the criterion for the epistemic objectivity of this categorial affective response is its congruence with, or fidelity to, the affective dimension of my transcendental notion of value. So, just as the drive to understand is satisfied only when all relevant questions have been adequately answered, and the drive to truth compels rationality to assent only when the evidence is sufficient, so also '[t]he drive to value rewards success in self-transcendence with a happy conscience and saddens failures with an unhappy conscience.'[31]

On this interpretation, for Lonergan a happy conscience refers to an experienced congruence between my categorial and transcendental affectivity. This is given in the experience of what Frederick Crowe has called the *mode of complacency*, which I suggest corresponds to the notion of connaturality described in chapter 3. By contrast, an unhappy conscience refers to the experience of some incongruity between my categorial and transcendental affectivity.[32]

Hence, the pivotal question becomes 'How do I know whether my conscience is trustworthy or authentic?' Lonergan's answer to this question is very Aristotelian. Such confidence is justified only if I am a morally wise or good person. This presupposes some degree of intellectual and moral development, such that I am capable of knowing the real and the concretely possible, and of discriminating among various values within this field of meaning. Moral development of this sort occurs in a context of moral progress where 'one's knowledge of human living and operating has increased in extent, precision, refinement and in which one's responses are advancing from agreeable to vital values, from vital to social, from social to cultural, from cultural to personal, from personal to religious.'[33]

Lonergan gives an example of this whole process of moral development by highlighting what moral teachers actually seek to do. They aim to foster in students a fidelity to achieving congruence between their concrete, affective responses to particular instances of the good and the affectivity of the transcendental notion of the good, which regards all instances. On this view, one's categorial affectivity remains fundamentally spontaneous, but it can also be educated to correspond more closely to the affectivity of my transcendental notion of value:

> [O]nce [feelings] have arisen, they may be reinforced by advertence and approval, and they may be curtailed by disapproval and distraction. Such reinforcement and curtailment not only will encourage some feelings and discourage others but also will modify one's spontaneous scale of preferences. Again, feelings are enriched and refined by attentive study of the wealth and variety of objects that arouse them, and so no small part of education lies in fostering and developing a climate of discernment and taste, of discriminating praise and carefully worded disapproval, that will conspire with the pupil's or student's own capacities and tendencies, enlarge and deepen his apprehension of values, and help him toward self-transcendence.[34]

Although some categorial feelings are transient, limited to the time and place of a value to which they respond, others have a much more permanent place in one's character. Consequently, a discussion about the validity of one's dispositions cannot but avoid becoming a very personal questioning of what one stands for, of the feelings that constitute one's habitual way of being and responding, that are congruent with one's core values. Lonergan emphasizes the power and importance of such feelings by noting that

> there are in full consciousness feelings so deep and strong, especially when deliberately reinforced, that they channel attention, shape one's horizon, direct one's life. Here the supreme illustration is loving ... [M]utual love is the intertwining of two lives. It transforms an 'I' and 'thou' into a 'we' so intimate, so secure, so permanent, that each attends, imagines, thinks, plans, feels, speaks, acts in concern for both.[35]

Lonergan also recommends that, in order to grow in moral authenticity,

> it is much better to take full cognizance of one's feelings, however deplorable they may be, than to brush them aside, overrule them, ignore them. To take cognizance of them makes it possible for one to know oneself, to uncover the inattention, obtuseness, silliness, irresponsibility that gave rise to the feeling one does not want, and to correct the aberrant attitude. On the other hand, not to take cognizance of them is to leave them in the twilight of what is con-

scious but not objectified. In the long run there results a conflict between the self as conscious and, on the other hand, the self as objectified. This alienation from oneself leads to the adoption of misguided remedies, and they in their turn to still further mistakes until, in desperation, the neurotic turns to the analyst or counsellor.[36]

Lonergan's terse summary claim is that epistemic objectivity is a matter of authentic subjectivity.[37] This statement holds for both the third and fourth levels. He does not consider genuine evaluations, even when they occur in works by historians, to be intrusions of an author's subjectivity into his or her efforts to speak objectively. What are intrusions of subjectivity, however, are false value judgments:

> There are true and there are false value-judgments. The former are objective in the sense that they result from a moral self-transcendence. The latter are subjective in the sense that they represent a failure to effect moral self-transcendence. False value-judgments are an intrusion of subjectivity. True value-judgments are the achievement of a moral objectivity, of an objectivity that, so far from being opposed to the objectivity of true judgments of fact, presupposes them and completes them by adding to mere cognitional self-transcendence a moral self-transcendence.'[38]

On my reading of Lonergan, any discussion of objectivity has to come back to intentional, cognitional subjectivity. In the effort to specify what objectivity consists in, Lonergan admits that one may not expect to discover 'some "objective" criterion or test or control.'[39] A key moment in the process of coming to know values is the cognitive act Vertin calls a *deliberative insight*. In this act my affective response to some content or entity plays a crucial role in grasping it as a value. This deliberative insight is authentic, and hence the content of my moral knowing is epistemically objective if the feeling in which I grasp this content *as* a value is self-transcending; and it is through my value judgment that I know the value. More precisely, the ultimate criterion for the self-transcendence of any categorial affective response is its congruence with the feeling that characterizes one's transcendental intention of value. Or as Vertin puts it, '[T]he pivotal element of an epistemically-objective value judgment is a *self-transcending* "value" apprehension, not just *any* "value" apprehension.'[40]

The question remains: 'Is not this whole approach that tries to interpret feelings as central to value judgments radically flawed because it is unreservedly subjective?' I take this to be an important objection that I need to address in this exposition of Lonergan's position. It is clear that Lonergan believes that it is possible to have subjective psychological acts that ground one's genuine knowledge of the real.[41] Perhaps some readers will be willing to grant Lonergan's account of judgments, but will be uneasy with the role he claims affect plays in evaluations. His position on feelings and value judgments is open to being rejected for purporting to ground an objectivist ethics but being unable to deliver. Other readers may object that he correctly bases ethics on feelings but that he is mistaken in arguing that such an ethics can or ought to be 'objective.'

The first line of criticism is apt to come from persons who identify themselves with one of the major traditions in moral philosophy. The Kantian or Utilitarian traditions, for instance, believe that there are, and indeed ought to be, general conceptual criteria for objectively determining the moral good. For them, feelings are far too subjective and variable to ever ground objective moral knowing.[42]

A second line of criticism is apt to come from those who identify with other less prominent ethical theories such as contractarianism. Following Hobbes's individualistic account of human nature, these thinkers would question the existence of any genuinely self-transcending response to values. For them, all feelings are perhaps unreservedly subjective and self-concerned. Nevertheless, they conclude that such feelings can and should be promoted by a social policy and morality that recognizes this true fact of human nature.

Besides such criticisms from moral philosophers, Lonergan's position is also apt to raise the concerns of representatives of broader non-moral families of thinkers. *Perspectivism, relativism,* and *scepticism* raise further methodological and epistemic issues that might become part of the discussion of the status of any ethical conclusion. These thinkers may argue that the good can never be known objectively, in the sense that Lonergan uses the term, because they deny either that there is such a thing or just that persons can ever know it. Hence, for them any attempt to articulate a normative ethic is fundamentally flawed. I will defer critically engaging these positions until the next chapter, though I would mention here that I have prepared the way for such an engagement in the earlier chapters.

An important goal of this chapter is to address directly the criticism that Lonergan's account of ethics is unreservedly subjectivist. I have been preparing a response to this question since chapter 4. And as Vertin points out, these questions have little to do with the specific issue of knowing values. Rather, they have much to do with the prior and more general issue of knowing anything at all. For this reason, I have addressed these prior, more general issues in chapters 4 and 5 before addressing the specific issue of knowing values in chapter 6 and here in chapter 7. Still, Lonergan claims that, at root, knowing the good involves this radically personal process of responding to values affectively. His position is in continuity with the account provided by virtue ethicists, which emphasizes the affective preparation of the moral agent through habituation to the good. It is also in continuity with his own account of knowing in general. For what he emphasizes in the fourth-level precept – Be responsible – is a commitment to being open to all relevant questions. My own reading of Lonergan's response to the charge that his account is irredeemably subjective is to note that his account purports merely to make explicit the already operative role of one's own cognitional subjectivity. Just as I can know facts through 'subjective acts,' such as insight and judgment, so also I can come to know values through subjective acts, such as affective responses to these facts. In both cases, the cognitive contents I achieve through judgment are objective or merely subjective 'inasmuch as they proceed or do not proceed from a self-transcending subject.'[43] The conditions for moral self-transcendence include knowledge of reality, an intentional response to values, and a judgment of value. An intentional response to values, in turn, is conditioned by my moral development and habituation to values. The objectivity of a value judgment is also conditioned by my willingness to raise all relevant questions and to act on my conclusions.

Lamentably, in one's effort to achieve moral self-transcendence this fourth-level process of knowing values may be derailed by the intrusion of one's *self-concerned* subjectivity. Fundamentally, my mistaken evaluations result from my own affective inauthenticity. This occurs when my deliberative insight is not in fidelity with the affectivity that characterizes one's transcendental intending of value.

A brief examination of the range of further or consequent errors may helpfully highlight other ways in which one can fail to make epistemically objective value judgments. It will also allow me to provide a taxonomy of ways in which my apparent knowing can indeed be merely subjective.

6   Some Ways That Evaluations May Fall Short of Epistemic
    ‹   Objectivity

The medical example of deciding how to treat Paul's chest pain illustrates how mistaken evaluations can arise concretely. In the process of correcting such mistakes, I engage in what Lonergan calls the *self-correcting process of learning*. This process complements his emphasis on insights by adding an equally important emphasis on reviewing how oversights occur. For my purposes here, I will presume that the cognitional processes on the first three levels have been authentic. I will therefore restrict my focus to the sorts of errors that are more specific to fourth-level operations of discerning values.

From Lonergan's perspective, the first and most significant source of false evaluations has to do with whether one bases one's decisions on responses to satisfactions or to values. The conflict that arises between Paul and myself as his physician illustrates this basic difference in orientations. Beyond this type of error, there remain problems with correctly applying the criterion of one's orientation to value to concrete determinations. In this task, there is a series of further possible errors that can arise. These fourth-level errors can be understood not only as logically distinct possibilities, but also as the consequence of certain biases that tend to undermine the efforts of even morally serious subjects to achieve epistemic objectivity in their evaluations.

To begin, how might one critically examine Paul's mistaken evaluation? Assume that my peers concur with me that Paul's decision to continue to insist on using cocaine, even in the midst of an AMI, was irresponsible. Just where, in Lonergan's terms, does this conflict between Paul's value judgment and mine arise? One interpretation of this conflict is that Paul's response is dictated by his attachment to the continuing satisfaction he derives from using cocaine.[44] If this is the case, the conflict between Paul's value judgment and mine involves differences in our respective orientations: his to self-concern, mine to moral seriousness.

On this interpretation, Paul bases his evaluation on conditions of mere satisfaction. He determines to continue to use cocaine on the basis of whether this prospect is agreeable to him. As with many addictions, the pleasure he seeks may even be bought at the cost of significant physical pain and social disruption. By contrast, in rejecting his conclusion I base my evaluation on conditions of value, that is, on my intending of the transcendental notion of value. I articulate this distinct orientation in the language of values, such as the vital value of promoting Paul's health and avoiding the risk of sudden cardiac death. Hence, Paul's mistaken value judgment can be considered as an intrusion of his current subjective, that is self-concerned, orientation. In this way, what he deems agreeable to himself prevents him from achieving moral self-transcendence in and through an epistemically objective value judgment.

This same difference in orientations also holds for dissatisfactions. One ancient story that illustrates this point depicts a man meeting a young boy while on a journey. The boy is carrying a smaller boy on his back as he plods along. The older man says to the young boy, 'That's quite a burden you have on your back.' Without hesitating, the young boy replies, 'He's no burden, sir, he's my brother.' Paul's considerations go no further than considerations of satisfaction; similarly, the older man's comments merely take into account apparent dissatisfactions. In contrast, my considerations and those of my medical peers go beyond this orientation to satisfactions and dissatisfactions, even if we acknowledge those issues. Similarly, the young boy's comments reveal that he is not oriented solely to the dissatisfaction that results from his brother's bodily weight, even if he might be brought to acknowledge that carrying his brother is indeed a heavy burden.

Even if I base my evaluations on the criterion of moral self-transcendence, my use of it can still be defective. That is, I may be morally converted, so that I habitually link my prospective value judgments to conditions of self-transcendence, and, nevertheless, still fail to achieve an epistemically objective value judgment or to decide to act appropriately on this knowledge. Moreover, I may fail to do this in a variety of ways.[45] For instance, even though I want to do something worthwhile with my life, I may fail to grasp that refraining from cocaine fulfils a necessary condition (i.e., is a value), when in fact it does. Or I may grasp that avoiding the expense for my family of hospitalization fulfils a condition for doing something worthwhile with my life (i.e., is a value), when in fact it does not. Again, I may correctly grasp that it would be good to change my lifestyle, but then fail to make some concrete move to admit to the destructive consequences of my addictive behaviour and obtain help to change it (i.e., simply not do what I know to be right). In all these cases, my errors result not from a lack of orientation to value, but from various cognitive mistakes, in particular value judgments.

Beyond this cognitive or logical account of my fourth-level errors, there are factors peculiar to the fourth level that result in misapplications of the correct criteria at all levels. Besides differences in native cognitive abilities and moral development, biases play an important role in mistaken value judgements. All persons, according to Lonergan, are subject to biases. Biases block or distort one's knowing in four principal manners. There are biases of unconscious motivation, and of individual egoism, biases that can arise from identifying with one's group, and a general bias that can be associated with common sense.[46] These biases undermine cognitive activities on all levels. On the fourth level, they interfere with the processes of raising questions for deliberation, of responding affectively to values, and of affirming values through value judgments.

Biases can be thought of as ways of escaping the exigence of one's orientation to value. Lonergan speaks of our efforts to dodge moral demands as falling into one of three categories. First, avoiding self-knowledge, which is to prefer illusion to a painful admission of moral failure. Second, rationalizing, which is to prefer self-deception so as to remove the inconsistency between one's moral knowing and action. A third is moral renunciation, which is to prefer giving up on the aspiration to making one's own living responsible.[47] He also speaks of biases as the psychological basis for certain patterns of recurring mistaken evaluations.

Paul's case illustrates how these biases affect fourth-level activities. Unconscious motives block Paul's raising questions for deliberation about his behaviour and choices. For Paul to raise questions about his own behaviour, he must be open to the possibility of finding it deficient and changing it. Openness to such personal questioning requires a number of strengths, such as courage and hope. By avoiding these critical questions, Paul need not face the possible pain of acknowledging his mistaken choices. He can drift along in this manner 'into an ever less authentic selfhood.'[48] This bias is 'unconscious' in so far as Paul fails to make his motives explicit by attending to, objectifying, and scrutinizing his resistance to his own or others' questions about his behaviour and choices. Addressing this bias is frequently the task of a psychologist or psychotherapist. Strategies they might use include supporting Paul's own strengths, as is the aim of supportive psychotherapy, or facilitating some insight into his behaviour by examining his intentional responses to values and their implicit scales of preference.[49]

The bias of individual egoism conflicts with the social good of the community. Paul's egoism, narcissism, or individualism blinds him and prevents him from considering his behaviour from any perspective other than his own. Not only does Paul disregard his impact on others, efforts by others to help him integrate into the life of the community are apt to be interpreted as intrusions on his rights and be met with hostility. Up to a point Paul can be countered by his community, the law, and the judiciary. But at some point, agents of the law, and ultimately the law itself, will have to become more tolerant. When a point comes that there are too many addicts in a society for the law to punish, the law becomes compromised and is no longer coincident with justice.[50] At its root, the problem of egoism for Lonergan is a problem of truncated moral development. Although egoists are not apt to become altruists overnight, perhaps one way of addressing this bias is to be more clear about what the good of the community consists in. I will explore this issue further in chapter 8.

Group bias is a more difficult bias to identify and address. It is not merely a matter of a group's own self-aggrandizement; it is also a group's attempt to justify itself by claiming that the misfortunes of other groups are due to their own depravity.[51] In Paul's case, there is apt to be a group or societal bias against persons with drug addictions, especially if they are poor and marginalized. Under the influence of such a bias, I may be apt to judge Paul harshly and overlook the social and human factors that condition his behaviour.

Finally, on the bias of common sense, Lonergan writes: 'Common sense commonly feels itself omnicompetent in practical affairs, commonly is blind to long term consequences of policies and courses of action, commonly is unaware of the admixture of common nonsense in its cherished convictions and slogans.'[52]

This bias could arise in answering the question about whether to treat Paul by providing him with a regular supply of cocaine. Such a question concerns important and complex issues of social policy. But according to the bias of common sense, such issues do not require an appeal to specialized knowledge of policy. Rather, they can and should be handled by Paul, as a private issue, or by myself, as his physician.

All these forms of bias lead, in one way or another, to mistaken evaluations. Lonergan contends that evaluations are felt to be true or false in as much as they generate a peaceful or uneasy conscience.[53] These biases are the intellect's attempt to quiet one's uneasy conscience by 'ignoring, belittling, denying, rejecting higher values.'[54] In the measure that Paul rationalizes his own behaviour, he will be blind to the real situation, and closed to argument and to other patterns of living.[55] He cannot be argued out of his self-destructive course, because the facts of his life are the absurdities that result from inattention, oversight, unreasonableness, and irresponsibility.[56] It is for this reason that one might expect that a strictly intellectual approach to Paul, as well as to larger social issues, will be unable to address the ethical issues at stake that are importantly affective.

In the example of Paul, I might conclude that it would be better to treat him with morphine as an outpatient rather than doing nothing, even though my peers disagree. Having made this evaluation, however, I might nevertheless fail to carry it through. The real reason for not giving Paul the morphine he requests might be that such an act risks entangling me in legal forms and scrutiny. The point of alluding to the various ways that I can fail to achieve epistemically objective evaluations is to highlight how fraught with difficulty this process is. Even my own hypocrisy 'is no more than the tribute paid by vice to virtue.'[57] Still, my efforts to dodge responsibilities, such as doing what I know I ought to do, themselves reveal this process to be thoroughly cognitive on the fourth level, and this cognitive process involves the affective side of my psychology.[58]

This discussion began with the assumption that in raising a question of value, I had already achieved *absolute objectivity* by successfully negotiating the prior cognitional levels. It is worth pointing out, however, that these evaluations are frequently made on the basis of uncertain outcomes of various courses of action. In addition, rather than achieving a firm and certain diagnosis, caregivers must often be content with a series of probable or *provisional diagnoses*. It is on the basis of such knowledge that plans are frequently made and evaluated. In Paul's case, for instance, I assumed that his chest pain was from his heart and that it was provoked by his use of cocaine. Even if this were the case, my recommendations for Paul were also based on what I thought would likely happen to him, following various courses of action. This type of knowledge, I discovered, is much less secure, and my conclusions can easily be shaped by my own optimism or pessimism.[59]

What, then, am I doing when I base my evaluations on future possibilities given certain courses of action? Note that what this judgment is about, its 'object' to which I intentionally respond after raising questions for deliberation, is manifest through some prior cognitive achievement. My value judgment sublates this prior achievement. My intentional responses 'answer to what is intended, apprehended, represented.'[60] They orient me 'massively and dynamically in a world mediated by meaning.'[61] As I mentioned in chapter 6, I can distinguish between my intentions of intelligibility, reality, and value. Categorial determinations are what result from the encounter of concrete data with my transcendental intentions.

These determinations can be distinguished as intelligibilities, realities, and values. In my value judgment concerning Paul, then, my decision purports to pronounce that one course of action is superior to the alternatives. If I decide to treat Paul with morphine as an outpatient, then I have concluded that this possible course of action is better than the other available possibilities, such as forcing Paul to stay in hospital or allowing him to leave the hospital without any narcotics.

Making a responsible evaluation presupposes that the 'object' that I am evaluating is not simply a fanciful image or bright idea, but an actual or possible state of affairs to which I am responding positively. In this value judgment, I sublate my achievements of the prior cognitional levels. My knowledge of a concrete value is a cognitional attainment that goes beyond the attainment of an actual or possible reality because it introduces something new and distinct to my fact knowledge. It adds to this fact knowledge by including everything that was achieved on the prior levels:

> [W]hat sublates goes beyond what is sublated, introduces something
> new and distinct, puts everything on a new basis, yet so far from
> interfering with the sublated or destroying it, on the contrary needs
> it, includes it, preserves all its proper features and properties, and
> carries them forward to a fuller realization within a richer context.[62]

Earlier, I noted that Lonergan's *principal notion of objectivity* emerges in a pattern of at least three judgments; for instance, that 'the typewriter is,' 'I am,' and 'I am not the typewriter.' In that context I also suggested that persons in the scientific community, such as physicians, are apt to presuppose that the distinction between self and non-self is fundamental, rather than derivative, as Lonergan argues. Consequently, scientists are apt to consider that in order to achieve epistemic objectivity, one must escape one's own subjectivity rather than seek to employ one's own subjectivity authentically.[63]

Prescribing a narcotic for Paul poses a further question regarding epistemically objective evaluations. The hypothetical dispute between my peers on the review board and myself was not so much a matter of differing evaluations on the value of opioids. We both agreed that Paul's continued use of narcotics was not the best option. We were more concerned with the prudential matter of *deciding* how best to proceed, given Paul's refusal to comply with what I first proposed as a reasonable treatment plan. That is, at issue is not merely the difference between knowing and doing the good. At a more basic level, it is between knowing *that* something ought to be, or ought not be, and deciding *how* best to promote this desired outcome. A decision to admit Paul to hospital against his will in order to treat his AMI and addictive behaviour is consistent with my evaluation that he is acting irresponsibly. Assuming that this evaluation is correct and that Paul is still, according to the criteria for capacity assessment, capable of consenting to or declining my proposed treatment, then my decision to admit him for treatment against his will remains problematic. This conflict requires the skills of a *mediator* who might better help Paul to achieve more authentic evaluations and decisions. An important feature of one's capacity to mediate is the ability to identify where disputants differ. Clarity on issues of cognitional and decisional subjectivity are of no small advantage to mediators.

Since any ethical discussion will involve issues regarding individual and societal goods, and how they relate to one another, I will conclude this chapter with an exposition of Lonergan's account of the human good.

7   The Social Dimension of Moral Development and the Human Good

The story of Sue Rodriguez, which I related in chapter 2, illustrates how social factors, such as one's attachments to others, can influence the development of one's character or personality. Conversely, contrasting her story with the story of Dennis Kaye, I pointed out how character or personality traits can influence one's experience of an illness. For both Sue and Dennis, their stories are part of larger stories about a family, community, country, culture, and religion. The themes of Sue's early life on which she focuses in her book, for instance, her family history, her relationship with parents and grandparents, and her father's illness and death from alcoholism, all give important clues about her adult character. Her character or personality, in turn, influence her experience of, and responses to, her terminal illness. Moreover, Sue's illness and death became part of her family's story, and one can safely assume that the public attention she

received will influence the attitudes and behaviour of others toward suffering and death. Indeed, Sue was surprised by the community attention and
debate that her request for physician-assisted suicide sparked. Despite these
evidently social contexts and implications, Sue insisted that her judgment
about what constitutes a 'good' death was strictly a private one.[64]

Although Lonergan would object to the notion that such decisions are
just private or individual, he does, nevertheless, focus on the personal or
autobiographical features of evaluations. In so doing, he emphasizes the
personal authorship and responsibility for the judgments one affirms or
denies. Part of such an autobiographical account includes attending to the
social conditions for personal moral development, as well as for the effective and sustained achievement of values by a community. I will now sketch
Lonergan's understanding of the social dimension of moral development
and of the human good, in order to indicate how he understands these
judgments, and the human good, to be both individual, or personal, and
social.

7.1 Socialization in Moral Development

In addressing the question 'How does one become a virtuous person?'
Lonergan refers initially to the work of child psychologist Jean Piaget.
Piaget analyses the acquisition of skills into elements and goes on to argue
that there is a sequence of age-specific development tasks. Applying this
notion to moral development, Lonergan argues that certain tasks in the
moral development of a child are importantly affective. He suggests that
this process of moral development begins with the achievement of infant
and maternal attachment, progresses through a series of stages, and culminates in what he calls the 'existential crisis.' More precisely, Lonergan
suggests that between the ages of one and three years, the infant achieves
an 'affective symbiosis' with her mother. From age three to six years of age,
good and independent adults aid the child's affective development by
providing him or her with what Lonergan describes as 'a fairly regular flow
of good advice.' By the age of six to seven years, children typically distinguish between right and wrong. This ability eventually gives rise to the
'existential crisis': '[O]ne comes eventually to the existential crisis, when
one discovers that one's deciding not merely affects other people and other
objects but also determines what one is to make of oneself. It is at that point
that you have the emergence of the existential subject in his authenticity.'[65]

Lonergan's notion of the 'existential subject in authenticity' links his
predominantly individualistic philosophical treatment of human cognition
with his psycho-social analysis. It also provides a context for understanding
how Lonergan might view the contemporary emphasis in applied ethics on

'moral autonomy' and the presuppositions of an 'individualistic' view of persons. By 'the existential subject in authenticity,' Lonergan means more than a child's capacity to have desires and act on them, which some take to be the criterion of moral autonomy. Rather, he has in mind a notion of 'moral autonomy' that involves some awareness of the significance of personal value and the meaning of personal responsibility. From this perspective, the issue of 'choice' becomes a moral issue in which one's value judgments, decisions, and actions are the door to one's fulfilment or one's loss.[66] The ability to navigate successfully these choices is, for Lonergan, the hallmark of the moral autonomy of a virtuous person.[67]

The activities of judging, deciding, and acting are, if undertaken freely and responsibly, radically personal. Still, we perform them in a social context of personal relations. That is, the emergence of a virtuous person is conditioned by a series of interpersonal factors, beginning in infancy with the affective bonding between mother and child. This account links the existential concerns of the moral philosopher with psychological and social issues that normally fall within the domains of other disciplines, such as child psychology and sociology. But if one grants affectivity a cognitive role in moral judgments, as Lonergan does, the findings of developmental psychologists become relevant to the philosopher's understanding of the moral life.[68] Moreover, if one conceives of individuals as essentially social, as Lonergan does, one will be at odds with the views of moral individualists, who deny the relevance of social context.[69] To highlight further the importance of the social order for an anti-individualistic account of the moral life, I will now outline how Lonergan conceives of the relationships among individuals and cooperating groups from the perspective of moral ends.

7.2 The Social Dimension of the Human Good

Lonergan insists that the good is both individual and social. His position is at odds with the view, sometimes expressed in the euthanasia debate, that the good of the individual obtains apart from, or in opposition to, the social good. Stories, such as that of Sue Rodriguez, supposedly illustrate an opposition between the individual and the social good. Moreover, on these presuppositions the role of public policy-makers is to formulate laws that will accommodate such individual requests without undermining the social good. On my reading of Lonergan, such an analysis merely distracts the discussion from the key ethical issue, namely, the individual's negative self-assessment of her life. Euthanasia is considered to be a 'benefit' on the basis of someone evaluating her life as not worth living. Once this claim is accepted, the discussion moves on to how society ought to respond to such a request. This is done on the assumption that it is not legitimate for society

Table 7.1 The structure of the human good

Individual		Social	Ends
Potentiality	Actuation		
capacity, need	operation	cooperation	particular good
plasticity, perfectibility	development, skill	institution, role, task	good of order
liberty	orientation/conversion	personal relations	terminal value

to assess critically an individual's self-assessment; rather society supposedly ought to accede to whatever an individual expresses as a wish. The real ethical issue, however, is to attend to, understand, and assess such an evaluation, and not to focus solely on the decisional issues.

Lonergan's account schematically relates individuals and groups to three main aspects of the human good, which he displays in a chart he calls 'The Structure of the Human Good.' This chart includes eighteen terms that are organized in three columns: (1) individuals and their potentialities and actuations; (2) cooperating groups; and (3) ends. Lonergan labels the ends one affirms through value judgments *terminal values*, which he distinguishes from *particular goods* that individuals desire and the common *good of order*. Thus, these three distinct ends impose a threefold division on the individual and social categories, as displayed in table 7.1.[70]

This chart indicates how Lonergan understands the human good to be both individual and social, and ultimately oriented to values. Relating the terms in the first line, individual members of a community actuate their capacities for operating and thereby fulfill certain needs through realizing *particular goods*. Because individuals live in community, much of this involes cooperating with others. Because individuals can learn and perfect their operating, there is a possibility of developing skills. The skills individuals decide to develop are typically those that their institutional role demands of them.

Now, the *particular good*, to which individuals direct their operations and cooperations, is whatever happens to meet their needs. It is what most people think about when they refer to the good: that which everyone seeks. The particular good regards the satisfaction of a particular appetite or need.[71] Such needs are to be understood in the broadest sense: 'By such an instance [of a particular good] is meant any entity, whether object or action, that meets a need of a particular individual at a given time and place. Needs are to be understood in the broadest sense; they are not to be restricted to necessities but rather to be stretched to include wants of every kind.'[72]

In contrast to these instances of the particular good is the concrete manner in which cooperation actually works out, which is what Lonergan means by the *good of order*. This good of order is the 'set-up,' or the basic order that is the framework for the circulation of such things as goods and services of any kind. It is distinct but not separate from instances of the particular good. Children argue about particular goods, adults argue about the set-up or good of order. The family, for example, is not a particular good, but a set-up for the flow of particular goods for father and mother and children.[73]

The good of order regards particular goods not singly and as related to individuals, but as recurring instances, and so as related to all members of some community. It is the concrete functioning or malfunctioning of a series of 'if-then' relationships guiding operators and coordinating operations so that there is a sustained pattern of recurring instances of particular goods. The good of order has its basis in institutions, such as industry, the economy, the polity. Institutions are a mechanism set-up to form a background for decision-making, and individuals are socialized through these institutions. This facilitates the flow of coordinated operations because individuals can count on others doing what is expected of them. Still, the successful functioning of any given set-up or good of order is, for Lonergan, the product of much more than its institutional base, for that is compatible with either success or failure. In addition, the success of the good of order requires 'all the skill and know-how, all the industry and resourcefulness, all the ambition and fellow-feeling of a whole people, adapting to each change of circumstance, meeting each new emergency, struggling against every tendency to disorder.'[74]

For example, I may become a physician to satisfy any number of needs, such as my desire for money or prestige, or to promote the health of others; that is, particular goods. As a family doctor, my medical performance occurs within a system of health-care professionals that involves an interdependence among persons with various roles and skills. I am part of this interdependence, and my performance is a cooperative performance. Because my role may also include providing specific services, such as emergency care, I develop additional skills in these areas. The point is that the set-up or system that promotes the health of all members of the community, or the good of order, is distinct from but related to my own individual good as a health-care provider.

Successfully improving the health of a community depends on fulfilling a number of conditions for healthy living. For instance, individuals need to band together to demand effectively a just and efficient system of health care. In addition, even the best system of health-care professionals needs to be complemented by individuals with good personal habits, including such things as knowledge of their health, a willingness to engage in activities that promote health, the ability to perform these activities safely, as well as an unpolluted environment.[75] The success of any system of health care is not automatic; rather it results from skilful and innovative people working together to meet one another's needs under changing circumstances.[76]

In the third row of his chart, Lonergan relates the remaining five terms: liberty, orientation/conversion, personal relations, and terminal values. By liberty Lonergan means not indeterminism, but self-determination. The processes of evaluation and deliberation previously described are not themselves decisive for one's self-determination. Because individual and group action is limited to some course among alternatives, each with risks and drawbacks, one exercises freedom by actively terminating deliberation, choosing a course of action that seems best, and then executing it. The key issue with regard to freedom is to use it responsibly by regularly opting not merely for the apparent good, but the true good. In this way, one brings about *terminal values*, namely, 'a good of order that is truly good and instances of the particular good that are truly good.'[77] In the process of using one's freedom responsibly, one achieves moral self-transcendence and constitutes oneself as an originator of values in oneself and one's society.[78]

One's exercise of liberty takes place within a matrix of personal relations that Lonergan says are normally 'alive with feeling.' These include 'common and opposed' feelings about qualitative values and scales of preference. There are also what Lonergan calls 'mutual' feelings by means of which individuals respond to each other either as ontic values or simply as sources of satisfaction. Beyond these feelings by means of which individuals grasp values, there is the 'substance of community.' A community is constituted not merely by the physical proximity of its members, but, more importantly, by common experiences, understandings, fact and value judgments, and orientations in life. Alternatively, the experiences, understandings, judgments, and orientations of members of a group may also be opposed. Hence, personal relations can vary to the extent that they can bind communities together or tear them apart.[79]

In chapters 4 through 6 I used the example of Paul, a patient with chest pain induced by his use of cocaine, to illustrate Lonergan's contention that the human good is both individual and social. Paul's particular 'good' corresponds to his desire to experience the agreeable effects of cocaine. In order to obtain cocaine on a regular basis, however, he needs to operate in some manner to obtain money to purchase cocaine. He also needs to enlist the cooperation of those who can supply him with the drug. In this way Paul establishes some set-up or 'good of order' to ensure that he is able to consume cocaine regularly. Although Paul enlists the cooperation of others, such as his suppliers, his personal relations with those who do not affirm his view that using psychotropic drugs is a terminal value are strained.

Paul uses others, such as the physicians who can prescribe narcotics for him, as a means of obtaining narcotics; but they typically respond to him by refusing to cooperate with his goal. The opposition between Paul and those in medicine, which this case illustrates, need not be considered as simply a conflict between the individual and social good. Rather, on Lonergan's analysis, the conflict involves a dispute over values. That is, Paul's caregivers deny what Paul affirms, namely that his particular good, and the good of order he establishes to support his habit, is worthwhile. In Lonergan's terms, they deny that it is a true good or a 'terminal value.'

On Lonergan's view, the orientation of individuals within a community, and the direction of their development, is related to the orientation of a community as a whole. Just as communities influence individuals and change them, so also individuals shape and change communities. By 'conversion' Lonergan has in mind a radical change in a direction of development that is for the better. This change may be brought about in individuals by a process of socialization. Again, individuals, such as great leaders, may convert or improve a community as a whole, through their fidelity to the transcendental precepts 'Be attentive,' 'Be intelligent,' 'Be reasonable,' 'Be responsible.' By contrast, Lonergan conceives of social decline as proceeding from violations of the transcendental precepts, that is, from recurring patterns of inattention, oversight, unreasonableness, and irresponsibility.[80] In Paul's case, for instance, there are two possible reorientations that could occur. First, Paul's community could encourage him to reflect critically on the value of his addiction to cocaine and so come to recognize that it is a false terminal value. Then they could take steps to help him overcome his addictive behaviour. Conversely, Paul's orientation to satisfactions could be met with the approval of others, and his influence might contribute to effecting a change in the set-up of the community such that they would gradually come to approve of cocaine use, legalize it, and allow everyone equal and regular access to it.

There are a number of points worth noting about Lonergan's account of the structure of the good. First, as merely a 'structure' or outline of the elements that constitute the human good, it is entirely open-ended. That is, this structure is merely an organizational scheme for thinking about relations between individuals, cooperating groups, and goods. This structure is compatible with the opposing trends of progress and decline; it can be used for understanding any human society, regardless of the content of the goods they affirm. In other words, although this structure allows one to distinguish between individuals, cooperating groups, and distinct ends to which they are oriented, it does not specify the content of the particular goods, the good of order, or the terminal values.[81]

Second, the three aspects of the human good are interlocking. A particular good, such as a meal, is only transiently satisfying. Because people are intelligent, they want to arrange things so that they have three meals a day, every day. This insistence on an assurance of regularity, security, and recurrence of particular goods leads to the aspect of the good referred to as the set-up or 'good of order.' Because whatever order one's group achieves is open to being questioned, evaluated, and criticized, unless one takes that order to be an idol, there emerges the notion of value: 'Is this particular good or good of order worthwhile?' This leads to the aspect of the good Lonergan calls terminal values. Hence, Lonergan expands his previous philosophical distinction between satisfactions and values to take into account the social dimension of the human good that involves the practical, political issue of some good of order within which individual needs and values can be met.[82]

Third, these three aspects of the good are parallel to other structures. Most fundamentally, they coincide with Lonergan's account of the structure of consciousness. Particular goods, the good of order, and terminal values are isomorphic with the cognitional activities of experiencing, understanding, and judging. Our acquaintance with particular goods is largely a matter of experience. Since experiencing, for Lonergan, is not the whole of knowing, particular goods are good just on the level of experience, as satisfying or dissatisfying. At this level it is ambiguous whether these particular goods are true values. The true good might be quite other than what is experienced as satisfying. Knowing this good requires more than just experiencing; it also includes raising and answering questions. One moves beyond mere experiencing to the level of understanding, for instance, by raising questions about the order that will achieve a regular and sustained flow of particular goods. This is a matter for intelligence, for insight into the set-ups that would allow particular goods to recur, and for formulating such insights conceptually. Through fact judgments, one affirms the possible occurrence of one's conception of a concrete good of order, as well as alternative orders. Through reflecting on different set-ups, one raises questions of value, such as which set-up is truly worthwhile or better than the others. Through a value judgment one affirms a particular good, and an order that will sustain it, as truly worthwhile, and hence as a terminal value. In this way, the three aspects of the good parallel the three levels of consciousness, namely, experiencing, understanding, and judging.[83]

With this overview of Lonergan's account of the structure of the human good, it is apparent that the human good is both individual and social, and that knowing the good has important social and historical dimensions. Although it is central to Lonergan's thesis that knowledge and value claims have authors (and dates), he also complements this emphasis on individual cognitive activities and achievements with his account of the social and historical dimensions of knowing the human good. These social and historical dimensions involve an interplay between individuals and cooperating groups oriented to various ends.

8   Summary

Lonergan's position on the objectivity of evaluations is continuous with his position on the objectivity of judgments. He insists that the human good is never some abstraction. Rather it is always a concretely intelligible actual or possible reality. Knowing values presupposes knowledge of reality, especially human reality. This includes 'knowledge of human life, of human possibilities proximate and remote, of the probable consequences of projected courses of action. When knowledge is deficient, then fine feelings are apt to be expressed in what is called moral idealism, i.e. lovely proposals that don't work out and often do more harm than good.'[84]

Just as I can transcend myself intellectually through a judgment that achieves genuine fact knowledge, so also I can transcend myself morally through an evaluation that achieves genuine value knowledge. The distinction fundamental to this whole discussion of value is that between transcendental intending of value and categorial evaluations. The most basic meaning of 'value' is that value is what I intend in my value questions, even before I actually grasp a value. Indeed, the source of such questions of value is my transcendental intending of value. Like the other transcendental intentions, it functions in an entirely general manner by prefiguring my every categorial determination. Moreover, even though the transcendental notions are broader than any category, they remain utterly concrete. For the transcendental notions of intelligibility, reality, and value *intend* the real under its every aspect and its every instance. The transcendental notion of the good, in particular, heads for a goodness that is beyond criticism, and this intending issues in concrete categorial determinations of values.[85]

When it comes to knowledge of values, one may speak of particular values, which are categorial determinations, and go on to make more general claims about the relations among different types of values, such as a scale of value preferences would suggest. For Lonergan, the most general norms governing even the content of my knowledge of values are based on how I constitute myself as an authentic subject. That is, I constitute my knowledge of values, actions, and my very self according to the norms by which I live authentically in fidelity to the transcendental precepts 'Be attentive; Be intelligent; Be reasonable; Be responsible.'[86]

The basic form of ideology, on Lonergan's view, is a doctrine that truncates my cognitional and decisional subjectivity, and so justifies my disregard of these precepts. From these basic forms of ideology, all others can be derived. As Lonergan suggests, for instance, moral idealism results from an ideology that justifies my being inattentive to concrete human realities. Again, Epicureanism, and perhaps some forms of Utilitarianism, stem from a view of knowing that considers it to occur at the level of sense experience. Such an ideology justifies my failure to be intelligent in my determinations of the human good. Lonergan would consider it to be a category mistake to determine in an a priori fashion precisely what constitutes the human good. Such determinations depend on knowledge of reality, especially human reality. Nevertheless, with Aquinas, he would insist on very general norms that refer primarily to methodological and dispositional stances, the most general one being 'Do good and avoid evil.'

The example of Paul serves as a concrete focus for summarizing Lonergan's position. If Paul's AMI is limited by my treatment, on Lonergan's interpretation I will have based my actions on an affective response by means of which I grasped this outcome, in the mode of complacency, as worthwhile. Note the distinction between the resolution of Paul's chest pain and my response to this in the mode of complacency. The chest pain is a feeling that is a first-level sense datum for Paul. My mode of complacency, by contrast, is a fourth-level affective harmony between the transcendental intending of value and my categorial response to the worthwhileness of Paul's improved cardiac status.

Contrary to what a Humean analysis might conclude, Paul's good is not simply identical with an improvement in his symptom of chest pain, which could be brought about by using morphine. It also includes the reasonable and responsible dimensions of the treatment decisions regarding hospitalization, monitoring, and thrombolytic therapy. Nor is it accurate to interpret this new situation as a value merely because of the pleasurable feelings of complacency I now experience, that is, that this decision is good just because it makes me feel good. Rather, in the complacency of my fourth-level, intentional, affective response to Paul, I apprehend that this possible change in Paul's condition would be worthwhile or good, and I decide to help Paul by suggesting and initiating treatments aimed at realizing this possibility.

In contrast to what the Kantian view might suggest, I do not grasp Paul's good, in the first instance, as a rationally abstract principle or intelligibility that I see or verify in Paul, for instance, as exemplifying the good of health. Rather, it is through feelings, by virtue of my response of complacency in the experience of a deliberative insight, that I grasp Paul's improved state as a value. This affective response provides me with my cognitive access to the value of Paul's possible new state, which I come to know through a value judgment. For Lonergan, by contrast to the Kantian, the good that I grasp is always concrete. My 'intellectual' cognitive light illumines the concrete intelligibility and reality of Paul's cardiac status; and my 'evaluative' cognitive light illumines the values of his status. In both the factual and evaluative moments, the real and the good are concrete. The main psychological difference between knowing facts and knowing values is that in knowing values, my light is distinctively and crucially affective.

Affective responses to objects, therefore, constitute the proximate grounds of an evaluation. It is 'in' these felt responses to actual or possible objects or events that I grasp their absolute or relative value. By means of a deliberative insight, I arrive at an evaluation. Through that evaluation I come to know the value of an object or event. These acts describe the cognitive, psychological grounds that culminate in ethical self-transcendence. The achievement of this process is knowledge of values, which is the content of one's evaluation. The epistemic objectivity of this evaluation is a function of the authentic subjectivity of the evaluator. Such authenticity involves my choosing and acting in fidelity with the affectivity that characterizes my transcendental intending of value.

PART FOUR

Ramifications of Lonergan's Stance on Evaluations for the Euthanasia Debate

8

A Critical Assessment of Lonergan's Account of the Role of Affect in Evaluations

Critically grounding knowledge isn't finding the ground for knowledge. It's already there. Being critical means eliminating the ordinary nonsense, the systematically misleading images and so on; the mythical account.

       Bernard Lonergan, 'An Interview with Fr. Bernard Lonergan, S.J.'

1   Overview of a Critical Assessment of Lonergan's Core Position

In this chapter I shall summarize and critically assess Lonergan's philosophical contributions to the global question of how and where feelings enter into evaluations. In the next chapter I will draw out some practical implications of his position for how one ought to understand and assess particular evaluations that prompt persons to consider euthanasia.

I will pursue the goal of assessing Lonergan's position in two ways. The first way will be to summarize his position as a response to a series of questions that regard the role of feelings in evaluations, and the consequent epistemic status of such evaluations. This will also involve summarizing Lonergan's position on some metaphysical questions regarding values such as the human good. In the second way, I will indicate what I take to be the strengths of Lonergan's position by highlighting the merits of the evidence that supports his stance, by indicating the importance and originality of his claims, and by responding to objections and difficulties that might be raised against his position.

2   Lonergan's Philosophical Position on the Role of Affect in Evaluations

The focal point of this discussion has been to interpret what Lonergan is claiming when he states that 'apprehensions of value are given in feelings,' and that these apprehensions are 'intermediate between judgments of fact and judgments of value.'[1] These terse statements raise a series of further questions. For instance, what does Lonergan mean when he says: (1) certain 'feelings' are cognitive; (2) 'apprehensions' of value are distinct from 'judgments' of value; (3) apprehensions of value are 'given *in* feelings'; (4) feelings that respond to values are 'intermediate' between fact and value judgments; and (5) feelings that respond to values, as distinct from satisfactions, do so according to a 'scale of preference'? In this section I will summarize my interpretation of Lonergan's answer to these phenomenological questions, which I have developed in the preceding four chapters.[2]

2.1 Phenomenological Question: 'What Cognitive Role Do Feelings Play in My Knowing?'

The first question concerns what Lonergan means by saying that there are feelings that are cognitive and enter into value judgments. On the interpretation I have advanced in chapters 4 to 7, a fundamental distinction that underpins his account of the role of affect in evaluations is that between the affectivity of my *transcendental* intending of value (i.e., 'transcendental feeling') and my *categorial* affective responses to values. Lonergan considers both types of feelings to be cognitive. In the case of my transcendental intending of value, transcendental feeling arises in response to some fact judgment. Such feeling plays a role in my raising value questions, and serves as a criterion for the adequacy of my answers to these questions.

Distinct from 'transcendental' feeling are my 'categorial' affective responses. What Lonergan refers to as categorial responses are not 'non-intentional' feelings, but rather 'intentional' affective responses to some entity. These responses regard two main classes of objects, satisfactions and values. Lonergan highlights the role of 'apprehensions of value,' or what Vertin has labelled 'deliberative insights,' as a central part of the cognitive-affective grounds for an evaluation. In brief, feelings enter into value judgments in two ways for Lonergan. 'Feeling' enters as the affective dimension of my transcendental intending of value, and distinct 'feelings' enter as deliberative insight, which is a categorial intending of concrete values.[3]

The preposition 'in' in Lonergan's claim that 'values are apprehended *in* feelings' refers to the fact that, for Lonergan, human knowing on the second and third levels is discursive. On the fourth level it is 'in,' 'through,' or 'by means of' certain affective acts (and their products) that one comes to know values. More generally, on the second to fourth levels certain acts produce an inner word that 'mediates' human knowing. In chapter 4 I described this discursive process by highlighting three distinct lines of elements that come together in Lonergan's account of human knowing. First, there is the grasp of the content of an insight, or of some 'unity in a diversity.' For instance, on the second level I grasp some content by means of a direct insight, and on the third level I grasp some content by means of a reflective insight. Correspondingly, on the fourth level, I grasp an evaluative unity by means of a deliberative insight.

Second, on the second to fourth levels I grasp some unity in a diversity that both partly brings about, and is expressed in, a follow-up product or inner word. On the second level, this product or inner word is a concept; on the third level it is a judgment; on the fourth level it is an evaluation.

Third, on the third and fourth levels, but not on the second, it is 'in,' 'through,' or 'by means of' this product that I come to know the real, as fact or value. On the fourth level there are three distinct moments in the discursive process of knowing values. First, there is the cognitional *act* of a deliberative insight that grasps some content or unity. Second, this content both partly brings about and is expressed in the product or inner word of a value judgment. Third, it is this value judgment that mediates my knowing a real value. This is how I would unpack Lonergan's terse statement that values are apprehended 'in' feelings.[4]

The feelings to which Lonergan's expression 'values are apprehended *in* feelings' refers, then, are first of all the affectivity of deliberative insights. These affective, fourth-level acts are cognitive. They grasp some evaluative unity in a diversity and constitute a pivotal moment in the process of knowing values. I interpret the preposition 'in' of this expression to refer to two stages in this process of evaluating. Affectivity enters into the evaluation during the first stage as a dimension of my deliberative insight. In the second stage, 'in' refers not to the affective dimension of the deliberative insight, but to its by-products, the content of the insight. It is in and through this content that I know values. In the first moment, '*in* feelings' refers to the fact that this deliberative insight provides key evidence for a subsequent value judgment. That is, my fourth-level affectivity apprehends values; it provides the grounds by which I achieve knowledge of values. It is 'in' these affective, fourth-level acts that I grasp some evaluative unity, which is part of the basis for my knowing a value. In the second moment, it is not so much 'in' the feeling itself, but more precisely 'in' the by-product of my deliberative insight, the content, in the inner word or evaluative unity I grasp in this insight, that I apprehend values. That is, Lonergan's use of the preposition 'in' is equivalent to 'through' or 'by means of,' and expresses the notion that the follow-up product of a deliberative insight, which is a value judgment, mediates my coming to know a real value through that judgment.

The main point here is to avoid misunderstanding Lonergan's expression that 'values are apprehended in feelings.' The 'feelings' to which he refers are not equivalent to first-level feelings or sensations. Nor does the preposition '*in* feelings' suggest that these feelings are data or agent objects in which one discerns values. Finally, by saying that 'values are apprehended in feelings,' Lonergan is not suggesting that feelings are themselves sufficient for knowledge of values, nor that knowing itself is somehow an immediate or unmediated process. The feelings to which he refers are the fourth-level feelings that are categorial responses to values, or deliberative insights. These deliberative insights are analogous to the acts of direct insights on the second level or reflective insights on the third level, not to the data in which these insights grasp a unity.

Hence, these fourth-level feelings are not to be confused with first-level feelings or sensations. Despite Lonergan's insistence on the role of feelings in the process of knowing values, it is important to emphasize that one does not attain knowledge of a value just by some first-level act of experiencing. More is involved, including the whole discursive process of raising and answering questions, as previously outlined. On the other side, a value is more than, perhaps sometimes even other than, the experience of an affective response. Although these fourth-level 'feelings' or deliberative insights are *necessary* cognitive conditions in the process of making a value judgment, of themselves they are not *sufficient* conditions for knowing values. This is a very different claim from the view that some X is a value because it induces in me good feelings. In Lonergan's view, one may affirm that some X is a value even though one finds X is personally dissatisfying or has distressing personal implications.

Fourth, Lonergan contends that these affective cognitions are 'intermediate' between fact and value judgments. Following my fact judgments, these feelings enter into my evaluation of these facts. That is, in the discursive process of evaluating, these affective cognitions move me beyond an already-achieved knowledge of facts to a not-yet-achieved knowledge of values. Lonergan spells this process out more fully by providing an account of the concrete phenomena of knowing values. In his account, he specifies how these affective cognitive acts sublate a series of prior cognitive operations whose affectivity, if any, is not yet centre stage. These prior cognitive acts include such acts as reflective understanding and fact judging.

2.2 *Epistemological Question: 'Do My Evaluations Ever Yield More than Just Subjective Knowledge?'*

Throughout this discussion I have endeavoured to separate the 'phenomenological' question, 'What am I doing when knowing facts or values?' from the subsequent 'epistemological' question, 'Why is doing this genuine knowing?' For Lonergan, the prior phenomenological issue is one of self-descriptive fact. It is distinct from, and should not be confused with, the further epistemological issue of the truth of one's cognitive achievements. The epistemological question concerns the contents of my cognitive achievements, whether they are epistemically just subjective or epistemically objective. His answer to this question adverts to the quality of my cognitive acts. Lonergan argues that genuine cognitional objectivity is nothing other than what results from the authentic performance of the previously described operations of cognitional subjectivity. He specifies four distinct precepts to guide my cognitive activities. In summary, 'authentically to know' is 'attentively' to experience, 'intelligently' to understand, 'reasonably' to judge, and 'responsibly' to evaluate.[5] Consequently, I can be confident in the content of my evaluations only if my performance is cognitively authentic. That is, I need to be operating authentically on all levels in my concrete cognitive performance. This means that to be confident in my knowledge claims, my cognitive performance must be faithful to the self-transcending transcendental notions of intelligibility, reality, and value, a fidelity that Lonergan expresses in terms of the transcendental precepts. Because my evaluations regarding either self or another can be epistemically objective, they have interpersonal significance.

2.3 Metaphysical Question: 'What Is the Human Good?'

Finally, Lonergan's phenomenal and epistemic account of how one makes value judgments serves as a basis for a 'metaphysics of values.' Lonergan's general position is that of a critical realist. When it comes to knowing values, he affirms that we do know 'real' values through evaluations, and that these values are either simple or comparative. A simple evaluation affirms that some X is (or would be) truly or only apparently good. A comparative evaluation involves comparing distinct instances of the truly good to affirm that one is better or more important or more urgent than the other.[6] Lonergan distinguishes his critical-realist position from that of the 'moral idealist,' whose knowledge of concrete human reality, that is, of human life, of human possibilities, proximate and remote, and of the probable consequences of projected courses of action, is deficient.[7] Critical realists base their moral choices, in part, on their affective responses to values. Such responses accord with some scale of preference among concrete options. In the usual cases, Lonergan suggests that one normally prefers vital values, such as health or vigour, to avoiding the work, privations, and pains (i.e., what he refers to as satisfactions/dissatisfactions) of acquiring, maintaining, or restoring them.[8] Based on such preferences, one orders distinct values according to a scale of preference. For Lonergan, such a scale involves recognizing that the structure of the human good is both individual and social.[9]

Thus, having affirmed that some X and Y are real (actual or possible) facts, my transcendental intending of value prompts me to ask whether this X is also good or better than some Y. My categorial intentional affective response to this X mediates the move from a fact judgment to a value judgment. Subsequent value judgments rank distinct values.[10] In as much as I proceed authentically, by being attentive, intelligent, reasonable, and responsible in my deliberations, I can be confident of the epistemic objectivity of my evaluations regarding either self or others.

To summarize, then, Lonergan's phenomenology of knowing provides a general account of what I am doing when I am knowing the real and the really good. This involves distinguishing and relating four levels of cognitive activities and achievements. The fourth level involves intentional affective responses, and the operations at this level sublate and integrate prior intellectual achievements. Lonergan's account of cognitional structure provides the evidential basis for addressing questions concerning the epistemic objectivity of the various operations involved in knowing. It also provides a basis for affirming an invariant structure of the really good, or a metaphysics of values.[11]

3   Summary of Lonergan's Philosophical Position as Answers to Six Core Questions

A convenient way to summarize the core claims of Lonergan's global position on the role of feelings in value judgments is to highlight what I take to be his answers to six key questions. I will use these answers to guide the remaining discussion in this chapter and the discussion to follow in chapters 9 and 10.

Lonergan's core claims, then, may be given as answers to the questions displayed in table 8.1. The question I will address in the next section is whether these core claims are correct. More specifically, is it true, as Lonergan argues, that (1) '[i]ntermediate between judgments of fact and judgments of value are apprehensions of value' and (2) '[s]uch apprehensions are given in feelings'?[12] In less technical language, does the heart really have reasons, as Pascal says, 'that reason does not know?'[13] Has Lonergan correctly explained some of the heart's reasons?

4   My Own Critical Affirmation of Lonergan's Philosophical Position

In offering here a critical affirmation of Lonergan's core claims on the role of feelings in value judgments, I shall argue that the evidence on which he

Table 8.1 Lonergan's answers to six core philosophical questions

---

Q.1 *Do feelings ever play a cognitive role in my knowing?*
A.1 Yes. Certain feelings are necessary cognitive elements of my knowing.

Q.2 *If some feelings are cognitively relevant, how do they relate to my knowledge of values?*
A.2 They are part of my cognitive grounds for knowing values. In themselves, they are not sufficient conditions for knowing values. They mediate my knowing of values, they do not give immediate access to those values.

Q.3 *Do such evaluations ever yield more than just subjective knowledge?*
A.3 Yes. Because values are grasped in affective responses, it does not necessarily follow that they are just subjective in content or epistemically subjective. The fact that I characterize these acts as 'affective' rather than 'intellectual' does not thereby render them merely subjective. Still, the only guarantee that my affective cognitions are trustworthy is if I am a virtuous person. My knowing is authentic or epistemically objective if my cognitive performance is faithful to the transcendental precepts.

Q.4 *How do evaluations relate to judgments? How do they relate to decisions?*
A.4 Evaluations sublate judgments, and decisions follow evaluations. The proximate basis for the distinction between facts and values is the distinction between reflective and deliberative insights. However, the ultimate ground for distinguishing between the third and fourth cognitional levels is the distinction between one's transcendental intending of reality and of value. The culmination of cognitional subjectivity is a value judgment, but such a judgment is incomplete without decision, which follows the value judgment on the fourth level.*

Q.5 *Is there a normative structure of the human good?*
A.5 Yes. The human good is both individual and social.

Q.6 *Is life a basic good? Is it an absolute good?*
A.6 Yes to the first question; no to the second.

---

*The source of the important distinction between cognitional responses that are intellectual and those that are affective is not made explicit by Lonergan in his writing. Rather, it is an interpretation and the result of an augmentation, based on certain key elements of Lonergan's own account, that Vertin has proposed. See his 'Judgments of Value,' 233.

bases his core claims is, in fact, the most basic type of evidence to which one can appeal. Moreover, I shall argue that Lonergan's account of this evidence is, in its main lines, accurate. Next, I shall contrast Lonergan's core position with the traditional Humean and Kantian accounts. Then I shall focus on each of his core claims and highlight how they are both important and original, even within his own Aristotelian tradition. Lastly, I shall raise and respond to three difficulties that I expect will have a bearing on whether the reader finds Lonergan's account, and my affirmation of it, convincing.

4.1 The Grounds of Lonergan's Philosophical Position

In critically affirming Lonergan's position, I will begin by highlighting the basic evidence or ultimate grounds for his core claims. I have already sketched this basic evidence in section 1, in response to the question of the role of feelings in value judgments. Affirming these core claims rests on one's acceptance of at least two further propositions concerning their justification. The first proposition is that the most basic evidence on which this, or any other, dispute rests is the self-evidence of one's own conscious-intentional cognitive operations. The second proposition is that Lonergan's account of his own conscious-intentional operations is, for the most part, accurate.

In my own name, I affirm both of these propositions. I also contend that Lonergan correctly justifies his core claims concerning the role of feelings in value judgments on the basis of his cognitional theory. I accept Lonergan's cognitional theory, in which he purports to articulate the self-evidence of one's own conscious-intentional operations. This is, I suggest, the most basic kind of evidence to which anyone can appeal in advancing a knowledge claim, including the denial of this claim. In the 'laboratory' of attending, qua philosopher, to my own clinical performance qua physician, I invariably verify the general structure of cognitional operations that Lonergan articulates in his cognitional theory. My explication of Lonergan's position in chapters 4 to 7, using an extended medical example, provides evidence that Lonergan's cognitional model adequately accounts for my own cognitive performance as a physician.

Still, I also admit that the degree to which Lonergan's account of how feelings enter into this cognitive process, if found convincing, ultimately rests on the reader's own autobiographical self-retrieval. The question is, 'Do feelings enter into these judgments in the way that Lonergan suggests?' The answer must be based on the reader's own experience of knowing and, more particularly, of making evaluations. In my own name, I cannot but affirm the broad outlines of Lonergan's account as holding true in my own experience of making evaluations. To deny Lonergan's account of evaluative human cognition would ultimately involve me in some form of operational self-contradiction.[14]

Whether or not the reader agrees with Lonergan's account, I would still argue that it is important that philosophers and ethicists contribute to articulating the normative structure invariably in operation when one attains accurate knowledge of values. Such an articulation needs to take a stance on the role, if any, that feelings play in this process. One way to contrast and assess the merits of alternative models of evaluating is to examine the basic evidence to which thinkers appeal in support of their positions. Aside from the different models of knowing that thinkers such as Hume, Kant, and Lonergan articulate, there are also important differences between them on the issue of what each considers as the most basic evidence in support of their views.

For instance, Hume bases his account of knowing on the model of ocular vision. For him, knowing is a matter of perceiving. By extension, knowing the good (or values) is equivalent to experiencing feelings of approbation in relation to these perceptions. I interpret Hume's answer to the epistemic question to be that, in principle, knowing is epistemically objective if my perceptions and feelings refer not just to me but to some other, external world. But these conditions for epistemic objectivity are never fulfilled for Hume. As I pointed out in chapter 3, this is because he calls into question belief in the continued existence of external objects, and even of the self, since, given his own assumptions, he has no secure basis on which to affirm them. Hume's final position is one of experiential atomism and cognitional agnosticism. He concludes that the only things one can legitimately believe in are 'fleeting ideas and impressions.' The basic evidence to which Hume appeals in support of his position is the self-evidence of the phenomena of his own knowing.

Although Lonergan's account of his own normative structure as an evaluator differs from Hume's, there is agreement regarding what counts as the most basic evidence for any position on this issue – the data of one's own knowing. On these grounds, then, readers can judge for themselves which account is most in keeping with their performance as knowers and evaluators. On these grounds, it is significant to note, as did Lonergan, that there is a tension between Hume the author and his statements: 'In Hume the *author* ... and in the knowledge he uses to give his account, we have *more* than a manifold of sense impressions linked by habit.'[15] One wonders, then, if Hume's reflexive account of his knowing actually does justice to his own performance as a knower.

Just as Lonergan would challenge Hume's own self-descriptive account of human knowing, so also he would challenge not only the model of knowing that Kant's position presupposes, but also what Kant takes to be the most basic evidence in support of his stance. Kant's position on knowing, and what counts as the most basic evidence for any claim one makes, illustrates another important alternative to Lonergan's stance. For Kant, knowing the real is a matter not of perceiving or affective experiencing, as in Hume's case, but of 'abstractly understanding.' Knowing the good involves understanding the moral law; and such understanding obtains apart from any moral experience or natural inclination and so is abstract. In answer to the epistemic question, Kant distinguishes between knowing appearances (*phenomena*) and things as they really are in themselves (*noumena*). Kant, it may be argued, accepts the reality of supersensible entities or *noumena*; but he denies that one can have any genuine knowledge of them. On the epistemic question, then, Kant, like Hume, is agnostic.[16]

From Lonergan's perspective, however, the model of knowing that Kant presupposes fails to recognize the third and fourth levels, namely, those of fact and value judgment. For Lonergan, it is only 'in,' 'through,' or 'by means of' a fact or value judgment that one *knows* being or the good.[17] Moreover, one can also contrast their positions on what each counts as the most basic evidence to which one can appeal in support of any claim. Kant appeals not to the self-evidence of his own moral knowing, as do Lonergan and Hume. Rather, I would interpret Kant's position to be that the most basic evidence in support of his claims is given in his answer to the epistemic question of the very possibility of genuine knowledge, that is, the distinction between *phenomena* and *noumena*.

At the most basic level of this dispute between differing models of evaluative knowing are alternative answers to a question of phenomenal or self-descriptive fact, 'What am I doing when I am knowing facts or values?'[18] Lonergan expressly addresses this question of cognitional phenomenology as the most basic one. He maintains that this 'knowledge of knowing' is, in a sense, privileged knowledge in that it provides the most fundamental evidence for any author's claims.

I will now review what I take to be Lonergan's answers to a series of questions regarding the phenomenology, epistemology, and metaphysics of evaluations. My aim is to specify how his position makes important and original contributions to some key concerns that contemporary philosophers and ethicists seek to address.[19]

4.2 The Content of Lonergan's Philosophical Position

(1) In answer to the question of whether feelings have any relevance to value judgments, Lonergan maintains that certain feelings are indeed relevant. In particular, the relevant feelings are intentional, affective responses to values, which he distinguishes from both non-intentional feelings and intentional responses to satisfactions. Lonergan claims that all my cognitive acts are both intentional and conscious. As intentional, they are acts in and through which I achieve knowledge, make choices, and implement those choices. As conscious, they are the basic means through which I

am present to myself. Now, on the basis of my own self-appropriation, I may distinguish intellectual, intentional acts, such as direct or reflective insights, from affective intentional acts, such as those I have called 'deliberative insights.' In both cases, the by-products of these cognitive acts mediate my achieving some knowledge content. My summary expression of Lonergan's first core claim, namely, that certain feelings are relevant to value judgments, refers to the fact that certain intentional, affective acts are part of the *evidence* for a value claim. This evidence is distinct from the content of the claim I achieve by means of these cognitive operations. That is, Lonergan's first core claim is that my intentional affective response to a value is relevant to my knowing values because it is a key element of the evidence for the value judgments through which I know values.

This first claim is important because it highlights the necessary and positive cognitive role of feelings in value judgments. It also suggests that certain feelings are an integral part of human cognition. Nor does Lonergan affirm that certain feelings are just 'relevant' to value judgments. Rather, they are *necessary*, though not sufficient, conditions for knowing values. He insists, with Scheler, that without the capacity for these affective, cognitive acts I would be unable to achieve knowledge of values. To advance beyond facts to values, then, I need to be able to respond affectively to values. Lonergan's position is also important because it explicitly connects his general cognitional theory with some account of how feelings enter into evaluations. In so doing, Lonergan is able to support the view that treatments of both intellectual and affective cognitive acts are essential components of a comprehensive account of evaluative knowing. In this sense, his position strikes me as an important addition to the one-sided Humean or Kantian accounts.

Moreover, the claim that feelings are relevant to value judgments makes an original contribution to understanding some of the limitations of the split between philosophy and psychology. This position challenges psychologists who fail to distinguish between non-intentional and intentional affectivity. It suggests that they risk reducing all of human psychology to a pre-moral level. They also risk misunderstanding human affectivity by examining it in isolation from the evaluative dimension of intentional-affective acts. Lonergan's position also offers an original challenge to those philosophers who are apt to dismiss all human affectivity as either non-intentional or else merely intentional responses to satisfactions. Such philosophers would side with those psychologists who likewise consider feelings to have no real 'cognitive' importance for value judgments. Lonergan's position offers an original challenge to the 'intellectualist' cognitive theories these views presuppose.

Although Lonergan's claim that affectivity is relevant to value judgments may be novel in certain philosophical and psychological circles, many people would support his view, and base their support on their own moral experience. Many people experience the relevance of their own feelings for their evaluations and decisions. For such people, feelings are at least part of the conscious data to which they typically attend in seeking answers to evaluative questions. It is commonplace, for instance, for persons to advise others to 'listen to your heart' when they are deciding something. In as much as Lonergan's position agrees with this common moral experience, it is not particularly original or radical. It merely highlights these affective elements of evaluative knowing that most people already acknowledge; and it relates these acts to other cognitive processes. What is original in Lonergan's account is that it goes beyond many of these common views in the precision with which he speaks of both feelings and knowing. Hence, I think that Lonergan's first core claim, that affective responses, though not intellectual, are nevertheless cognitive acts relevant to evaluations, offers an important and original contribution to contemporary concerns in philosophy and ethics.

(2) Lonergan's answer to the epistemological question regarding whether such affectively based evaluations are just subjective in their content addresses the claim that any affective intentional act is epistemically just subjective. Understanding the force of this epistemological question helps one to appreciate the importance and originality of Lonergan's answer. What this claim of epistemic subjectivity for affectively based evaluations presupposes is a model of knowing that is based on an analogy with the visual act of looking. On this ocular model of knowing there arises the view that in order to 'see' correctly just what is 'out there' one needs to escape one's own subjectivity. On this model, short of such an escape from one's subjectivity, one's knowing is inevitably just subjective, rather than epistemically objective. So if value judgments are based in part on evidently personal affective responses, as Lonergan contends, the model dictates that such judgments cannot possibly achieve knowledge of anything beyond one's own subjective feelings. That is, it would seem that if these affective responses are merely psychological phenomena, the derivative value judgments will be irredeemably just epistemically subjective.

From Lonergan's perspective, however, on such suppositions one could also raise an objection about any intentional cognitive act, not only about those acts that are characteristically affective. The philosophical label for this issue is 'the problem of the bridge.' I have already outlined Lonergan's response to this problem in chapter 5. Since this problem has been such a basic one for modern philosophy and ethics, his response to it is of fundamental importance.

Lonergan rejects the view that all affective responses, and their derivative value judgments, are epistemically merely subjective. He denies the presupposition that is behind the problem of the bridge, namely, that the explicit distinction between self and other is primordially given in consciousness, rather than emerging as a subsequent cognitional achievement. This dispute really comes down to a question of phenomenal or self-descriptive fact. The question is whether or not one can adequately understand what one is doing when one is knowing by appealing to an analogy with the visual act of looking. Lonergan criticizes those whose positions presuppose such an analogy, and the derivative view of objectivity that this ocular model of knowing suggests. By contrast, he stresses that knowing is a discursive process that culminates with judgments that mediate one's knowledge of the real. In and through such judgments one affirms the real. If Lonergan's account of knowing is accurate, then the 'problem of the bridge' disappears. Whether the contents of knowledge I affirm regard self or others is no longer a key issue. Also, the further move from fact to value knowledge is not problematic for Lonergan because he recognizes that intentional affective acts, in part, ground evaluations of facts. From this perspective, he can speak about cognitional theory as an objectification or description of one's own knowing, which includes both intellectual and affective cognitive acts.[20]

Lonergan's rejection of the contention or presupposition that the distinction between *self* and *non-self* is utterly fundamental removes a key justification for the claim that one can dismiss the affective elements of knowing because such acts would inevitably render one's knowing just epistemically subjective. His position insists that affective responses, like intellectual insights, can legitimately ground evaluative claims that are epistemically objective. Such epistemically objective claims can be about either oneself, such as claims about features of one's own phenomenal subjectivity, or about something other than oneself. His stance challenges the position that one should suppress, distrust, and dismiss affective data because they are irredeemably epistemically just subjective. For him, there is no reason why one cannot achieve epistemically objective knowledge of values, even if this knowledge depends, in part, on acts that are characteristically affective.[21]

Part of the originality of Lonergan's contribution to the problem of the bridge is his introduction of several key categories. For instance, he distinguishes a series of related cognitional levels. Again, he distinguishes between one's cognitive acts and one's cognitive achievements. These categories also allow him to articulate a unity in the diversity of cognitive acts. Within this unity, he highlights those acts that are characteristically affective, such as deliberative insights, as against other, more intellectual, insights. From this perspective, all my cognitive acts are 'subjective' in the sense that I am conscious of them as my own. This stands in contrast to the intentional contents I achieve by means of these acts. Consequently, Lonergan argues convincingly that one should not distinguish between epistemically 'subjective' and 'objective' contents merely on the basis of whether the underpinning cognitive acts are affective or not. All my intentional acts are 'subjective' in as much as they are acts of a conscious subject. The methodologically prior issue is that of one's phenomenal, cognitional subjectivity. This is what I objectify as embodying the distinct and related operations of my cognitive performance. The methodologically subsequent issue involves achieving epistemic objectivity. I will treat this in reviewing Lonergan's fourth core claim.

(3) Lonergan's answer to the question regarding what grounds the distinction between facts and values, that is, what one addresses in 'is' or 'ought' questions or claims, contributes to a notion of ethics as an enterprise that entails 'ought' questions. One concretely generates an answer to 'ought' questions in a way that is quite distinct from the concrete process in which one generates answers to 'is' questions. Lonergan's account highlights a unique way of distinguishing fact and value claims by moving backwards from these *abstract* claims to the *concrete* processes that generate them. That is, his account moves from abstract conceptual and judgmental products, which are 'inner words' I express as the results of some insight, backward to the concrete insights that generate these inner words. In this way, Lonergan's account demonstrates a real difference between fact and value claims.

Lonergan's stance also challenges Hume's view that the distinction between facts and values must find its basis in logic, a view that denies that an 'ought' can be logically derived from an 'is.' According to Lonergan's intentionality analysis, one may indeed distinguish facts and values as cognitive achievements that address different questions and result from different cognitive processes. That is, they are categorial achievements that follow from third- and fourth-level cognitive operations. These distinct levels originate in the transcendental intentions that give rise to fact and value questions.[22] The transcendental intention of reality, in the case of fact questions, and the transcendental intention of value, in the case of value questions, are contained in my questions even prior to my answering them. The move from a fact judgment to raising a value question, however, is more than just a logical one. It is really part of the dynamic unfolding of my conscious intentionality. In summary terms, the concrete process that generates a fact judgment involves a reflective insight, which is quite distinct from the deliberative insight that generates a value judgment. Although Lonergan's analysis is consistent on this point with the Aristotelian tradition that I sketched in chapter 3, it provides original grounds for this tradition. Rather than grounding his analysis in metaphysical categories and faculty psychology, Lonergan expressly grounds his account of knowing facts and values in an intentionality analysis.[23]

An important contribution of Lonergan's analysis is his differentiation of logical, rational or reasonable, and responsible issues, all of which play a role in the enterprise of ethics. In his view, ethics focuses on questions of value. Answering these questions involves cognitive acts, such as deliberative insights, that depend on and sublate the achievements of the prior levels. For instance, one's third-level achievements attain knowledge of what is rational and reasonable, sublating the logical and conceptual achievements of the second level. One's success as an evaluator, then, depends not only on one's fourth-level performance, but also on one's performance on the prior levels. This philosophy has personal implications, for it offers some insight into features of one's own cognitive capacities that one might otherwise overlook. These are the clearly articulated, distinctive features of moral consciousness that mistaken philosophies are apt to obscure or dismiss. Lonergan's emphasis on the distinctiveness of evaluations provides an original basis for criticizing mistaken attempts either to downplay the importance of the prior levels in relation to fourth-level evaluations, or to reduce any questions of value to questions that are proper to prior levels. On the one side, for instance, the moral idealist tends to obscure the importance of knowledge of concrete human reality for value judgments. On the other side, a rationalist account of the moral law arguably inflates a part or component of moral knowing to the status of the whole.

Again, Lonergan's account makes an important contribution by undercutting Hume's problem of moving from an 'is' to an 'ought' claim. Hume presupposes, for example, that the only warrant for the move from facts to values is a logical one. Since Hume is unable to find the requisite warrant for this move in logic, he rejects its validity, and even the distinction. For Lonergan, by contrast, this move is simply part of the unfolding of intentional consciousness. His intentionality analysis does not imply that the move from facts to values is a strictly logical one. In fact, this move is analogous to the move from the first level of experiencing to the second level of understanding. Lonergan's position is that efforts to reduce questions of value to one part of the process of knowing, such as intelligent operations of understanding the intelligible or rational acts of fact judging, are mistaken because they inflate a part of the process to the status of the whole. Although this is a very basic philosophical point, it has enormous consequences. One need only consider some of the historical implications of mistaken cognitional theories.[24]

(4) Distinct from the question regarding whether the contents of my evaluations concern only self, rather than both self and what is other than

self, is the question regarding the epistemic objectivity of any fourth-level evaluation. A core feature of Lonergan's global position on the role of affectivity in value judgments is that such judgments, like fact judgments, can be epistemically objective. A condition for attaining this epistemic objectivity, however, is not the impossible task of escaping from my own phenomenal subjectivity. Instead, my attaining epistemic objectivity depends on the quality of my phenomenal, cognitive activities. Lonergan's whole project helps me to improve the quality, and hence the results, of my own phenomenal cognitive performance. It does this by heightening my attention to my phenomenal and epistemic performance, especially when my results are mistaken, as I engage questions of fact and value and proffer answers to these questions.

Lonergan expresses his fourth core claim in the formula 'Objectivity is simply the consequence of authentic subjectivity.'[25] In chapters 4 to 7 I provided some evidence from my own experiences of knowing in medicine that supports this claim. In chapters 4 and 6 I appropriated my phenomenal subjectivity in answering fact and then value questions in medicine. In chapters 5 and 7 I addressed the epistemological question that asks what made the difference between my correct and mistaken medical judgments. I concluded that the epistemic objectivity of my answers varied with the quality of my cognitive performance. That is, my medical judgments were 'epistemically objective' if my phenomenal performance was a matter of experiencing 'attentively,' understanding 'intelligently,' judging 'reasonably,' and evaluating 'responsibly.'

The view that my transcendental intention of value is the ultimate criterion for the epistemic objectivity of my value judgments makes an important contribution to ethics, for it places non-intellectual elements, such as affectivity, conscience and virtue, at the centre of the evaluative process. On this view, I grasp the correctness of my evaluations affectively, in the correspondence between my categorial and transcendental affectivity.[26] Although this may occur rapidly and easily, discerning may be difficult and take place gradually, perhaps even over many years.

Lonergan's account also emphasizes, correctly I think, the central importance of individual virtue and conscience. It rejects the view that there is some automatic guarantee of epistemic objectivity, either of fact or of value judgments. Like Aristotle, Lonergan is not concerned with the Kantian question of discovering necessary and universal conditions of all human knowledge. In fact, according to Lonergan's account, I can only be sure of the genuineness of my evaluations if I am a morally virtuous person, and I follow my conscience. According to this view, 'moral virtue' is the habit of operating in fidelity to the transcendental precepts or, more fundamentally, in fidelity to the transcendental intentions. In particular, it concerns the transcendental intention of value that leads to the fourth cognitional level, but it is also relevant to my fidelity to the other transcendental intentions. Hence, transcendental and categorial feelings, virtue and individual conscience, are all key elements in the process of moral discernment of what is a true, and not merely an apparent, value.

On Vertin's interpretation of Lonergan, which I am affirming, the affective dimension of the transcendental intention of value is the ultimate criterion for my categorial value judgments.[27] In some ways, this claim is not particularly original or novel. It is merely a technical way of speaking about something most traditions of thought are already familiar with. One might express the same claim as the affective demands of love. Even those people who are unfamiliar with Lonergan's categories or terminology are, I expect, personally familiar with the demands of love in interpersonal relationships. It is because of this familiarity that a mother recognizes, for instance, that certain concrete words or deeds are inconsistent with the general intending of value she has for her child. Even so, the traditional philosophical categories within which thinkers typically address moral questions are frequently incapable of appealing to, or of accommodating, the affective dimensions of human experience. By contrast, Lonergan's account of the role of feelings in value judgments helps to narrow the gap between moral experience and theory. In so doing, he has made an important contribution to key concerns in contemporary philosophy and ethics.

Finally, the distinction between Lonergan's first basic question, which seeks the phenomenal features of the cognitional process, and the second basic question, which seeks the epistemic features of the cognitional process, provides an original and clarifying response to some historical disputes that conflate these two issues. The philosophical concern that sets the context for the debate between Hume's and Kant's accounts of the moral law, for example, is an epistemic one. Hume concludes that passions do and ought to rule reason. He then concedes, however, that values and facts are epistemically merely subjective. Kant, by contrast, grounds morality in a necessary and universal moral law that is accessible to all rational beings. He does this, however, at the expense of rejecting the moral relevance of human affectivity or inclinations. Lonergan's contribution to this debate, I think, is to distinguish clearly Hume's methodologically prior phenomenal concerns from Kant's subsequent epistemic concerns. In response to Hume, Lonergan would affirm that certain feelings play an important role in value judgments. But he also challenges Hume's conclusion that such judgments are always just epistemically subjective. In response to Kant, Lonergan would affirm that we do sometimes achieve epistemically objective evaluations. In so doing, he challenges Kant's view that *noumena* are unknowable and Kant's oversight of judgments, and especially his oversight of the cognitive affective elements in concrete moral deliberations, and not merely aesthetic judgments. Even though an important element of evaluations involves affective cognitive operations, Lonergan maintains that such evaluations can reach beyond what is phenomenally just subjective, or epistemically just subjective, to achieve epistemically objective evaluations.

(5) Lonergan affirms, correctly I suggest, that although his account of value judgments emphasizes feelings, it nevertheless provides a basis for a 'metaphysics of values' or the invariant structure of the human good. An important contribution here is Lonergan's distinction between satisfactions and values. Lonergan helps one to be attentive to the affective grounds of evaluations and to distinguish judgments that are based on responses to satisfactions rather than to values. Yet even if one's judgment is based on a response to values, Lonergan also points out that these responses accord with some scale of preferences. The key point concerns disputes at the level of evaluations that have ramifications for alternative public policies. These may hinge on different affective responses underpinning the judgments. To be aware of these differences, then, may be a first step toward the goal of accurately identifying the basis of these disputes. This will ultimately help one to reach a judgment about the merits of the evidence supporting opposing views.

I will defer discussing some of these metaphysical issues to chapter 9. Before leaving my present effort of highlighting the importance of each of Lonergan's core claims, however, I will suggest that the strength of his overall position is greater than that of the sum of its parts. What Lonergan has elaborated is a cognitive theory that integrates the affective dimension of human cognition into his previously well-developed intellectualist cognitional theory. The later Lonergan expands his earlier account of human knowing to include not merely direct and reflective insights, but also those insights that Vertin has labelled 'deliberative insights.' The key point is that, in contrast to direct and reflective insights, deliberative insights are distinctively and crucially affective. This makes an important contribution to philosophy by providing the grounds for reintegrating the discussion of human affectivity, now largely confined to psychology, back into the philosophical sphere. Besides philosophy's understanding of its task as one of educating 'minds,' Lonergan's account insists, correctly in my view, on the further and complementary task of educating 'hearts.' Both intellectual and affective educations are crucial to a complete moral education. One implication of Lonergan's position is that philosophers interested in morality may need to educate themselves in psychology, and work more closely with persons specializing in it.

Finally, Lonergan's insistence on distinguishing responses to satisfactions from responses to values offers an original framework for considering the process of deliberation. People frequently speak about having 'mixed feelings' about some moral proposition. Lonergan's theoretical framework helps us to identify and label feelings that may result in conflicting evaluations, either in oneself or in others. Values that I affirm or seek to achieve may nevertheless be dissatisfying to me. For instance, taking chemotherapy may make me feel ill and leave me hairless, both of which I may experience as dissatisfying. Still, I may affirm the value of this arduous course of action as a means of restoring my health. Although feelings play a key role in moral deliberations for Lonergan, he also acknowledges the mixture of opposed feelings I may have about particular values; for instance, athletes often speak of accepting short-term pain for long-term gain. The fact that we do experience mixed feelings concerning particular questions of value is a reason that value questions require deliberation. Moral discernment is, on this view, the process of concretely 'sorting out' opposed affective responses. For Lonergan, a key task of this 'sorting out' is to distinguish between one's responses to values and one's responses to satisfactions, in order to base one's evaluations and rankings on the former.

5   Difficulties regarding Lonergan's Philosophical Position, and Some Responses

There are three key difficulties or objections that readers are apt to raise regarding Lonergan's global position on the role of affectivity in value judgments. These difficulties or objections involve questions readers may have about Lonergan's account of the phenomena of the affective life as it relates to value judging, his interpretation of these phenomena, and the normative and universal conclusions he draws from his interpretation.

First, some readers might object that Lonergan does not delve into the phenomena of the affective life deeply enough. Consequently, they may charge that Lonergan gives us an overly optimistic and intellectualized account of the role of feelings in value judgments. Second, some readers may object that the distinctions shaping Lonergan's discussion of feelings, such as his distinction between responses to satisfactions and to values, cause Lonergan to project these categories onto the reality of the moral life. This objection might be most evident to those readers for whom this distinction does not resonate with their own experience. Third, some readers might object that Lonergan goes too far in concluding that there is an invariant cognitive structure in human beings that underpins a normative scale of preferences among values. Indeed, they may be uneasy with some of the theological implications of Lonergan's view of human nature, which they may see as merely a different way of expressing what has traditionally been expressed as the 'natural law.' Again, philosophers might object to Lonergan's notion of an invariant cognitive structure by charging that he attempts to draw extremely general conclusions about knowing and the known based merely on his own cognitional self-retrieval. For each of these three global objections, I will identify their force and suggest how I would respond to their challenge in defending what I take to be Lonergan's position.

5.1 Is Lonergan's Retrieval of the Data of Feelings Too Selective?

The first objection to Lonergan's account of the role of feelings in value judgments is that he fails to discuss the full range of feelings. In particular, he seems to neglect those feelings, of which readers may be acutely aware, that seem to have a detrimental effect on one's own evaluations. Lonergan's position, then, seems open to the charge that his positive account of the role of feelings in value judgments results from this selective attention to a restricted range of affective data. In the objector's view, in *Method in Theology* Lonergan attends mainly to those feelings that are 'intentional.' His focus on intentional feelings overplays the cognitive importance of feelings with respect to value judgments. For instance, Lonergan would frame a decision by a fourteen-year-old homeless girl to have a child according to the categories of responses to satisfactions or values. But it also seems plausible that such a decision could really be based on feelings that are non-intentional, such as an instinctive drive to procreate, depression, anxiety about being alone, or pressure to do what one's peers are doing.[28]

The focus of this objection concerns the classification of feelings as either non-intentional or intentional. For this distinction, Lonergan expressly follows Scheler. He defines 'non-intentional feelings' as feeling 'states' (e.g., anxiety) or 'trends or urges' (e.g., hunger). These feelings are often what persons spontaneously think of when the issue of affectivity is raised. But Lonergan insists that distinct from these 'feelings' are the intentional, affective acts he calls 'intentional responses.'[29] Non-intentional feelings (e.g., fatigue) have some physiological basis (e.g., lack of rest). Still, they do not arise out of any cognitive achievement (e.g., I first feel tired, then I diagnose the problem to be a lack of rest). By contrast, intentional, affective responses are in a distinct class of feelings because they answer to some cognitive content, to what I intend, apprehend, or represent. These intentional feelings relate me not to some cause or goal, as with non-intentional feelings, but to some object.

Even granting this distinction, some readers might still object that the feelings Lonergan labels 'non-intentional,' such as anxiety, depression, hunger, or sexual discomfort, are the ones that are most prominent in their own evaluations. They may wonder why Lonergan de-emphasizes the role of these non-intentional feelings in his account, and why he focuses instead on feelings that are 'intentional.' Part of the force of this objection is that it challenges Lonergan's position regarding the basis of his phenomenological retrieval of the affective life. The objection suggests not only that Lonergan's retrieval is too restricted, but also that the pre-intentional dimension of affectivity is also relevant to the moral philosopher seeking to provide an adequate account of moral evaluations. To the extent that this objection is consistent with Lonergan's own insistence on the methodological priority of cognitional phenomenology, it challenges him to return to the phenomena of the affective life and of value judging. One implication of this objection is that one may need to revise or expand Lonergan's own position to take better account of the role of non-intentional feelings in value judgments.

Part of the difficulty I face in addressing this challenge is identifying genuine examples of evaluations on which to reflect. Further tasks involve labelling, locating, and understanding the function of the various types of feelings that enter into these evaluations. This challenge is greater than the terminological difficulty of labelling affective data that characterize the processes of heart, and are distinct from those of mind. It also involves the further difficulties of articulating how these affective responses relate to evaluations, and evaluations to judgments, on the one hand, and to decisions, on the other. But the fundamental challenge is to generate examples of evaluating that occur concretely in one's own life. Such a starting point is preferable to beginning merely by constructing 'intellectual' dilemmas, which is what students typically do in moral philosophy classes.

The challenge of finding moral examples on which to base one's phenomenological account of evaluating is even greater than the one Lonergan encountered in his early career when he focused on the intellectual cognitive acts of understanding. In *Insight* Lonergan took pains to draw out various facets of acts of understanding and to relate them to other cognitive acts. The strategy of the early Lonergan was to provide his readers with a series of examples in which they could experience themselves understanding something. By this method, readers could identify, label, and distinguish, in their own experience, the acts of experiencing, understanding, and judging. By contrast, the later Lonergan does not provide the relevant examples of evaluations for readers to appropriate their own affective responses to values or deliberative insights. One reason for this might be, as Frederick Crowe suggests, that one requires personal examples of moral problems and decisions in order to have access to the relevant existential, affective dimensions of evaluations. In this sense, examples are of limited usefulness when it comes to elucidating the role of feelings in evaluations. This is because any 'practice' of evaluative decision-making, by the very fact that it is merely practice, paradoxically is no practice at all.[30]

The focus of Lonergan's discussion of feelings in *Method in Theology* concerns the affectivity of intentional responses to values. By contrast, many of the historical thinkers I reviewed in chapter 3 focus on that aspect of human affectivity that falls under Lonergan's category of non-intentional feelings. When they speak of 'feelings,' they are referring primarily to affective data that are non-intentional, such as feelings of hunger or anxiety. These data are neither properly intentional nor cognitive, but are feelings that are caused (and may be countered) by physiological or pre-conscious mechanisms (e.g., a depression induced by a low level of thyroid hormone). So, is Lonergan's whole discussion, then, seriously flawed by his inattention to non-intentional feelings?

I would concede the phenomenological point that lies behind these objections. That is, in *Method in Theology* Lonergan may not have attended sufficiently to the influences of non-intentional feelings on evaluations. Indeed, he may have deliberately prescinded from attending to non-intentional, affective data for a number of reasons. Some of these reasons might be similar to the reasons many of the philosophers mentioned previously prescind from all affective data. That is, Lonergan may have considered them to be not *immediately* relevant to a discussion of evaluations. Whatever his reason for this omission, I think further contributions to understanding the relationship between non-intentional and intentional affectivity are important. I suspect not only that non-intentional affectivity conditions my evaluative processes, but also that my evaluations, in turn, condition my non-intentional affectivity.[31] For instance, in reflecting on my own life decisions, such as decisions to study medicine and philosophy, I recognize that they have a lot to do with personality traits. These, in turn, were substantially shaped by factors such as my position in a large family, early life experiences, friends, and so forth. Although I admit that these issues are very much affective, they still have little to do with the sort of cognitive processes that Lonergan explicates.[32]

This being said, Lonergan was aware of the effect of non-intentional feelings on evaluations, and he did think that these effects are philosophically important. In *Insight*, for instance, his negative tone toward feelings as concerns value judgments emerges in his discussion of the biases.[33] Still, he did not attempt to exhaust the phenomenal issues in his analysis of value judgments in *Method in Theology*. In fact, as I note in chapter 1, Lonergan acknowledges that value judgments have many facets to them, but he thought the fruitfulness of analysing all these facets is limited.[34]

5.2 Does Lonergan Foist His Categories onto Reality?

Readers may also make the twofold objection that not only does Lonergan project his own categories onto reality, but also those categories are themselves questionable. For instance, readers may find Lonergan's distinction between feelings that are intentional responses to satisfactions and to values to be problematic. Moreover, they may also question Lonergan's ranking of values, and therefore object that he foists his own ranking of values onto reality. That is, where in the prior objection Lonergan seems unaware of affective phenomena that are evident to some readers, in this case other readers object that Lonergan sees things in his own affective life or that his account of the moral life is one that does not register with them.

To take the first part of this objection, as I have frequently mentioned, Lonergan maintains that intentional affective responses regard two main classes of objects: 'on the one hand, the agreeable or disagreeable, the satisfying or dissatisfying; on the other hand, values, whether the ontic value of persons or the qualitative value of beauty, understanding, truth, virtuous acts, noble deeds.'[35]

Responses to satisfactions are ambiguous as regards values, for what is satisfying may or may not also be a true good. That is, it may happen that what is a true good is also disagreeable. This distinction is important since only those feelings that are intentional, affective responses to values are helpful guides to my knowing true values. But if I am unable to distinguish my affective responses to satisfactions from those that regard values, all my feelings will be ambiguous guides to values. Furthermore, to take the second part of this objection, Lonergan claims that I do not simply respond to values in isolation. I also relate them to one another according to some scale of preferences. In ascending order, he distinguishes vital, social, cultural, personal, and religious values. Some readers may rebut these distinctions and claims and, consequently, charge that Lonergan is foisting his mistaken categories not only onto his own affective life, but also onto reality. In the previous example of the fourteen-year-old homeless girl who wishes to have a child, the feelings that underpin this decision seem to be too complex and mixed for one to categorize them neatly as non-intentional or intentional; intentional, affective responses to satisfactions or to values, or responses predominantly to either vital, social, cultural, personal, or religious values. Even if Lonergan's categories are correct and the ambiguity of feelings that arise in this particular case could be sorted out, the further question remains as to whether it is legitimate ever to 'impose' or 'project' such categories onto reality. Is such a projection ever justified?

In response, I would acknowledge that there is an ambiguity that enters into a philosophical discussion of the affective life as it relates to the cognitive life. This ambiguity makes speaking of feelings more difficult than speaking about the intellectual aspects of human cognition. Part of the ambiguity of the affective life occurs because one only rarely has either an entirely positive or an entirely negative affective response to some object. Rather, one's affective responses are typically 'mixed' with simultaneously occurring contrary responses to a given object. It is for this reason that Lonergan suggests that the image of 'uni-dimensional time' does not do justice to the complexities of the life of feeling. For him, a better image is that of music, which expresses a 'multi-dimensional now.' The affective life finds expression in the rhythms of music, and conversely music provides one with an auditory image of the affective life.[36] Consequently, it should not be surprising if some readers fail to grasp certain distinctions that Lonergan draws concerning the affective life. What I would urge, however, is that just because some readers do not identify Lonergan's categories in their own self-awareness, that does not mean that their own position is invulnerable, as their question seems to suggest.[37]

Consider the objection that Lonergan is projecting his own categories onto reality in distinguishing satisfactions and values. One way that I might respond to this challenge is by considering some examples. I have sought to illustrate one side of this distinction by means of the example of the drug addict who bases his decisions on responses to satisfactions rather than to values. To illustrate responses to values, one might consider the war hero whose acts of self-sacrificing love for his comrades or country are motivated by something other than responses to satisfactions. In more traditional terms, Lonergan's distinction expresses the difference between the sensible and the intellectual appetites, or between one basing one's decisions either on what is sensibly gratifying or on what conforms with right reason.

The key issue that Lonergan seeks to highlight here, I think, is really a methodological point, rather than some metaphysical claim. The point is that if all human knowing is discursive, the epistemic objectivity of any claim is a function of its relation to its ground and ultimate criterion. When it comes to evaluative claims, one needs to move beyond the content of the claim to ask whether its author arrives at the conclusion on the basis of his or her response to values rather than to satisfactions. To base one's evaluation on responses to satisfactions is to adopt an ambiguous criterion. Such a criterion may answer the question of whether something is agreeable to me. But it cannot answer the question of whether it is truly worthwhile, that is, is it a value? This is not to say that the fact that something is dissatisfying, or even aesthetically unpleasing to me, is irrelevant to its value. The point here is merely that the evidence for judging whether something is worthwhile should be whether the conditions demanded by my intending of transcendental value are fulfilled. In other words, the ultimate criterion for a value judgment ought to be whether something satisfies one's transcendental intending of value.[38]

To illustrate the issue more fully, consider four possible combinations of objects that are satisfying or dissatisfying, and/or values or disvalues. One possibility would be those objects that are evidently good in as much as they are both satisfying and values; for instance, the vital value of tasty red apples. A second possibility would be those objects that are evidently bad because they are both dissatisfying and disvalues; e.g., the vital disvalue of foul-smelling rotten apples. A third possibility are those objects that, though satisfying in some sense, are disvalues; e.g., cigarettes or cocaine. Finally, a forth possibility are those objects that, though dissatisfying, are nevertheless values; e.g., some forms of chemotherapy.[39]

Whether one's ultimate criteria for judging something to be choiceworthy are satisfactions or are values seems to be a key issue in the euthanasia debate. In this debate the question arises whether the ontic value of life may be undermined by the fact that this life has become excessively dissatisfying. This becomes an especially persuasive consideration if the dissatisfaction someone experiences cannot be remedied, such as intractable pain in an individual whose life is nearly over. Still, on Lonergan's account, whether one's life is more dissatisfying than satisfying is an ambiguous criterion for determining its true value. So if one affirms the ontic value of someone's life based on a response to values, this sets the context within which one makes decisions about how one ought to respond to a person who expresses suicidal ideas.

Still, an objector might counter that basing one's choices on responses to values rather than to satisfactions is fine for some people, but why should others follow this procedure? Moreover, what right does Lonergan have imposing this view on others? Although I will return to this issue again in chapter 9, I will briefly outline the personal thrust of Lonergan's claim. In making this objection, Lonergan contends that the objector is overlooking an aspect of their own performance. Hence, the issue is one of 'self-insight' or 'self-discovery,' rather than an issue of Lonergan or others 'imposing' alien standards on other people.

It is helpful to begin with the objector's insistence that what one means by values are those things that one finds satisfying in some sense. On Lonergan's own account, 'particular goods' are objects that are satisfactions insofar as they meet the needs of a particular individual. He understands such needs in the broadest sense to include wants of every kind.[40] One might avoid some of the difficulties of making a sharp distinction between satisfactions and values by expressing distinct human goods as the satisfaction or fulfilment of various desires of the human person. Accordingly, I may experience a range of yearnings, the ranking of which becomes evident when some desires conflict with others. Then, I must choose between them. Conceived in this manner, one might do better to avoid the categories of faculty psychology, which result in the tendency to regard sensitive goods as always being opposed to intellectual goods. One might say that some things, such as cocaine, though temporarily 'satisfying' certain desires, fail to be choiceworthy as terminal values because they impede or destroy the deepest desires of human persons for achieving meaning, truth, and value in their lives, desires that Lonergan articulates in terms of the intending of transcendental intelligibility, reality, and value. I would submit that some such assessment by individuals and communities regarding what is 'truly worthwhile' is behind laws and public policies. One may express such an assessment in absolutist language when what is being considered are things that clearly threaten the good of the community as, for example, the 'satisfying disvalue' of certain recreational drugs like cocaine.

But what if the objector does not experience the affective dimension of their own evaluations in a way that agrees with Lonergan's analysis and therefore complains that Lonergan is foisting his own categories onto the real? I would respond, first, by emphasizing that the objector correctly identifies the issue as an autobiographical one. The objection arises, I contend, because there are differences between Lonergan's and the objector's cognitive self-retrieval. I submitted evidence in support of Lonergan's account from my own self-retrieval as a physician in chapters 4 to 7. The challenge for readers who hold a contrary view is to provide more convincing evidence for their claims. If they agree with Lonergan that the most basic evidence to which anyone can appeal is the evidence of one's own cognitive processes, then differences are reducible to differences in one's cognitive self-retrieval. These differences may occur if one party is either overlooking, or indeed fleeing from, further relevant data or questions. In the measure that I would welcome such critical input from readers, and be prepared to change as a result of it, I assume a similar commitment on the part of objectors. Of course, some philosophers may object that this sort of cognitive self-examination is too personal and is not 'real' philosophy, at least as they understand it in some modern, analytical sense. I would argue, however, that there is an ancient warrant for such an autobiographical view of philosophy. It can be traced back to Socrates and is given in the sage's wise advice to 'know thyself.'[41]

It is also worth pointing out Lonergan's own response to the general objection of some thinkers that one 'projects' certain intelligible unities, relations, or necessities onto the real. Lonergan counters that such an objection illustrates a basic counterposition to his own cognitional theory.

For him, the distinction that this objection presupposes is between imma-nent and projected intelligibilities. He argues that this is a distinction that is necessarily made by an 'empiricist' or 'naive realist.' For these thinkers, 'immanent intelligibility' is the one you know by taking a good look at what really is out there. By contrast, 'projected intelligibility' is the one you think out in your own mind but do not see in the object. Since Lonergan disclaims the presuppositions of both the empiricist and the naive realist, he also rejects the importance of their distinction between immanent and projected intelligibilities. The distinction that is significant for him is be-tween intelligibilities that one affirms in true judgments and those that one does not affirm. On this issue, he concludes: '[F]rom one viewpoint of the nature of knowledge a distinction between immanent and projected intelli-gibilities may be plausible, but if one's criterion of the real is truth then the only relevant division of intelligibilities is between those truly affirmed and those not affirmed or able to be affirmed.'[42]

In responding to the challenge that Lonergan is foisting his categories onto the real, then, I would face the objector's own cognitive self-retrieval. I would also critically examine, or, better yet, ask the objector to examine, the adequacy of the cognitional model that he or she presupposes. For that is what is at the heart of this objection to Lonergan's position.

5.3 Does Lonergan Imagine That There Are Transhistorical Features of Human Subjects?

One might also object to Lonergan's claim that there are 'transhistorical' constants in the cognitional operations of the human subject. A specific form of this objection might run counter to the claim that 'feelings' are a transcultural element of human moral deliberations. Some readers may accept that feelings are somehow relevant to personal evaluations. But they may reject the further claim Lonergan makes that one sometimes goes beyond one's feelings in affirming true evaluations. More generally, they may counter that all one's cognitional operations are ultimately and radi-cally contingent on such things as one's psychology, social background, culture, or other historical factors. On this view, not only do one's particu-lar feelings dictate one's evaluations, but one's particular feelings are entirely dependent upon or dictated by cultural and historical influences. Hence, there is no such thing as a basic cognitional method that one can generalize to include all instances of human knowing that occur across historical and cultural contexts.

To support this counter-claim, such readers might invoke the evidence of history. They could point out that the whole attention to 'method' is a relatively modern phenomenon. Only with the development of modern science in the seventeenth century did thinkers emphasize methodological issues and make them thematic. Such readers might further claim that there are numerous examples of persons within one's own time and culture who operate according to, and even articulate, distinct cognitional models. How can Lonergan presume to speak of the existence in every human subject of an invariant cognitional structure? When it comes to evaluations, what about those persons whose deliberations consistently answer to conditions of mere satisfaction rather than of value, as the case of the drug addict seems to illustrate? If Lonergan is correct in claiming that the desire to know the good, which one expresses in questions for deliberation, is a universal human experience, how does one account for those who maintain that such questions never seem to arise in their experience, or who insist that Lonergan's account does not apply to them?

Before I respond to these objections, it is important to be clear about what Lonergan is claiming, and what he takes to be the ultimate evidential basis for his claims. Lonergan's fundamental claim is that there exists a multi-levelled subject. He characterizes these levels according to the distinct cognitive operations of experiencing, understanding, judging, and evaluating. On the fourth level of evaluating, the subject engages in certain intentional, affective acts that are distinct from the intentional, intellectual acts, such as reflective insights, that occur on the third level. In addition, affectivity enters into evaluations on the fourth level in two ways. It enters in the subject's intending of transcendental value, which is the affectivity that characterizes one's fourth level transcendental intending. It also enters by way of one's categorial intentional responses to, or intending of, values, which I have been referring to as deliberative insights. Lonergan's basic claim is not merely that the account of such a multi-levelled subject accurately expresses the results of his own cognitional self-retrieval. He proposes that such an account also holds true for his readers; and he invites his readers to verify this account by attending to their own cognitional performance. Accordingly, he would suggest that those who bring forward the present objection are overlooking or truncating an aspect of their own self-retrieval of their performance. In other words, they are inadvertently overlooking some aspect of their conscious data.[43]

By contrast with the possible objection of some readers that their manner of arriving at value judgments is at odds with Lonergan's account, Lonergan argues that there is an invariant structure of the human subject that is a transhistorical, transcultural constant. One may discover such an invariant structure of the human subject operative and expressed in evaluations that have been made throughout the ages of recorded human history. To those who object to this thesis, Lonergan counters that, in their very attempt to deny verbally this claim, they inevitably invoke operationally the very structure they verbally reject. Finally, although Lonergan insists that this is a question that one has to answer for oneself, he does not think that the answers are in serious doubt:

> Not even behaviorists claim that they are unaware whether or not they see or hear, taste or touch. Not even positivists preface their lectures and their books with the frank avowal that never in their lives did they have the experience of understanding anything whatever. Not even relativists claim that never in their lives did they have the experience of making a rational judgment. Not even determinists claim that never in their lives did they have the experience of making a responsible choice. There exist subjects that are empirically, intellectually, rationally, morally conscious. Not all know themselves as such, for consciousness is not human knowing but only a potential component in the structured whole that is human knowing. But all can know themselves as such, for they have only to attend to what they are already conscious of, and understand what they attend to, and pass judgment on the correctness of their understanding.[44]

Thus, the most fundamental evidence to which one might appeal for or against Lonergan's claim that this multi-levelled subject exists is the self-evidence of one's own cognitional operations. I affirm that even in the specialized field of medicine, I proceed according to this general structure. Hence, I must also affirm that what holds true in Lonergan's own self-retrieval also holds true for myself. By extension, I would also maintain that the same holds true for others who may have never seriously attended to, understood, or tried to make thematic their own successful cognitive performance. As for the apparent counter-evidence advanced by those who affirm radically different cognitional structures, I grant I must remain open to the possibility that they are highlighting elements of myself that I may have overlooked. But it is not likely I would be convinced of their claims unless they were able to point out what I had overlooked. That is, their arguments would only be convincing to me if, besides rejecting Lonergan's thesis, they provided an alternative cognitional theory. Moreover, their own theory would need to be based on an appeal to the fundamental evidence of the data of consciousness that better articulates how they, and I, actually operate as successful knowers. If one were to undertake such a project, however, one would need to grant the central claim of Lonergan's philosophy, which is that knowledge of one's cognitional and decisional subjectivity is key to any philosophy.[45]

A further practical question remains for me to address: namely, how

Lonergan's stance on the role of affect in evaluations contributes to understanding and assessing and, ultimately, facilitates evaluations with regard to issues that may arise in medical ethics. I will begin to answer this important question in the next chapter by reflecting on the evaluations that arose in the end-of-life stories that I discussed in chapter 2.

9

Ramifications of Lonergan's Position for the Euthanasia Debate

Medicine has perennial moral problems, two of which are particularly serious in the present age: insensitivity to suffering and abuse of power. The distancing produced by our abstractions makes us especially prone to the first; our greatly enhanced prognostic and therapeutic power makes us especially liable to the second. Reforming our clinical method has at its deepest level a moral purpose: a restoration of the balance between thinking and feeling and a renunciation, or at least a sharing, of the enormous power modern technology has given us.

Ian McWhinney, 'The Importance of Being Different'

1   Introductory Remarks

The goal of the present chapter is to engage the polemical euthanasia debate and to make a positive and original contribution to the debate itself. I hope to highlight how accepting Lonergan's account of cognitional and decisional subjectivity has important ramifications for understanding and appraising key evaluations that are at the centre of medical-ethical debates such as that on euthanasia. More specifically, I will highlight some ramifications of Lonergan's position for the euthanasia debate on three distinct levels: first, for understanding and assessing particular stories from which requests for euthanasia might arise; second, for the ethical debate concerning such requests; and third, for the public-policy discussion about how society ought to respond to such requests. I shall attempt to show how presuppositions about the role of affect in evaluations shape the debate and how Lonergan's philosophical position and categories help to clarify the distinct types of questions that are being raised at each of these levels.

To illustrate some of these ramifications concretely, then, I will turn again to the stories of Sue Rodriguez and Dennis Kaye. In the earlier discussion, I adopted a 'bottom-up' approach by starting with particular stories as a basis for identifying the questions that were being asked and for reflecting on more general philosophical issues. Now, however, I am in a position to use Lonergan's answers to some of these general philosophical questions in a 'top-down' approach. (Cf. table A.1, p. 310.) The aim is to demonstrate the fruitfulness of this methodological experiment to those who regard these two approaches as somehow mutually exclusive.[1]

2   Interpreting the Positions of Sue Rodriguez and Dennis Kaye

In chapter 8 I sought to pin down Lonergan's position by specifying what I took to be his answers to six core questions that relate affect and evaluations, and I articulated and defended his answers to these questions. In this section, I will respond to these same questions on the basis of what I have gathered from the life stories of Sue Rodriguez and Dennis Kaye. Since neither Sue nor Dennis were professional philosophers, this will require that I interpret and extrapolate from their stories answers that are most consistent with their words and deeds. In the end, I acknowledge that the answers I construct, based on the available information, might not accurately reflect their actual historical positions in every respect. Nevertheless, the main point of this exercise will not be entirely lost. By comparing and contrasting what I take to be their stances on these questions I hope to show how persons on opposite sides of this debate can have similar as well as differing answers to these questions about cognitional and decisional subjectivity. I will also show the relationship of these answers to Lonergan's. In so doing, I hope to be able to attend better to some of the concrete, human dimensions of the life stories of Sue and Dennis. Their stories include not only the previously explored psycho-social, cultural, and religious areas, but also their philosophical presuppositions concerning cognitional and decisional subjectivity and how these relate to their stances on euthanasia.

Part of the importance of attending to these stories is that they suggest the possibility that the debate might be focusing on points that are not problems for persons such as Sue and Dennis, such as the distinction between killing and allowing to die. Conversely, the larger ethical and legislative debates might also be overlooking crucial ethical issues that Sue and Dennis did in fact face. For example, little attention has been given to Sue's concerns about the effects of her illness on her son, or to Dennis's deliberations about artificial respiration as he became weaker. In addition, as Dennis's story illustrates, little ethical attention has been given to the impact of this whole ethical discussion on people in situations similar to the situations of Sue and Dennis. For instance, Sue's contention that her life would not be worth living if she became as incapacitated as persons like Dennis raises the issue of the generalizability of such self-evaluations. Only by attending to such stories can one begin to wonder what impact society's apparent agreement with Sue that such a life is not worth living must have on others who are similarly disabled.

2.1 Do Feelings Ever Play a Cognitive Role in My Knowing?

In chapter 8, I argued that Lonergan answers this question with an unambiguous 'Yes.' He distinguishes between feelings that are non-intentional states or trends and intentional, affective responses.[2] Indeed, for Lonergan, affective responses are not only cognitively important; they are *necessary conditions* for knowing objects as satisfactions or values. This places Lonergan's philosophical stance on the relation between reason and emotions within what in chapter 3 I called the 'heart' tradition. It also places Lonergan's stance outside of other families of thinkers who would reject outright the cognitive relevance of feelings.[3]

In chapter 2, I provided evidence from the stories of Sue Rodriguez and Dennis Kaye for the view that they both consider feelings to be cognitively relevant. On my reading of their stories, there is ample evidence to support the claim that Sue and Dennis's common-sense answer to this question, if they were to formulate it, would agree with Lonergan's philosophically formulated answer. They both presuppose in effect that at least some feelings are relevant to their cognitive processes. Moreover, they appear to regard certain feelings as *necessary* conditions for making certain knowledge claims.[4]

Let me provide an example to support this interpretation. Both Sue and Dennis express the cognitive importance of *personal* involvement in order to understand the issues that persons who are dying face. This is an important clue that leads me to conclude that both would agree that some feelings are relevant and necessary components of human cognition. I would suggest that what such a personal involvement adds to an intellectual or theoretical engagement of such issues is a necessary emotional dimension. Both Sue and Dennis contend, for instance, that a *necessary* condition for making a meaningful contribution to this discussion is that one needs to have some personal experience of dying. Sue, for instance, is dismissive of apparent 'experts' who speak on this issue from merely a theoretical perspective. She speaks of the deficiency of the views of those who are healthy and in the midst of life and who 'chose not to enter that world [of the dying] with open hearts to see the realities.'[5] What does she think might be added to their merely theoretical perspectives if they were to have some concrete, particular experience of dying? What I think she is referring to in her recommendation that others 'open their hearts' is that their views need to be supplemented by being attentive and sensitive to the emotional elements of her experience of ALS.[6]

The deficiency both she and Dennis are highlighting in these experts, I suggest, is the denial of the cognitive relevance of feelings. In this respect, I would think Dennis and Sue represent what I would call the 'common sense' view. Note that they are not suggesting a deficiency exists in these experts at the level of intellect or reason. Nor is it simply a matter of restricted life experience. The problem lies elsewhere, at the level of what Sue refers to as 'heart.' The remedy for this problem is not to draw finer distinctions or demand greater logical rigour, at least not initially. In other words, the problem is not that these experts have lost their reason. Rather, they have lost or at least are not engaging something other than their theoretical reason, something symbolized by 'heart.' Hence, both Dennis and Sue seem to agree with Lonergan on this point, that personal affective responses are necessary conditions for human knowing. As will become more evident, one's answer to this first question sets the stage for, and in some way shapes, one's answers to the following core questions on this list. Indeed, different answers to this first question seem to me to be at the centre of the euthanasia debate.

2.2 If Some Feelings Are Cognitive, How Do They Relate to My Knowledge?

Lonergan's answer to this second question is that feelings that are intentional responses *partly* ground my cognitive access to satisfactions or values. That is, affective cognitions are never sufficient grounds for my knowing. Combining his answers to these first two questions, one can say that Lonergan's claim is that some feelings are *necessary* cognitive conditions for knowing well, but they are not *sufficient*. I interpret Sue's position to be that at least some feelings are both *necessary* and *sufficient* conditions for certain knowledge claims.[7] For Sue, there seems to be some *immediate* relation between certain feelings and knowledge claims. In comparing the answers of Sue and Dennis to this question, it appears that Dennis's position agrees with Lonergan's in as much as he recognizes that feelings partly ground knowing, but are themselves open to development, just as knowledge claims are open to further questions and discernment.[8]

Some evidence for Sue's view that feelings are sufficient for knowledge claims is her resistance to having her claims challenged, as if any such challenge would, in principle, be unfair. That is, a possible consequence of Sue's presuppositions regarding the sufficiency of feelings for knowing is that this position tends to make her excessively defensive toward anyone who challenges her conclusions. Since such a challenge is, on Sue's presupposition, intrinsically flawed or philosophically wrong-headed, for it seems to her that any such challenge had to be motivated only by the desire of others to 'meddle in her personal life.'[9] As Hobbs Birnie relates, Sue regards any such critical comments of her views as evidence of a lack of compassion by others toward her.[10]

2.3 How Are Cognitive Feelings Related to My Knowing Values or Evaluations? Do Such Evaluations Ever Yield More than Just Subjective Knowledge?

Lonergan's short answer to this third, two-part question is that feelings that are affective responses to values relate *mediately* to evaluations, and that such evaluations, based in part on affect, can be *epistemically objective*. Sue's short answer seems to differ from Lonergan's on both points. I would argue that, for her, feelings are related *immediately* to evaluations, and that 'most' evaluations are *epistemically just subjective*.[11] On both questions, I would argue that Dennis's position is compatible with Lonergan's.[12]

This contrast becomes clear in a key interchange between Dennis and Sue, which Dennis reports in his book. The interchange was sparked by an interview Sue gave in which she reported that she did not want to linger in life until she was reduced to 'a mere biological existence.' In a letter to Sue, Dennis wrote: 'I know it wasn't your intention but coming from someone in much better shape than me, it was a painful thing to hear.'[13] To make the point that feelings are necessary elements of knowing, that they partly ground knowledge claims, that they are related to evaluations, and that such evaluations are not epistemically just subjective, it is important to grasp why Dennis was personally 'pained' by this perceived slight from Sue. I would interpret him to have inferred that Sue's negative self-assessment was relevant to himself in that by extension she would have to conclude that *his* present life was not worth living. That is, he considers Sue's personal revulsion at the prospect of a 'mere biological existence' to be relevant to the worthwhileness not merely of *her* life, but also of his own. His response acknowledges that although her feelings are personal (i.e., her own and about herself), they also affect him personally. He draws attention to Sue's 'unintended' oversight of the fact that frequently even a strictly personal self-knowledge claim can easily be generalized so that it has implications for others, such as himself. As Dennis interprets Sue, she was maintaining that if her life became as physically restricted as his own, she would judge such a life to be not worth living.[14] I would express Dennis's objection to be that although he agrees with Sue that feelings are relevant to evaluations, he challenges her assumption that such judgments are epistemically just subjective.

On the question of the objectivity of such evaluations, Sue's story suggests that she regards almost all evaluations as merely subjective utterances. That is, she understands almost all evaluations to be ultimately private and idiosyncratic. The reason why I interpret her stance on the objectivity of evaluations to apply to *almost all* of her evaluations is that she does insist on at least one public value that is more than just epistemically subjective: respecting the values of other people when they differ from one's own. This claim allows her to argue against imposing one's private and personally held evaluations on others. As Sue expresses it, 'Why on earth would anyone want to impose their own value system on me? I've got mine, they've got theirs.'[15]

At issue is not only Sue's objection to the apparent intolerance of others to her values. A more fundamental issue is the possibility of any epistemically objective evaluation, at least beyond the value of tolerating diverse values.[16] On these grounds, Sue rejects the legitimacy of others affirming a normative stance regarding physician-assisted suicide. She seems to regard such a stance, and any legal constraints that might be consistent with it, as being in violation of the absolute moral norm of tolerance. Without wanting to hold Sue to too great a demand for consistency, it is worth making explicit an inconsistency in her position. On the one hand, her main objection is that a law against euthanasia is flawed because such a law would *legally constrain* her from acting on her values, and therefore violates the absolute norm of tolerance of others' values. On the other hand, she does not refrain from affirming values, in her own name, that are *morally constraining* on others. That is, any positive, general evaluative claim, such as the social value of tolerating values, will *morally constrain* anyone who affirms some other value.[17]

It seems, therefore, that Sue's position on the objectivity of evaluations can be interpreted in two ways. If the question is whether she thinks that evaluations are *ever* more than just subjective, I would have to answer 'Yes.' If the question is whether she thinks evaluations other than the value of tolerance are ever more than just subjective, I would have to answer 'No.' The fact that she does maintain that at least one value is more than epistemically just subjective, as in the case of the value of respecting or tolerating the evaluations of others, is philosophically important. But since she would argue that she comes to know the value of tolerance *immediately* in her feelings, the philosophical approach of pointing out this inconsistency in her position would likely be unpersuasive. For to be open to the possibility that this evaluation is mistaken would mean that she would also have to abandon her answer to the second question, that feelings are sufficient grounds for any evaluation. Hence, having grasped the value of the norm of tolerance, she expresses it as one that is also binding on more than herself alone. In fact, she believes it ought to inform and constrain certain critical words and deeds of others with regard to herself.

2.4 How Does Value Judging Relate to Choosing?

In chapter 6 I spelled out Lonergan's answer to this fourth question. On the relationship between those elements that constitute 'value judging' and 'choosing,' Lonergan's short answer is that the distinction is between knowing the good and doing it. That is, it is a distinction within the fourth level between cognitional and decisional acts and achievements. This distinction and relationship is worth highlighting because there seems to be an important verbal difference in emphasis on the relative importance of these acts, which comes to the fore in the euthanasia debate. With Lonergan, I have emphasized the cognitive elements of fourth-level value judgments, particularly those affective cognitions labelled deliberative insights. I have also argued that value judgments can be either epistemically just subjective or epistemically objective. In either case, these cognitive acts are methodically prior to decisional acts of choosing and executing one's choice. Some attention to what these decisional acts entail and how they relate to value judgments brings to light an important difference in emphasis on these acts between Sue and Dennis.

The act of choosing what one deems to be an actual or possible value ends the fourth-level evaluative process of knowing, and raises a series of decisional issues. First, one's choosing can be positive or privative. Since I can still choose not to do what I know I ought to do, my knowing does not entirely determine my choosing. When my knowing and choosing are consistent, the choice is a positive one. By contrast, when I choose not to do as I know I ought, the choice is privative. Second, my choosing can regard some actual good or some possible good. In the case of an actual good, I can choose positively to enjoy it or privatively not to enjoy it. Similarly, in the case of a concretely possible good, I can choose positively to do it or privatively not to do it. In the case of an actual good, my choosing is passive or in the mode of complacency, and in the case of a possible good my choosing is active or in the mode of concern. A further privative choice is choosing not to choose, or merely to drift. Third, my choosing to do some possible good is completed by my doing or executing it. Hence, my fourth-level evaluations are characterized as responsible not merely because I achieve knowledge of some good or some value, but also because I choose positively to enjoy passively or actively to execute what I deem to be choiceworthy.[18]

The main point to highlight here is that acts of choosing do not involve some further cognitive achievement. To express this point in more traditional terms, the entire fourth-level process correlates with *will*, with the cognitive elements on the fourth level being a dimension of affectivity. By contrast, cognition on the second and third levels is intellectual. The distinction between evaluating and deciding corresponds to the distinction between knowing the good and choosing to enjoy or actualize that good.[19] Put negatively, there are two distinct forms of moral failures, those resulting from *ignorance* or failures to know the good, and those resulting from *sin* or failures to choose to enjoy or, if pertinent, to actualize the good.

Given these distinctions between value judging and choosing, how does this cast some light on what is going on with Sue and Dennis? As I interpret Sue, she tends to emphasize verbally the act of choosing, at least in some key instances, thereby suggesting that it is the key act on the fourth level. I qualify this as a 'verbal' emphasis because on a closer reading Sue's own choosing was positive in the sense that it was consistent with her knowing what she deemed to be her good. In other words, she was not arguing for the freedom to choose to do what she deemed to be a disvalue. Rather, she insisted that physician-assisted suicide was choiceworthy because it was a concretely possible value in her case. Despite her emphasis on the act of choosing, the real fourth-level issue regards not the act of choosing, whether it be positive or privative, but rather the act of value judging and whether it is epistemically objective or merely subjective.

Sue's emphasis on the act of choosing has the consequence of distracting attention away from the content of her value judgment. On Sue's own account, her choice to die by physician-assisted suicide was not always, or even primarily, because she judged her life to be 'not worth living.' A key argument for her choice seems to have been the negative one that, as a free choice, it needed no argument or justification. By expressing her position as merely a matter of free choice, Sue suggests that any choice, not just one about the worthwhileness of one's life, is strictly personal. So any effort on her part to justify or even explain her choice is gratuitous or unnecessary. Consequently, Sue resented those who sought to attend to and question her value judgment, as if such attention and queries are not legitimate. When pressed, however, she admitted several revealing reasons and feelings that underpinned her view that physician-assisted suicide was choiceworthy. For instance, she referred to such things as the negative effects of her dying on others, or that she was merely agreeing with others who had already judged her life to be 'not worth living.'

I suggest that Sue's emphasis on the act of choosing is a merely verbal one because her actual choice is positive, rather than privative, in the sense that she actually wills what she deems to be good. Her position seems to rest on the view that there is no epistemic objectivity with respect to value judgments, which is essentially the position of ethical voluntarism. A noteworthy exception, however, are those choices that impose one's values on others, which for Sue are always privative.[20] The key value question is whether or not her life really was worth living, and if not, why not.

One can better appreciate the content of Sue's value judgment by expressing it in terms of the major premise of a syllogism. For instance, if Sue chose physician-assisted suicide because she deemed the burden of her care was too great for others to bear, the major premise of her deliberative syllogism would have been something like the following: 'If one's dying is or will cause others undue burdens, then one should take one's life.' Such a form of expression is helpful because it focuses attention on the content of the value judgment rather than merely on the act or content of the choice. It is this value judgment that is really at issue, even for Sue.[21]

Sue concluded that her life would, at some point, not be worth living because it would be a 'merely biological existence.' This view expresses an *instrumentalist* account of her moral status. It implies that she holds her moral status to be conditioned by her ability to do certain things, and such conditions would not be fulfilled if she deemed her life to be a 'mere biological existence.' On this view, when she deemed the quality of her life had declined to one that was a merely biological existence, she would request assistance with committing suicide. Given her view of the conditions she placed on her moral status, one could agree that her decision to die by physician-assisted suicide was a fitting one and that her choice positively expressed her value judgment. However, if one does not accept the major premise of her deliberative syllogism, which expresses an instrumentalist or comparative view of moral status, then her argument becomes much less convincing. What seems to be going on here is that Sue conflates the distinction between ontic and qualitative values. Moreover, even though she insists that her self-evaluation is particular to herself, at least Dennis recognized that such an instrumentalist evaluation of the worth of her life had ramifications for others in similar contexts, including himself.

In Dennis's story, several examples illustrate that he was less prone to truncating the fourth-level operational process by verbally emphasizing merely the act of choosing. For instance, consider his response to the suffering of Aleza and her husband that resulted from her caregivers thinking that she was mentally disabled. Dennis judged that if these caregivers had understood ALS better they would not have mistreated Aleza the way they did. Further, he thought that he could help to avoid similar harms being done to other ALS patients by adding a chapter to his book on the 'nuts and bolts' of ALS. In this example of a fourth-level process, one can identify the distinct and related elements of (1) a question of value,

(2) deliberative insight, (3) value judging, and (4) choosing and executing this choice.[22] The key moment in this fourth-level process is the deliberative insight, which is a matter of affective cognition, the content of which issues in a value judgment. That is, the deliberative insight grounds the value judgment, or provides the cognitional reason for asserting the value judgment. By choosing to write this chapter and then writing it, Dennis actively willed and executed, in the mode of concern, what he deemed to be a concretely possible good. His choosing followed immediately from his value judgment, and his choice was a positive rather than a privative one. By contrast, Sue's case illustrates a hasty attenuation of what Lonergan would locate as the crucial steps in the deliberative process, which includes correctly grasping not only the fulfilling conditions of the major premise of one's deliberative syllogism, but also the initial 'if ..., then ...' link of the major premise. Sue obscures the content of what she grasps in her deliberative insight by placing all her emphasis on the subsequent volitional act of choosing. A similar overemphasis of the decisional act of choosing also occurs in some of the subsequent ethical and legal analyses, as I will point out in later sections.

2.5   Is There a Normative Structure of the Human Good? If Yes, Does It Involve Both the Individual and Social Good?

As I explained in chapter 8, Lonergan's short answer to the first part of this fifth question is 'Yes, there is an invariant structure of the human good.' His short answer to the second part of this question is 'The human good is at once individual and social.' Moreover, since social values condition the vital values of the whole community, they are to be preferred to the vital values of individual members of the community, such as health, strength, grace, and vigour.[23] On my reading of their stories, I would argue that the positions of both Sue and Dennis are roughly compatible with Lonergan's on this question. To interpret Sue's position to be roughly compatible with Lonergan's, however, one has to pay attention more to what she does than to what she says.

   In Sue's story there seem to be inconsistencies between some of her more public claims and some of her ideas, concerns, and behaviours that Hobbs Birnie articulates in her book. For example, one might argue that she bases her decision to kill herself by physician-assisted suicide on the criterion of a negative response to the dissatisfactions of her current and projected life. In chapter 2, I highlighted some of the negative affective context within which Sue makes this evaluation and decision. Of particular note are her feelings of anger and resentment toward others. In fact, these responses were always such a prominent part of Sue's character, even prior to her illness, that it led her psychotherapist to conclude that anger is *foundational* to her personality.[24] But I wonder whether it is fair to say that her main reasons for requesting physician-assisted suicide had to do with issues of self-concern, that is, about her individual good without regard to the social good.

In the previous section I mentioned three different lines of thought that seem to have led Sue to her decision to die by physician-assisted suicide. However, if one presses her reasons, it would be inconsistent with the facts to conclude that her concerns were entirely for her individual good. For instance, one reason Sue thought her life was not worth living is that she believed that her status in the eyes of others would decrease along with her increasing disability from ALS. She anticipated that, at some point in her decline, others would eventually treat her as *a non-person*, and she would merely be a burden on everyone.[25] In support of this view she interpreted certain probably unintended slights by others as evidence that, because of her disability, she no longer mattered to them. Hence, at least some of Sue's negative self-evaluations cannot be interpreted fairly as stemming from a view of the human good as entirely individual. Moreover, some of the considerations that underpin Sue's decision for physician-assisted suicide actually express her moral seriousness and concern for the social good (e.g., avoiding being a burden or psychologically traumatizing her son). Her decision to commit suicide could be at least consistent with a view of the primacy of the social good.[26] Examining Sue's story, then, it may be unfair to say simply that it illustrates a life conducted on the plane of self-concern rather than moral seriousness. But it also may be inaccurate to suggest that she had faced the fundamental question of whether to be oriented to satisfactions or to values and had decisively resolved it.[27]

Dennis's story provides a moving illustration of the concrete functioning of the human good, and of the relation between individual and social goods. He described his intimate community, for instance, as his 'life-support system,' in which there was no essential opposition between his individual good and the social good of his community. He also related a story of the lasting effect that a small act of kindness had on him. This act subsequently inspired in him similar selfless acts, such as publicizing his experiences with ALS, raising funds for ALS research, and being a kind and loving father and husband.[28] His efforts to raise public awareness and promote research in the area of ALS bear witness to his grasp of the relation between individual and social goods, that is, that the former are conditioned by the latter. Conversely, his story is a testimony to the personal meaning and fulfilment he discovered through promoting the social and cultural good of caring for vulnerable members of society. Hence, effectively, there seems to have been little doubt in Dennis's mind about the reality of a normative structure of the human good. Nor do his words or deeds suggest that he thinks there is an essential opposition between the individual and his community, or that individual goods ought to take preference.[29]

2.6 Is Life a Basic Good? Is It an Absolute Good?

Lonergan's short answer to the first part of this sixth core question is 'Yes, life is a basic good.' To the second part of the question, Lonergan answers, 'No, life is not an absolute good.' If pressed to elaborate, Lonergan would clarify the first part of his answer by distinguishing the basic good of the *ontic value of persons* from other *qualitative values*, such as those attributes of persons like beauty, understanding, truth, virtuous acts, and noble deeds.[30] He would also want to distinguish the ontic value of life from those *absolute values* that rank highest on one's scale of preferences, which for him are religious values.[31]

Among Sue's 'mixed feelings' toward physician-assisted suicide are some positive responses to certain values. For instance, the act of choosing the time and mode of her death, and acting on this choice, seems to have met Sue's need to control her dying.[32] To die by physician-assisted suicide also has a certain aesthetic appeal for Sue in comparison with dying a possibly unsightly and uncomfortable death from ALS. Such a death would be quick, clean, painless, and timely.[33] Another compelling value that this choice leads to is the opportunity for Sue to contribute to the political debate on euthanasia. Her decision in favour of physician-assisted suicide gives the final chapter of her life a goal, namely, to increase what I would interpret as 'the social good of effective freedom.' On her own testimony, this final goal conferred meaning and significance on her whole life.

I would argue that, by claiming that 'the quality of life is everything' and that a life without a certain level of quality is not worth living (e.g., having ALS and being unable to speak), Sue presupposes value preferences that are inconsistent with Lonergan's. That is, I would interpret Sue's scale of preferences to rank certain social values, such as the qualitative value of speech, whereby one is able to express oneself to others verbally, as conditioning the ontic value of her life. That is, behind Sue's decision to kill herself is the effectively operative assessment that the value of her life is fundamentally conditioned by her ability to speak. Hence, when on top of all her other losses she is deprived of her ability to communicate by speaking, she would evaluate her life as 'not worth living.' By contrast, Lonergan would want to affirm the ontic value of Sue's life, as well as the many qualitative values that she exhibited (e.g., her understanding, grasp of truths, noble deeds, and virtuous acts). His position would be that moral status ought not be considered as conditioned by certain qualitative values. He would also be sympathetic to her own assessment that this phase of her life is indeed significant to the meaning of her life as a whole, and perhaps point to the irony of this self-assessment and her decision to opt for physician-assisted suicide.

By contrast, I would argue that Dennis's position on this two-part question is compatible with Lonergan's view that life is a basic good but not an absolute one. For example, Dennis rejects the possibility of prolonging his life by the use of an artificial respirator. However, for him, life is a basic good because it conditions all other human goods. For instance, he relates his apprehension of the goodness of 'just being alive' (e.g., witnessing the beauty of a sunset). A further question is whether Dennis regards human moral status as *instrumental* or *comparative*. That is, does he accept the view that, in Sue's case, her moral status would decline in some manner corresponding to her declining physical condition? I would argue that Dennis's negative reaction to this opinion suggests that his own position is that moral status is stable, not based or dependant on comparison with others, and non-instrumental – which is another way of expressing the value of life as a basic *ontic* good.

3   Comparing and Contrasting the Philosophical and Empirical Positions of Sue Rodriguez and Dennis Kaye

3.1   Philosophical Positions of Sue and Dennis

By *philosophical*, I mean that I will be referring to differences that arise at the level of cognitional and decisional subjectivity, such as different views on the cognitive relevance of feelings. By *empirical*, I mean I will be referring to the achievements that result when my cognitional and decisional subjectivity encounters data.

Sue's philosophical position is compatible with Lonergan's on at best points 1, 5, and 6. On point 1, which regards the phenomenological role of feelings in knowing, Sue agrees with Lonergan that feelings are cognitively relevant, indeed necessary, for knowing. On point 5, which is a point regarding the metaphysical structure of the human good, Sue agrees with Lonergan that the human good is both individual and social. There is some evidence that her decision favouring euthanasia is, in part, an expression of her desire to promote not just what she took to be her individual good, such as the avoidance of what she expected would be a dreadful death. Even more importantly, she expressed her decision as an effort to promote certain social goods, such as concerns for her son, family, caregivers, and society. If this is true, it suggests that she was not oriented fundamentally by self-concern. Rather, her decision for physician-assisted suicide is an expression of moral seriousness. On point 6, which is a point regarding the metaphysical value of life, it seems that Sue also agrees with Lonergan that life is a basic good that conditions other human goods, but that it is not an absolute good.

Besides agreeing with Lonergan's position, as Sue does on points 1, 5, and 6, Dennis also agrees with Lonergan on points 2, 3, and 4. On point 2, which is a further point regarding the phenomenal role of feelings in knowing, I interpret Dennis to consider feelings *partly* to ground his cognitive access to knowledge, specifically, knowledge of values. That is, although he considers feelings as *necessary* conditions for generating certain knowledge claims, he still regards them as *not sufficient conditions* for generating such claims. In his estimation, the fact that they are necessary renders those opinions of certain 'experts,' whom he found lacking in this regard, inherently invalid. The insufficiency of feelings for him, however, is evidenced by his challenge to Sue's evaluation. For despite Sue's immediate access to such feelings, Dennis nevertheless objects to the conclusion that his is a 'merely biological' life and not worth living. On point 3, which concerns both phenomenology and epistemology, Dennis agrees with Lonergan that affects are related *mediately* to evaluative knowing, and that claims arrived at by means of affective responses can be *epistemically objective*. On point 4, which concerns the relation between evaluation and decision, Dennis seems to agree with Lonergan that these are distinct but related steps in the evaluative process. Although they are related, this relation is contingent rather than necessary. Hence, on these philosophical points, Dennis's position on euthanasia is sound, according to Lonergan's analysis.

It remains for me to highlight the significance of the philosophical differences between the positions of Sue and Lonergan on points 2, 3, and 4. On point 2, Sue regards feelings as entirely grounding her cognitive grasp of certain knowledge claims, namely, those regarding values. That is, not only does she regard them as *necessary* conditions for knowing values, as does Lonergan, she also takes them to be *sufficient* conditions for knowing values. From Lonergan's perspective, Sue's position is vulnerable to the charge that it overstates the role of feelings because it does not distinguish the relevant affects (i.e., intentional responses to values) from other feelings (e.g., intentional states or trends). Moreover, her position seems to place insufficient emphasis on the role of other cognitive acts in knowing.[34]

On point 3, which concerns the relation of feelings to evaluations and the consequent epistemic status of those evaluations, a crucial difference arises. Sue seems to regard the knowing process by means of which feelings grasp values as analogous to the immediacy of sense experience, rather than as a mediated process. Consequently, she seems to regard her knowledge claims, based on her feelings, as privileged but also restricted to herself. They are privileged in the sense that they give her access to values that others could not grasp for lack of the relevant feelings. They are restricted, however, because their content regards only herself. It seems that the price of Sue's position, which emphasizes in a certain way the role of feelings in knowing, is that the contents thus known are never more than epistemically just subjective. It is for this reason that she is able to claim that others have their values, and she has hers (although this did not hold for the value of tolerance).

Finally, on point 4, Sue's position seems to presuppose some necessary connection between evaluation and decision. That is, her cognitive achievement, which culminates in an evaluation, seems to have some immediate or necessary connection to her decision. Another way of expressing this is to say that, from Lonergan's perspective, her position seems to place undue stress on the decisional issue at the expense of the cognitive issue.

3.2 Empirical Positions of Sue and Dennis

Besides these philosophical differences between the positions Sue and Dennis espouse, there are other differences between their views that are not of a philosophical nature. My aim here is to highlight the distinction between their concrete or empirical performances and their philosophical or methodological presuppositions, which I have been discussing. This is important because significant differences between their positions may lie more at the level of concrete cognitional and decisional issues than at the level of strictly methodological ones. Although I would argue that clarity on the methodological issues may be of some advantage to one's concrete performance as a knower, it is not a necessary condition for skilled performance.[35]

Consider first a point of similarity between the positions of Sue and Dennis on what I would call an empirical evaluative issue. Both decided against the option of respiratory support, such as a tracheostomy and portable respirator, to maintain their respiratory status as each of them weakened from their disease. I would consider these decisions to be important for each of them, but one that has received almost no attention in the debate. The question is, 'Would such a device, which would likely be of some physical benefit, be worthwhile?' Both Sue and Dennis answered this question negatively. What is not apparent from their stories is what determined this response. Inasmuch as this evaluation is an empirical matter, which it surely is, it would be important from Lonergan's perspective to know that they each did their 'homework' prior to arriving at their decisions, that is, that they went through a process of experience, understanding, judgment, and evaluation that informed their decisions.[36]

A point of difference between the positions of Sue and Dennis on what I would also call an empirical evaluative matter is their opposing decisions concerning euthanasia. In Dennis's story, it seems that he never seriously entertained the option of suicide and that this was because he thought that his life, at least on good days, was more than a 'merely biological existence.' His story seems to confirm the view of various ethicists that a decision in favour of euthanasia would only be entertained on the basis of the self-evaluation that one's life is not worth living. Even so, there is no evidence from Dennis's story that he explored the issue of suicide, or knew of others who had ended their lives, or considered the effects this had on their families, or tried to dissuade others.

Sue's opposing position on euthanasia helpfully points to some underlying judgments and evaluations that made this option appear attractive to her, and which seem to be overlooked as empirical matters in the larger debate. The most surprising discovery is that several evaluations, either individually or collectively, seemed to justify her decision. In the previous section I described what is perhaps the standard account of her decision, that once her disease diminished her to a 'mere biological existence,' her life would no longer be 'worth living' (i.e., what I referred to as an instrumentalist view of moral status). But if one reads her story carefully, there are at least two other lines of thought that appear to have underpinned her decision to commit suicide, neither of which involved the evaluation that her life was 'not worth living.'[37]

One line of thought was the prospect of a torturous death. I take this to be a version of the classic 'life-boat' dilemma, in which there are limited available options (e.g., starvation or cannibalization). Sue expresses concern to avoid the type of death from which she assumed people with ALS commonly die. She gathers that such a death results from suffocation and choking. For her, such a death would be psychologically unbearable. That is, her reason to exit from life early was to avoid this experience of dying *in extremis*, as those in medicine call it. On this view of the matter, Sue's decision appears to be proportionate to or fitting for her negative evaluation of the prospect of a dreadful experience of dying. That is, her decision is connected to her evaluation, in the manner described by Lonergan. But according to the ALS expert I cited in chapter 2, there might have been a problem at the level of her fact judgment. For this expert claimed that the type of death she feared was *not* the sort of death most people with ALS actually have. If this is true, the problem is an empirical one of getting the facts straight. There is no evidence from her book that she explored these facts (she attended only one meeting of the ALS Society), or considered other possible ways of avoiding this dreaded end, all of which involve issues of empirical cognitional skill.[38]

A further, distinct reason for Sue's choice of euthanasia was that she was convinced that, by so doing, she was acting in a way that would be good for others, especially her son. Her decision to die by physician-assisted suicide followed, in part, from her answer to the question 'What would be best for her son Cole?' It appears that she thought it best to protect him from the possibly negative consequences of seeing her in an extremely poor physical condition at the end of her life. That is, she wished to protect him from the psychological trauma or harm of witnessing the final stages of her physical decline. One way of understanding this is from the perspective of a good mother trying to protect her child. Although she realized that she could not ultimately protect Cole from the fact of her mortality, she seemed to think that it was her duty to protect him from witnessing this reality. It seems that she considered her death to be a private matter, and she was concerned to set limits on how much of this, and how much of her own vulnerability, she ought to share with her son. Sue's desire to shield her son from her death figured prominently in her decision and is surely an empirical issue. This protective motivator for euthanasia is something that neither the most prominent ethicists currently addressing the euthanasia issue nor the legislators who study the issue from a legal point of view seem to recognize.

The step between judgments and evaluations involves the cognitive skill of considering empirical evidence. There seems to be no indication that Sue critically questioned the view that the risks of negative long-term consequences on her son's psychological health would be greater from his being present with her in her vulnerability and decline than from the trauma of dealing with the fact of her suicide. If she had the opposite view on this empirical question, she might have reached a different conclusion regarding the need to request physician-assisted suicide.

The key concern here is the epistemic issue of whether one's empirical evaluations are true, that is, epistemically objective. For one might act tolerantly by treating persons with sympathy and understanding and yet not act in fidelity to the truth. One acts in fidelity to truth by treating as true the claims persons make only if one has sufficient evidence for those claims. For example, one can be supportive and understanding of the drug addict even while challenging claims about the value of a life oriented to psychotropic drugs. It seems to me that a clear-headed person can be sympathetic and understanding toward a sufferer (e.g., a drug addict) without agreeing that what the sufferer says is true or what the sufferer wants is good. Wise and loving parents of teenagers face a similar challenge daily. Since the objects are distinct, the responses to them need never be in conflict. Concretely, of course, it takes a clear-headed person to make this distinction in the first place. And getting the sufferer to grasp it is a further challenge. But neither of those requirements undercuts the validity of the point itself. Similarly, in Sue's case, there seems to be no inherent conflict between being sympathetic and understanding toward her, and disagreeing with her that what she wants is good. Moreover, I would add that it is an issue of moral integrity that one ought sometimes to refuse to collaborate with what one judges to be wrong-doing, especially if such collaboration places one at odds with one's core values. I suspect that somewhere in the euthanasia debate is an awkwardness that is shared by many regarding the task of setting limits and saying 'no.'

3.3 Summary of Ramifications of Lonergan's Position for the Euthanasia Debate at the Level of Concrete Life Stories

What can one conclude from this comparison and contrast of the *philosophical* positions of Sue Rodriguez and Dennis Kaye in relation to Lonergan's philosophical position? First, Lonergan's attention to the role of affect in evaluations seems to address an important matter that arises concretely in the experience of individuals like Sue and Dennis. Second, it is precisely on matters concerning the *role* that affect plays in knowing values that Sue's position diverges from Dennis's. Hence, their opposing conclusions regarding euthanasia may be related to this underlying philosophical difference. More generally, if a person requests euthanasia, some attention to their position on the role of affect in knowing values may help one to understand why they do so. Third, the differences in philosophical positions between Sue and Dennis, as I have interpreted them, are on phenomenal and epistemic issues, not on metaphysical ones. This may be important for understanding not only why some persons request euthanasia, but also how to assess and address their concerns. Finally, I want to stress that although this analysis has uncovered significant philosophical differences between the positions of Sue and Dennis, one should not think that the issue is settled by addressing these differences. Even if both Sue and Dennis were to agree with Lonergan on the philosophical issues concerning cognitional and decisional subjectivity, there may still be significant differences between them on an issue like euthanasia. Still, it is helpful to locate these differences as empirical ones rather than philosophical ones.

Similarly, what can one conclude from the comparison and contrast of the *empirical* positions of Sue and Dennis? First, although they both said that they would not make use of mechanical devices, such as a respirator, there is no discussion in their books about how they came to this decision. Since it is an empirical issue, and possibly as important a decision as those about other treatments, or even those about euthanasia, this lack of detail suggests to me that this option was not seriously considered either by Sue or by Dennis.

The most important point of difference between the empirical positions of Sue and Dennis is on the matter of euthanasia. What emerged from this comparison was the issue of concrete cognitional and decisional skills. Sue's decision seems to have been influenced by several claims, many of which lacked adequate empirical grounds.

To be fair to Sue, it also seems that Dennis did not always base his decisions on well-evidenced claims. On the issue of euthanasia, for instance, there is no suggestion that he actually looked into the matter himself (although this may have been so incongruent with his core values that no such investigation was needed). Perhaps the most important discovery from contrasting the empirical stances of Sue and Dennis is that, in both cases, several key evaluations were based on very little evidence. I am eager not to be overly critical of either Sue or Dennis. Still, Sue's cognitional skills are relevant to the larger debate precisely because her evaluations frequently are presumed to be invulnerable to critical reflection, or at least out of bounds. The fact that Lonergan regards these issues as empirical ones is important for the larger debate. This is especially so since key proponents of euthanasia base their position on the empirical assumption that *the person in question* is in the best position to make the evaluation as to whether his or her life is worth living, and they assume that such a person can also make this evaluation well.[39]

My interpretations of the philosophical stances of Sue and Dennis were necessarily tentative, given the limitations of the available evidence from their stories. Neither Sue nor Dennis were professional philosophers; neither expressly address in their books the precise questions I have posed to them. Still, the main point of this exercise is to engage the debate using Lonergan's philosophical categories and his position on the role of affect in evaluations. I would regard such an engagement as successful if it brings to light important questions to which others currently engaging this debate are not attending. Even if further evidence should come to light and force a revision in my interpretations, this exercise would still be valuable in raising certain questions and highlighting points of similarity and difference between Sue and Dennis's respective philosophical and empirical stances. In particular, do differences between Sue and Dennis on philosophical issues relating to the role of affect in evaluations (whatever these may have been) help account for their decisions for and against euthanasia in a way that other analyses have missed? On the practical level the question is, 'If Sue's request for euthanasia follows from an evaluation that I was unable to affirm on either philosophical or empirical grounds, does this have any bearing on how I ought to respond to her request?' This raises the further question of one's obligations to Sue and Dennis and how, if at all, it depends on whether one affirms their evaluations. For instance, if Dennis requested mechanical ventilation, and I affirm his evaluation and decision on philosophical and empirical grounds, would my obligations toward him differ significantly from my obligations to Sue's request for euthanasia, which I cannot affirm on philosophical or empirical grounds?

The discovery of, and explicit philosophical attention to, these points of similarity and difference is, I would argue, an important and original contribution to this debate. It is important because it provides some clues to what I take to be the two key questions posed by all the members of the Special Senate Committee on Euthanasia and Assisted Suicide in their recommendations to the Canadian parliament. Despite differences among committee members on the issue of euthanasia, all recommended that more information be obtained on these two issues: 'Why are persons requesting euthanasia?' and 'Are there any alternatives that might be acceptable to those who request euthanasia?'[40] On the basis of Lonergan's stance on the philosophical issue of the role of affect in evaluations, highlighting these points of similarity and difference between the positions of Sue and Dennis (as well as those of ethicists involved in this debate) offers some insights that may help to answer these questions. It also locates differences between Sue's stance and Dennis's stance on euthanasia at the philosophical and empirical levels. Hence, empirical research might be able to answer the committee's questions 'Why are persons such as Sue requesting euthanasia?' and 'What alternatives might be acceptable to them?' Still, one would not expect empirical research to identify or to handle critically the sort of cognitive philosophical issues on which the present discussion has focused, or to address adequately the normative evaluative issue of whether Sue's life really was not worth living.[41]

This contribution, I suggest, is also original in the context of contemporary philosophical engagement of the debate. In chapter 2 I reviewed the debate as it moves forward in several contexts. I pointed out that in medical discussions there is an emphasis on somatic pain and other physical or psychiatric symptoms that persons experience when dying. One study to which I referred raised the issue of the possible relevance of affective elements for such requests. This was in a study by Chochinov et al. who, from a psychiatric perspective, studied the desire for death in the terminally ill. These researchers pointed out that there is a small population of individuals for whom the desire for death was stable and unrelated to medical needs, such as poor pain management or depression.[42] Although this study raised the issue of affect as possibly being behind such requests, the authors did not provide an analysis of the precise role that affect might play in these requests, nor would I expect such a psychiatric analysis to address or handle well these philosophical issues.

Even less attention to and analysis of the role of affect in evaluations emerges from subsequent levels of the euthanasia debate. Despite nods to notions such as mercy and compassion in the ethical and legal discussions, ethicists and legislators typically focus on conceptual matters, such as 'killing and allowing to die.' Though such distinctions are critically important, at least in the two cases I examined, this distinction was neither a conceptual nor a practical problem. That is, everyone clearly identified Sue's request for euthanasia as the ethical issue, regardless of their position on the normativity of this decision or of society's response to it. It clearly involved what most people would call 'killing.' By contrast, there was no debate over what I would identify as a key ethical question for both Sue and Dennis, which was whether to use the technology of an artificial respirator as their own respiratory status declined. Although powerful voices insist that the issues of 'killing' and 'allowing to die' are ethically similar or equivalent, such a view seems to be at odds with the facts of at least these two stories.

As I will elaborate in the next section, although there is some mention by Beauchamp of the advantage of the *person in question* making an evaluation, Beauchamp does not seem to identify this expressly as an affective issue or provide an analysis of what this advantage might be. At the legislative level of the discussion, besides attending to issues of individual liberty and justice, both proponents and opponents of legalizing euthanasia refer to the importance of *compassion*. Here again, they provide no analysis of what compassion is, or how precisely it functions in evaluations. What controls or conditions need to be met, for instance, to distinguish between compassion as a response to an individual and a critical response to that individual's orientation to satisfactions as distinct from values? Nor do they ask whether those value judgments and choices that issue from some compassionate response are open to interpersonal verification or are epistemically never more than just subjective.

In chapter 2, I made the role of affect in evaluations an issue by reporting some affective themes from Sue and Dennis's life-stories. Novel though this approach may have been for a work in philosophy, it now strikes me that attending to these affective features of real stories is crucial to an ethical analysis. Nevertheless, such attention does not guarantee that one will identify the philosophical issues that Lonergan's account brings expressly to light. For instance, even though both Sue and Dennis agree that 'feelings' are somehow necessary in 'knowing,' they would likely be hard pressed to answer the sort of questions that Lonergan addresses, such as: 'What feelings (i.e., intentional/ non-intentional)?' 'What knowledge (i.e., facts/ values)?' 'What is the status of this knowledge (i.e., subjective/objective)?' To the extent that these are important questions to raise, and to the extent that the current discussion either overlooks them or deals with them only in a cursory or confused manner, I regard the ramifications of Lonergan's account for this debate to be important and original.

I have been attempting to point out only *some* of the ramifications of Lonergan's position for the euthanasia debate, not necessarily all. And I have been indicating some of the more important and original ramifications of Lonergan's philosophy for what I regard as the most fundamental level of the debate, and how in light of those ramifications one might engage this debate. As an ethicist, I feel obliged to continue the analysis by addressing related ethical and legislative discussions. In the next two sections, then, my focus will be on highlighting some ramifications of Lonergan's position for these subsequent levels of the debate. In particular, I will consider whether there are consistent stances on the underlying philosophical issues among the proponents and opponents of euthanasia at the ethical and public-policy levels of the debate.

4   Comparing and Contrasting the Philosophical and Empirical Positions of Tom Beauchamp and Richard McCormick

It is with some trepidation that I employ Lonergan to engage critically the arguments of Tom Beauchamp and Richard McCormick. Not only are they first-rate thinkers, they have also made important ethical contributions to the difficult and controversial issue of euthanasia. And not only did Lonergan not address the issue of euthanasia himself, his position on the role of affect in evaluations seems to bear no immediate relation to either the ethical or to the public-policy debate. It is important, therefore, that I begin by qualifying the remarks I will be making in the next two sections.

First, one must bring together the perspectives of the particularists, who are content to reflect on the life-stories such as those I have discussed, and the generalists, who are happy to confine themselves to philosophical issues. When I reviewed the literature, it became apparent to me that there is significant confusion about the types of questions that are being posed, and this is reflected in the sort of evidence that is proffered in response to them. Claims that Lonergan would identify as philosophical are advanced as if they were empirical ones, and vice versa. Hence, my goal in the next two sections is to highlight examples of this confusion and, in the final section, to clarify Lonergan's account of the distinction and what results from it for this debate.

Second, I have found this debate to be far too complex and wide-ranging for any one person to engage it in both a general, comprehensive way and in a way that is concrete and practical. In part this testifies to the genuinely interdisciplinary nature of the debate, which is one reason I chose to write on it. It also strikes me that the debate is *slippery*, for frequently the author of the claims being made is not identified. This might not matter so much in some areas, or from some perspectives, but it is vitally important when it comes to analysing ethical claims from Lonergan's perspective. This is because Lonergan places the responsibility for the objectivity of claims squarely on the shoulders of the subject who advances them. For Lonergan, 'objectivity is but the fruit of authentic subjectivity.' Consequently, my strategy in the next two sections is to try as best I can to relate the key claims that are being proffered on either side of this debate to the individuals or groups of thinkers who are making them.[43] (See table A.2, p. 311.)

For the ethical level of the euthanasia debate, I have chosen to compare and contrast the views of Tom Beauchamp and Richard McCormick. And one of the reasons I have chosen these two thinkers is that Richard McCormick has publicly distinguished his own views from those of Tom Beauchamp.[44]

I wish also to acknowledge and address some of the concerns that Lonergan scholars are likely to have. I anticipate that one of their main concerns would be that I not misapply Lonergan to some controversial issue in a manner that would allow others to discredit his legitimate philosophical contributions. It is with this in mind that I have chosen to use Lonergan's categories to challenge arguments on *both* sides of the debate, rather than to use him to argue for just one position. My main aims are to highlight issues that may easily be overlooked in this debate, and to demonstrate the relevance of Lonergan's stance on the role of affect for both sides of the debate. By the end of the discussion, it will become clear which side of the debate I think is more convincing on philosophical grounds. Further, drawing on Lonergan's work, I will also argue that since this debate concerns an empirical matter, one should not expect it to be settled by mere philosophical arguments.

4.1 Philosophical Positions of Beauchamp and McCormick

In chapter 2 I provided a brief sketch of Beauchamp's position on euthanasia and summarized his stance on the normative ethical question. I also highlighted his philosophical and methodological commitments, which expressly underpin this stance.[45] My aim here is to identify some ramifications that Lonergan's philosophical stance might have for Beauchamp. As regards Beauchamp's position on the role of affect in evaluations, I begin by highlighting the prominence he seems to give to the personal grounds of any evaluation.

First, it strikes me that Beauchamp would agree with Lonergan on some points. Beauchamp seems to be claiming that if I am *the person in question*, I would have some cognitive advantage over others when making the self-evaluation that my life is 'not worth living.' A plausible interpretation is that my advantage is personal access to the grounds or basis of my value judgments, such as my feelings. Since these feelings relate to something at the core of my being, which only I can access, I have some evaluative advantage over others. If this is correct, then it seems that Beauchamp would at least agree with Lonergan that feelings are cognitively relevant, and even that they play some necessary and crucial role in evaluations.[46] Second, Beauchamp and Lonergan also seem to agree that life is not an absolute good. Still, it is unlikely that Beauchamp would accept Lonergan's distinction between the ontic value of persons (i.e., the basic good or worth of persons) and the qualitative values attributed to them, or if he did accept the distinction, understand it in the way Lonergan does.

Aside from possible areas of agreement, there are some important differences between the stances of Beauchamp and Lonergan. First, I wonder how Beauchamp understands the relation between affect and value judging, and whether he thinks that those value judgments made by *the person in question* are always epistemically just subjective. This point, I think, is close to the centre of the whole debate. On the one hand, Beauchamp recognizes (rightly according to Lonergan) that personal cognitive elements, possibly feelings, play an important role in evaluations. But having admitted this, he seems to leave unexamined such key questions as: 'What feelings are cognitively relevant?' 'How do they enter into evaluations?' and 'Do such value judgments ever transcend one's own affective subjectivity?' By contrast, Lonergan has argued that not only do certain feelings play a crucial role in my value judging, but also that to the degree that they are the fruits of authentic subjectivity, such feeling-informed evaluations can be epistemically objective.[47]

Second, Beauchamp's apparent agnosticism on the question of whether one can ever make an epistemically objective value judgment leads him to overemphasize the subsequent act of choosing, much as occurred in the case of Sue Rodriguez. Beauchamp argues that passive euthanasia (allowing to die) and active euthanasia (killing) are morally indistinguishable choices because they can both follow from the value judgment that my life is 'not worth living.' This differs from Lonergan's analysis by driving a wedge between value judging and choosing and by failing to distinguish choices that involve actual goods from those that involve future possible goods. On Vertin's clarification of Lonergan's analysis, 'passive willing' pertains to choosing to enjoy some actual good in the mode of complacency. By contrast, 'active willing' characterizes one's choosing to actualize some future possible good in the mode of concern. According to this terminology, active euthanasia refers to the choice to actualize or bring about someone's death. The question is whether such a choice is positive or privative, the answer to which involves some evaluation of a life, whether by the one whose life it is, or by some other.

Finally, Beauchamp's position differs from Lonergan's by supposing some essential opposition between the individual's good and the social good. For instance, although Beauchamp locates the key evaluation in the debate to rest with me as *the person in question,* Lonergan might rightly ask about social elements that shape one's evaluation that one's life is 'not worth living.' Moreover, might this evaluation not be more readily made in a culture and context where, for instance, a work ethic devalues any 'idle stillness' (i.e., passive choosing to enjoy some actual good in the mode of complacency) or where a pragmatism and emphasis on economic efficiencies press one not to 'linger in life'?[48] Conversely, even if, entirely in isolation from the influences of others, I reached the evaluation that my life was 'not worth living,' might not this evaluation also have implications that extend beyond myself, as did Sue's self-evaluation for Dennis?

Beauchamp sidesteps this crucial evaluative issue by seeming to admit, at least in principle, that he is unable to specify what a normative evaluation would be in a case of my request for euthanasia. One might press him on this point, as I did in Sue's case, to see if this holds generally for any evaluations (e.g., tolerance in Sue's case) or just for evaluations about whether my life is worthwhile. His position is vulnerable on this point: if he admits that his inability to make any normative statement about this type of evaluation is not a purely philosophical issue, he then needs to specify the conditions that would make my negative self-evaluation normative. That is, in the same way that I would rebut his claim that his life is 'not worth living,' I would expect him to mount a similar rebuttal of my claim that 'my life is not worth living.' To admit that he could not critically assess my self-evaluation would be absurd.

I turn now to Richard McCormick's position on the role of affect in evaluations. My comments here are based on a lecture that McCormick gave, entitled 'Killing and Allowing to Die: Is There a Difference?' McCormick addressed the euthanasia debate on this distinction and expressly distinguished his own position from Beauchamp's. He articulated the view that there is an important ethical difference between killing and allowing to die. He also argued that this was a (if not the) crucial issue in the ethical and public-policy debates on euthanasia in the United States at that time.

In the lecture, McCormick rejected acts of killing by physicians such as those being proposed by proponents of euthanasia. He did so on the grounds that such acts should not be normative responses by society to those of its members who are suffering. Like Beauchamp, he argued that the important ethical issue was the underlying value judgment. By contrast to Beauchamp, however, McCormick argued that what is crucial about the subsequent choice is not whether one actively or passively caused death, but rather one's culpability.[49] Although he confined most of his critical comments to matters of logic, he did conclude with some personal reflections on the values at stake in the debate. For example, he considered a future in which euthanasia was legal and widely accepted and reflected on the disvalue of his elderly mother having to wonder if it was time for her to request euthanasia.

On the basis on this lecture, it seems to me evident that McCormick and Lonergan are in agreement on most, if not all, points of comparison. I take from his example that 'authentic' feelings regarding his mother worrying about having to ask for euthanasia can partly ground his negative evaluation of a normative public policy. Moreover, I interpret him as regarding such personal responses to values as more than epistemically just subjective, at least sometimes. He was also clear on the distinction between such cognitive elements as fact judging, value judging, and choosing, and I would judge these distinctions to be more or less compatible with Lonergan's distinctions. Finally, he expressly located his own position on the value of life as one who would affirm it as a basic good, but not an absolute one.

McCormick's engagement of the euthanasia debate, however, was almost entirely on Lonergan's second level of understanding. This made me wonder whether he takes the intellectual-cognitive processes of understanding and fact judging to be importantly distinct from the affective-cognitive processes of evaluating and choosing.[50] The other reason I raise this as a possibly helpful point to ponder is McCormick's critique of the public debate as overemphasizing some notion of autonomy. Thus he writes:

> The offshoot of this absolutization [of autonomy] is that very little attention is given to the values that ought to guide the use of autonomy. The fact that the choice is the patient's is viewed as the sole right-making characteristic of the choice ... Choices, however, can be right or wrong [positive or privative], and unless we confront the features that make choices right or wrong, autonomy usurps the evaluation.[51]

For McCormick, this reflects the cultural bias he would label *individualism.*

Lonergan's emphasis on the positive importance of an individual's feelings would have challenged McCormick to reconsider the grounds for his own evaluation concerning the future possibility of his mother having to ask for euthanasia. Reflecting on this example, it would be helpful to know what, in his own value judging, is the relative importance of logic and affect. This example also strikes me as one that illustrates an autonomous, personal evaluation that is not primarily self-concerned. Hence, it is an expression of what Lonergan might characterize as an individual's *authentic* autonomy, which is not just individualistic. Perhaps what is needed is an account of autonomy that could incorporate some notion of *authentic subjectivity* as articulated by Lonergan. Indeed, I would argue that Lonergan's account of subjectivity has ramifications for all ethicists, whose role might be conceived as helping others to discover, in their own experience, the responsibilities of moral agency.

4.2 Empirical Positions of Beauchamp and McCormick

Distinct from differences between these two thinkers on what Lonergan would identify as philosophical matters, there are also differences on empirical matters that are worth highlighting.

By *philosophical* matters, I am referring to what might more accurately be labelled *purely* philosophical matters that regard the structural, heuristic, a priori elements of cognition. These are distinct from *relatively* philosophical matters that involve some categorial knowledge claim having to do with objects, such as the difference between particular and general approaches to ethics, or between killing and allowing to die. The former regard my cognitive acts and the latter the cognitive achievements that result from my engagement of these structural elements with data.

What I mean by *empirical matters* here is simply this: how close to the stories of persons like Sue and Dennis are the questions and analyses that thinkers like Beauchamp and McCormick consider? In addition, I wonder if some of the issues they raise as philosophical ones are actually empirical matters and would therefore best be investigated as such.

Beauchamp focuses on what he takes to be the fundamental issue behind requests for euthanasia, namely, the evaluation that one's life is 'not worth living.' But there can be *many* different evaluations that lead one to decide to request euthanasia. In Sue's case, she did not request euthanasia primarily because she thought her life would not be worthwhile. She articulated her request in terms of her inability to fulfil what she considered to be the duties of *a good mother, friend, patient,* even *citizen.* If this observation is borne out by further empirical research on many cases of requests for euthanasia, this would make Beauchamp's analysis vulnerable to the charge of not addressing the real-life questions.

I would add some further considerations on two other empirical issues on which Beauchamp's argument in favour of euthanasia rests: (1) the distinction between killing and allowing to die and (2) the impact on the human good that such a policy would have. As for (1), both Sue and Dennis's stories seem to me to illustrate the distinction, both as a matter of fact and as involving two distinct evaluative issues. As I noted earlier, no one argues that Sue and Dennis were ethically culpable for not agreeing to use an artificial respirator. It is also interesting that this distinction plays such a prominent role in legal analyses. McCormick reported that not only did the U.S. Court of Appeals for the Ninth Circuit deny the distinction between killing and allowing to die, it also placed the burden of proof on *opponents* of euthanasia to demonstrate that such a distinction is 'real.' Presumably, they are expecting a philosophical argument rather than an invitation to examine the empirical evidence themselves. As for (2), it is interesting in Beauchamp's own account of the euthanasia debate that he highlights how considerations have become more restricted. He reports that the traditional debates (e.g., in Aquinas) centred on whether suicide violated one or more of three types of obligations: to oneself, to others, or to God. He also reports that David Hume's famous argument for the permissibility of autonomous suicide responded to only two of these traditional obligations, namely, to oneself and to others, but not to God. Finally, it seems that Beauchamp has provided an argument that responds to only one of the traditional obligations, namely, to oneself. Such an argument is at odds, it seems to me, with even Sue's experience of the importance of her perceived obligations to others as at least partly motivating her suicide.[52]

In McCormick's case, I would regard the concrete role of affect in evaluations as, in part, an empirical matter. Similarly, Lonergan considers attending to data of consciousness, which includes one's own cognitive processes, to be part of a *generalized* empirical method.[53] Important as it is for McCormick to focus on the logical issues that are being raised by others in this debate, I wonder if he is sufficiently attentive to the affective features of the stories of individuals, such as Sue and Dennis. In chapter 2 I reported how prominent the affective dimension was in Sue's story and in Dennis's. Sue seemed to make explicit the need for others to attend to more than the mere medical facts when she invited others to enter into the lives of the dying with 'open hearts' in order to see the realities. Similarly, Dennis rejects as 'inherently invalid' the views of experts who have no personal (i.e., affective) experience of issues connected with dying. Given that affect seems to play such a prominent role in these stories, and given my own reading of McCormick's positive stance on the relevance of feelings for his own evaluations, I wonder if Lonergan's analysis might fruitfully challenge anyone who holds a position similar to his to attend more closely to this dimension of the concrete stories and to engage the debate by addressing the level at which people experience their own mortality in the face of serious illness.[54]

4.3 Summary of Ramifications of Lonergan's Position for the Ethics of Euthanasia

What can we conclude from the comparison and contrast of the philosophical positions of Beauchamp and McCormick from a Lonerganian perspective? I suggest that, as with the positions of Sue and of Dennis, this analysis has brought to light two especially important points. First, both thinkers regard affect as somehow philosophically relevant to knowing values. Second, crucial differences between them arise on the issue of the role of affect in knowing values. Most fundamentally, they differ on the epistemic objectivity of evaluations that issue from affective cognitions or deliberative insights. It seems to me that the main reason Beauchamp is a proponent of euthanasia is because of the limitations, in principle, of any critical challenge of another's negative self-evaluation. That is, he is unable to engage critically the 'person in question' who concludes that his or her life is 'not worth living.' Although his philosophical position gives the appearance of prescinding from critically assessing another's self-evaluation, it nevertheless commits him to an instrumentalist view of moral status, that is, to accepting the view that the ontic value of a person's life is conditioned by certain qualitative attributes, which are to be judged by the person in question. For his part, McCormick seems to accept affect as relevant to evaluations. But he neither makes this role explicit nor suggests that it is a crucial issue in grounding and assessing the different value judgments that arise in this debate.

It was also especially revealing to examine the empirical positions of Beauchamp and McCormick, as distinct from their philosophical positions. A contribution here was to recognize their claims as empirical ones, and hence relevant to the issues and concerns that arise in particular stories from which requests for euthanasia can, and frequently do, arise. Engaging the ethical debate from this perspective was quite revealing. There is a series of claims concerning euthanasia that seem widely accepted, despite the fact that these claims have little to do with the concrete issues that arose in the two stories I have examined. Beauchamp, for example, advances two important claims that seem to be at odds with the experience of Sue and of Dennis: first, that the ethical issue at stake in the debate concerns the negative self-evaluation that one's life is 'not worth living'; second, that there is no relevant ethical difference between killing and allowing to die. Both claims drive a wedge between value judging and choosing. Moreover, since Beauchamp's claims are categorial and empirical ones, he needs to support them by appealing to some empirical evidence. He does not, however, present any such evidence. From the two cases I examined, I have shown that neither of these claims do justice to the experiences of Sue or Dennis. Again, McCormick's position on these empirical issues in the euthanasia debate also strikes me as needing some further development. My concern is with his lack of attention to the affective dimension of the stories of individuals, such as Sue and Dennis. Consequently, not only does he overlook psychologically important features of such stories, he also overlooks philosophically crucial data that are important to reflect on if one truly is to understand and assess requests for euthanasia.

5   **Comparing and Contrasting Philosophical and Empirical Positions of the Minority and Majority Members of the Senate Committee on Euthanasia**

To complete this sketch of the ramifications of Lonergan's position for the euthanasia debate, I will now highlight some potentially fruitful issues on which to engage the debate at the legislative level. Again, I will distinguish between philosophical and empirical issues that might account for differences between proponents and opponents of euthanasia. Since many of these issues already arose in the preceding analysis, I will confine my comments mainly to those issues not already discussed.

5.1 Philosophical Positions of the Minority and Majority Committee Members

Let me begin with the view of the minority members of the Special Senate Committee, which favoured changing the law to allow euthanasia (I will refer to them as the proponents).[55] On my interpretation, their philosophical stance agrees with Lonergan's mainly on the cognitive relevance of feelings for knowing values. They agree to some extent with the view that the human good is both individual and social, although they tend to frame the euthanasia question as one in which the two goods are in opposition. Finally, they appear to agree that life is not an absolute good, and might also agree that life is a basic good. (See table A.3, p. 312.)

The agreement, however, may not be a firm one. For instance, the report indicates that committee members were consistently confronted with the question of how to balance two different interests: individual rights and the interests of society. On this issue, it appears that the minority voted to protect 'the individual's rights of autonomy and self-determination,' even at the risk of compromising society's interest in upholding the principle of respect for human life. The proponents also considered 'allowing to die' to be ethically equivalent to intentional killing or euthanasia.[56]

As for the points of disagreement between the proponents and Lonergan, the main one concerns the epistemic status of affectively based evaluations, as was the case for both Sue Rodriguez and Tom Beauchamp. Another point of disagreement is on the relation between value judging and choosing. Note that the perspective of the proponents differs from those of Sue and Dennis, and even from the perspectives of Beauchamp and McCormick. The question addressed by these latter individuals was whether, or on what grounds, an individual could responsibly choose euthanasia or physician-assisted suicide. By contrast, the proponents focus primarily on the question of whether one could justify society's positive response to such requests (presumed to be responsible) through authorizing physicians to accede to them. Their analysis penetrates only as far as an individual's express *wish* to die. So long as such an individual is able to make a 'competent' request, by which they mean the individual knows the *facts* and alternatives and is free to choose his or her preferred option, then they are prepared to admit that euthanasia 'can be a merciful and appropriate response to suffering, in cases where it cannot be relieved by other means.'[57]

From Lonergan's perspective, the proponents' formulation is consistent with a substantive general moral claim. They merely admit that such a claim is not to be taken as a pre-empirical generalization. Hence, for any such general claim one must concede that one cannot predict in advance all the particularities of cases that might arise, so that one can absolutely rule out this response to suffering.[58] Still, it seems that the proponents have focused no further than someone's express wish for euthanasia, and do not seem to appreciate that, or how these wishes might be connected to diverse evaluations, as I suggested was the case with Sue. The question, as interpreted by these legislators, is importantly different from the one on which Beauchamp and McCormick focus their ethical analysis. For the proponents, the central issue is not whether my or some other *individual's* choice of euthanasia is a normative or justified one. They seem to assume that such a determination cannot be made. Rather, their question regards the normativity of *society's* response to the fact that there are such requests (responsible or not), on the assumption that what is being requested is a genuine benefit for the person in question. If it is a benefit, society (through its physicians) is assumed to have a duty to distribute this 'benefit' according to some measure of fairness or justice. Hence, the issue becomes one of equality when it is framed, as Sue's lawyers framed it, as a matter of society providing benefits to some persons and being unwilling to provide them for others. Lonergan's challenge to the proponents' position is to penetrate further than the express choice/wish to ask whether it is positive or privative. If I were the one requesting euthanasia, then, they would need to address my question 'What about the evaluation that my life is not worth living?' 'Do you, as legislators, affirm or deny this?' 'Or can you never, in principle, challenge my negative or positive self-evaluation?'[59]

As regards the opponents' philosophical position, it seems to agree with Lonergan's on all points. In their express deliberations they highlight a number of issues I have already dealt with, such as the importance of affect. They note, for instance, that 'dignity exists when one faces the final stages of life with a feeling of self-worth and with the care, solicitude, and compassion to which all human beings are entitled.'[60] One of the opponents, however, favoured a change in the law that would allow assisted suicide, and then, in a step-by-step approach, the gradual adoption of adequate safeguards to allow euthanasia.[61] From Lonergan's perspective, this view is prone to the charge of unfairness because it distinguishes society's differing responses to persons before and after this change on ethically irrelevant grounds.

Finally, regarding the relation between the individual and social good, opponents appear to agree with Lonergan's view that not only are these two not in opposition; they also agree that the social good conditions the vital goods of the individual members of society. The opponents concede that '[w]hile disallowing assisted suicide may seem unfair or harsh in an individual circumstance, this is outweighed by the negative impact that decriminalization would have on the popular conscience.'[62] From this statement it seems that the opponents were prepared to accept that persons like Sue might rightly conclude that their lives are 'not worth living,' which would make euthanasia a positive choice. Even so, they would still resist changing the law because of the risks of such a change to society as a whole. From Lonergan's perspective, one might challenge this view because it accepts the negative self-assessment of persons like Sue at face value without actually investigating the grounds of such an assessment. And if one were to investigate such cases as Sue's, Lonergan's view would recommend that one consider their claims in light of the inner norms of authentic subjectivity, which ought to characterize not only the deliberations of Sue but also those of her peers, including Dennis.

5.2 Empirical Positions of the Minority and Majority Committee Members

On the empirical side, the proponents' stance reinterprets the ethics of common medical practice. My own view is that their interpretation equivocates on the value of life. That is, since they correctly point out that medical practice is inconsistent with the view of life as an 'absolute' good, they conclude that neither ought it be regarded as a 'basic' good.

Let me explain how they use the empirical evidence of medical practice. Following James Rachels's argument, taken from his article 'Active and Passive Euthanasia,' which first appeared in a medical journal in 1975,[63] the proponents consider both (1) withholding and withdrawing life-sustaining treatment and (2) providing treatment aimed at alleviating pain that may hasten death as 'similar to' voluntary euthanasia. The ethically relevant point of similarity for them is that in all these cases the foreseeable outcome is death (i.e., they block out entirely from their ethical considerations the data of intention or motivation).[64] But as McCormick rightly pointed out, the ethical issue is not one of *causality* in the face of the foreseeable outcome of death, but rather of *culpability*, which regards all of one's choices in this setting.

In my view, the ethically relevant evaluations are those of individuals who request euthanasia, and those of a society that responds to such requests. On the former issue, the proponents equivocate on the value of life, which leads to ironic consequences. If I am the *person in question* who has ALS, and if I choose, as did both Sue or Dennis, not to go on a respirator as my status declines, how would the proponents interpret this choice? It seems that if they hold that 'allowing to die' is equivalent to intentional killing, they would need to judge my refusal of life-sustaining technologies to be suicidal, and me as culpable for not choosing such treatment. But surely there are situations in which I need not do everything to sustain my life; and if that is so, life is not an absolute good.[65] On the other hand, there are surely situations in which I ought to choose some life-saving or life-sustaining treatment; for instance, if I developed a simple chest infection and knew I would succumb without readily available antibiotic treatment. In such a case, the proponents would rightly argue that my choice not to take such treatment is privative and that I am culpable of a reckless disregard for the value of my life. By the same reasoning, I could also be culpable for choosing euthanasia. But they conclude that if one finds the first case acceptable (allowing death), then one must also accept euthanasia as ethically equivalent.

If this fairly represents the proponents' interpretation of common medical decisions, then they are equivocating on what they take to be the value of life. I would be culpable in the first case for not choosing a respirator only if life were understood as an *absolute* good, which they surely deny. But if life is a *basic* good, then I am not necessarily obliged to choose any means whatever to promote or prolong it. In the second case, I would be culpable for choosing not to take antibiotics if life were regarded as a *basic* good that I could easily secure. But proponents seem to deny not only that life is an absolute good, but even that it is a basic good, since they are arguing for euthanasia, which would seem to violate the value of life understood even as a basic good.

The irony of the proponents' position, which focuses exclusively on the ethics of society's response to an individual's request for euthanasia, is that by their reinterpretation of 'empirical' medical practice they risk undermining the very values they hope to promote. Their fundamental concern is with physicians' hesitation to treat adequately their patients' pain and other symptoms. To this end, they hope to remove from these 'hesitant' physicians any legal concerns regarding public accountability for their actions in this regard, concerns that can cause them to be overly cautious in treating symptoms. Instead, they hope this legal change will encourage physicians to alleviate 'suffering' by all means possible, even if this includes active killing. In equating this common medical response to patients requiring pain relief near the end of life with killing them, the proponents may have removed some legal barriers, but they have surely erected more ethical ones. Their efforts to enhance patient care may well have the opposite effect of making physicians more reluctant to provide sufficient pain relief for fear that they are violating, or would be perceived by others as violating, the basic good of a patient's life.

I am suggesting that fundamentally this is an empirical issue of interpreting the normative responses of individuals and caregivers to illnesses. What I want to insist upon is not the conceptual problems of this interpretation of practice, but the fact that it is an empirical issue, and that the interpretation of medical practice that they are offering is superficial at best.

As for the consideration of empirical issues by opponents of euthanasia, I note that they (i.e., the majority members of the Senate committee) were the only ones to appeal expressly to any empirical evidence, and this appeal regarded the experience of the practice of euthanasia in the Netherlands. Opponents also made certain claims that could be empirically confirmed or refuted, such as claims about the effect of euthanasia on the public's conscience and the infrequency of requests for euthanasia. But they cited no empirical evidence to support such claims. One ramification of Lonergan's insistence that these questions are fundamentally empirical is that further research is needed on both sides of the euthanasia debate. Indeed, it is surprising to me that there were no detailed references to any cases in the report, or even in the submissions to this committee. Looked at from the point of view of an empirical science like medicine, the type of empirical evidence that was relied upon by both sides in their deliberations was expert opinion. This is generally considered to be among the weakest types of empirical evidence.

6   Summary

On what I take to be the first and most fundamental level of the euthanasia debate, the level of the concrete life-stories, such as those of Sue Rodriguez and Dennis Kaye, Lonergan opens up and takes seriously the complexities of responsible human moral agency, both of individuals regarding themselves, and with a view to the good of all members of a society. Moreover, he regards the individual and social components as both crucial for any concrete realization of the human good. Lonergan's position is not some ideal formula that no human could possibly live up to: Dennis Kaye's *common-sense* stance seemed to me to be compatible with Lonergan's own position. I also discovered that there was agreement on at least three of six points of comparison between Sue Rodriguez's position and Lonergan's. That is, they seemed to agree that (1) feelings are cognitively relevant; (2) the human good is both individual and social; and (3) life is not an absolute good. Identifying such points of common understanding was important because it allows one to begin the process of dialogue on common ground. I would add that if I were to enter into genuine dialogue with someone who held a position such as Sue's, I should be willing to offer her my reflections on possible inconsistencies in her position (e.g., both affirming that value-claims are always epistemically just subjective and concurrently claiming to know that the value of tolerance is not epistemically just subjective). I should also be open to the possibility of the reverse and be willing to change my own position as a result.

This contrast of positions also revealed points of differences between how each of them understood the role of affect in evaluations. It was helpful to discover a number of differences between the positions Sue Rodriguez and Dennis Kaye held. First, for Sue, feelings related to value judging in some *immediate* way, rather than *mediately*, as for Dennis. Hence, for Sue, feelings were *sufficient* grounds for an evaluation, rather than *partial* or *insufficient* grounds, as for Dennis. Second, the resulting evaluations that Sue grasped affectively were purported to be *epistemically merely subjective*, rather than *epistemically objective*, as for Dennis. Third, as a consequence of Sue's agnosticism regarding the epistemic objectivity of any evaluation, she seemed to drive a wedge between value judging and choosing, and, at least verbally, she emphasized the ethical importance of choosing. By contrast, Dennis's main concern was with the basis for Sue's negative self-evaluation, and particularly with the ramifications of this evaluation for others, including himself. I also argued that Dennis's position was compatible with Lonergan's on each of these points of comparison.

If I were to highlight what I regard as the most important discoveries resulting from this analysis, I would mention three. First and perhaps most importantly, regardless of one's stance on the role of affect in evaluations, one cannot do justice to the stories of either Sue or Dennis without attending both to their ideas *and* to their feelings. Stated generally, the point is that one needs to attend to both intellectual and affective-cognitive elements in oneself and in others. Again, these stories cannot be adequately understood without attending to the concrete medical and human realities of the *whole person* who experiences some illness. That is, regardless of one's response to Sue's request for euthanasia, one still needs to attend to and understand her experience by accepting, in some sense, her invitation to enter her world with an open heart and see the realities of herself and her situation. These realities are relational and cognitive, the latter being importantly affective. Hence, to engage this debate from a strictly individualistic or logical perspective would be to miss these fundamental issues. Finally, these concrete empirical examples are important for philosophers and legislators to consider. Thinkers or experts who engage subsequent questions from the diverse points of view of such fields as medicine, ethics, or public policy need to ground their reflections and recommendations in *real* stories, such as those of Sue and Dennis. That is, one needs to consider Dennis's challenge that what 'experts' recommend is bound to be invalid unless they have some personal knowledge of the experience of dying. I would add that they also need some capacity to reflect critically upon such experience, to which their recommendations are meant to apply.

I indicated how one might begin to explore the ramifications of Lonergan's position on the second level of the euthanasia debate by briefly contrasting the philosophical presuppositions of Tom Beauchamp and Richard McCormick on the role of affect in evaluations, and I related the position of each of them to Lonergan's position. Again, I could summarize my most important discoveries under three points. First, on the purely philosophical issues, the positions of each of these two authors exhibit different tendencies, which make their positions bear some family resemblance to positions other than Lonergan's. For example, I raised the question of whether Beauchamp tends to restrict his attention to affective-cognitive subjectivity, and whether he is less attentive to intellectual-cognitional subjectivity and less open to the possibility of cognitional self-transcendence than is Lonergan. In McCormick's case, I wondered if he tended to the opposite extreme by restricting his ethical attention to logical or intellectual-cognitive elements, and if he is less attentive to the cognitive role of feelings in evaluations than is Lonergan.

Second, a further philosophical issue concerned the moral relevance of the distinction between passive and active choices. Like Sue Rodriguez, Beauchamp also seems to have driven a wedge between value judging and choosing, and to hold that value judgments concerning the worth of one's life are epistemically merely subjective. Although he emphasized the ethical relevance of value judging over choosing, he uses this contrast to make the further distinction between choosing to kill (i.e., actively willing the future possible death of someone) and allowing to die (i.e., passively willing the actual death of someone) ethically irrelevant. Although McCormick does not understand the passive/active distinction as equivalent to judgments about actual and possible goods, nevertheless he countered Beauchamp's analysis by pointing out that the real issue is not one's causal implication in the death of a person by either passive or active choices, but rather one's culpability. This move seemed effectively to challenge the wedge Beauchamp had driven between value judging and choosing.

Third, on empirical issues, I discovered that both exhibit a tendency to short-circuit the empirical side of the stories on which they need to be reflecting. Though they are far from someone like James Rachels, I raised as a question whether they exhibit a milder version of the same tendency of philosophers to invent cases and thereby pass over too quickly what Lonergan would regard as a crucial stage of attentiveness to data and to the questions that arise from concrete, lived experiences and stories.

Finally, I engaged the third level of the euthanasia debate by reflecting on some ramifications of Lonergan's stance for public-policy recommendations. Let me summarize what I consider to be my most important discoveries in three final points. First, the public-policy question about whether it would be wise to relax the legal prohibition of physician-assisted suicide is, in the first instance, a *societal choice.* As such, the decision regards the normativity or responsibility of a *society*'s set of responses to an individual's suicidal request, presumably following a negative self-evaluation by that individual that his or her life is 'not worth living.' More fundamentally, however, a responsible and prudent public-policy decision must also address, and take a stance on, the normativity of the individual's self-evaluation that his or her life is not worth living, which seems to be the most convincing grounds for voluntary euthanasia. Lonergan's account of the role of affect in evaluations highlights the fact that the internal norm of authentic subjectivity has a bearing upon such value judgments. For him, a responsible public policy cannot avoid taking a stance on the epistemic objectivity of such evaluations. On this issue, his position was in sharp contrast to those legislators I examined who were on either side of this issue. Proponents and opponents of euthanasia both assumed that such negative self-evaluations were so personal that they could not be critically assessed.

Second, philosophers can be most helpful to this debate by articulating an adequate account of cognitional and decisional subjectivity, and by challenging rival views. On all three levels of the debate, the most consistent difference between proponents and opponents of euthanasia was not over whether they thought feelings were cognitively relevant to evaluations. This was typically a point of agreement between disputants. Rather, the key issue was whether such evaluations were ever more than epistemically just subjective. If these evaluations were deemed to be just subjective, thinkers then emphasized choosing over value judging. For legislators, these choices are to be guided by the application of legal notions of autonomy and equality. Although similar issues and stances were taken on all three levels of the debate, the legislative discussion among both proponents and opponents of euthanasia rarely benefited from either concrete stories or any explicit attention to the ethical analyses and discussions.

Third, for Lonergan, once one addresses and takes a stance on the philosophical issues regarding cognitional subjectivity, the euthanasia question becomes essentially an empirical one. The issue is whether a system of caring for those at the end of life that includes euthanasia would actually be better than the present system. Hence, it is on the basis of empirical evidence, not philosophical arguments, that evaluative questions, like the distinction between killing and allowing to die, need to be settled. Consequently, one would not anticipate that a substantive ethical claim would reach the level of generality of a pre-empirical claim. At most, it could be a categorial, empirical, transcultural, general proposition.[66]

To their credit, members of the Special Senate Committee raised some empirical-medical questions concerning the efficacy of symptom control at the end of life. Still, members paid very little attention to other important empirical questions concerning, on the one hand, systems that involve euthanasia and, on the other, systems that involve a vitalistic approach that insists on aggressive medical interventions for all people at the end of life.

At this point I believe I have come full circle. I began with two concrete life-stories that illustrate opposing responses to the question of euthanasia in the context of the same disease. I then worked through a series of philosophical questions to end up at the question of a public-policy recommendation for the issue of euthanasia. An underlying theme that I have carried through this discussion is a concern to be explicit about my own cognitive and decisional agency. It was for this reason that I have deliberately identified myself as the author of any claims that I made, rather than using the passive voice which obscures such authorship. One reason for thinking that this would be helpful is that the issue of autonomy has become such a prominent one in ethics, even to the extent of trumping any other ethical consideration.

To spell this out more fully, I invite the reader to proceed to chapter 10, in which I will state my own position on the euthanasia debate.

Ramifications of Lonergan's Stance on the Eye of the Heart for Philosophy and for the Euthanasia Debate

Moral feelings and moral judgments are occurring all the time – there is nothing recondite or rare about them (e.g., 'What a brute he is!' or 'What a nice person!'). Most human conversation is praising or blaming somebody or something. One could possibly work out an analogy with judgments of fact or possibility, in terms of the virtually unconditioned, but this is a little removed from the actual process. In the actual process it is like knowing you have an insight ('Gee, I've got it!'). The moral judgment on a particular issue is something that can come about very slowly, be maturing over a long time – people make retreats and elections, and so on. One's moral being is satisfied when one comes up with a sound judgment, just as one's intellectual being is satisfied when one understands.

Bernard Lonergan, 'Milltown Park Lectures on *Method in Theology*'

1   An Overview of Personal Ramifications of Lonergan's Stance

I began this discussion with two questions that have motivated my research: 'What role does affect or *heart* play in value judgments?' and 'What are some implications of Lonergan's stance on the role of affectivity in value judgments for the euthanasia debate?' With these two questions in mind, then, I shall now attempt to draw together the various strands of the discussion by first recapitulating Lonergan's theory of value judging, which affirms both the role of affect in evaluations and the possibility that such evaluations, like fact judgments, can be epistemically objective, and then go on to specify in my own name some ramifications of Lonergan's philosophical position for the euthanasia debate.

There were three patterns in the form of the argument that have shaped this discussion. The first was an emphasis on a 'bottom-up' methodology (parts 1 to 3), which was later brought to some closure with a 'top-down' analysis (part 4). This methodology allowed me to consider the nuances of certain cases in which the question of euthanasia arose and also to bring to light larger philosophical issues on which one's assessment of these cases rests. The second pattern was to treat the issue of what one is doing when knowing *facts* prior to the question of what one is doing when knowing *values*, and then to consider under what conditions each of these cognitive achievements results in valid knowing. This allowed me to illustrate in some detail Lonergan's claim that epistemic objectivity is the fruit of authentic subjectivity, a claim that applies to *both* fact judgments and value judgments. The third pattern was to provide a first-person analysis of cognitive operations. This involved attending not only to the circumstances under which I make good judgments, but also involved analysing my own misjudgments in order to root out the sources of my mistakes. Ultimately, the reader's assessment of the success of this project will itself involve the very type of first-person evaluation that I have tried to elucidate.

On this basis, I questioned the usefulness of the particularist/generalist distinction for clearly separating methodologically distinct approaches to bioethical issues. Moreover, I argued that differences among thinkers on specific topics in bioethics, such as euthanasia, rested on more fundamental cognitional issues. What seems most evident in the euthanasia debate are disputed notions about the worthwhileness of someone's life under certain circumstances. That is, concrete evaluations are involved. But thinkers differ on the question of whether one can ever make a true evaluation. I proposed that the answer to this pivotal question depends on one's stance regarding whether one can make true fact judgments. Those thinkers, like Hume, who deny that fact judgments are ever epistemically objective also reject the possibility of making objective evaluations. By contrast, thinkers such as Kant, who affirm the practical possibility of epistemically objective value judgments, do so by denying that feelings have any apprehensive function.[1] In so doing, these latter thinkers dismiss what I have argued is the key distinctive feature of the fourth level of conscious intentionality, namely, any affective cognitions such as deliberative insights.

I argued that differences among thinkers on the question of how one knows values correspond to differences on how they think one knows facts. I provided an account of Lonergan's most basic stance on how insights enter into one's knowing in chapter 4, where I explained his account of how one understands and knows facts. The most basic evidence to which I appealed in support of this account was the self-evidence of my own performance in knowing medical facts. By focusing on the phenomenal/epistemic and the fact/value distinctions that underpin the euthanasia debate, I gave a mainly positive argument about how one knows values. I did this by way of an exposition of how Lonergan's categories might serve as useful tools for analysing and assessing methodologically distinct positions in bioethics.[2]

2   Lonergan's Stance on the Role of Affect in Value Judgments

Lonergan's position on the relation between 'affect' and 'evaluation,' which I articulated in chapters 4 and 6, and affirmed in my own name in chapter 9, is that certain affective responses play a cognitive role in value judgments. According to Michael Vertin's development of Lonergan's position, the relevant feelings are of two distinct kinds, 'transcendental affectivity' and 'categorial affective responses.' I depicted categorial affective responses as a posteriori affective intentional responses. These can be responses to either values or to mere satisfactions. I argued that it was to these feelings that Lonergan referred when he wrote that 'apprehensions [of value] are given in feelings.'[3] It is *in* or *by means of* such feelings that one grasps objects as concrete values. That is, such feeling responses function as part of one's cognitive *access to* or *grasp of* values, through what one might label a 'deliberative insight.' Such insights function like 'direct' and 'reflective' insights in as much as they are acts of grasping some unity in a diversity. Although each of these distinct insights is a pivotal act for subsequent cognitive achievements, deliberative insights enter into one's cognitive process as an intermediary between fact and value judgments. Deliberative insights are also distinct from direct and reflective insights because they are 'affective' and not just intellectual acts.

By contrast with categorial affective responses, 'transcendental affectivity' refers to those a priori feelings that are an aspect of one's transcendental intending of value. This is the affective dimension of the transcendental notion of value that is the source of one's value questions and the ultimate criterion for the correctness of one's evaluative achievements. In chapter 7, following Vertin's interpretation of Lonergan, I characterized a true value judgment as one in which there is a 'felt' correspondence between one's categorial affective response to a possible value and the transcendental affectivity of one's orientation to value.

On the basis of this account, I depicted feelings as *necessary but non-sufficient* conditions of value judgments. They are part of the evidential grounds on which one who is morally developed bases his or her affirmations of values.

Subsequent to value judging is deciding or choosing to enjoy or implement, if appropriate, what one affirms to be good or worthwhile. This act of choosing brings the deliberative process to a close. I argued that this view of the role of affect in value judgments or evaluations rounds out a comprehensive cognitive theory that includes in its account of moral knowing both intellectual and affective cognitive elements (i.e., 'head' and 'heart'). It also provides a basis for a critical-realist (or axiological-objectivist) theory of values by rejecting the model of knowing that the main rival theories presuppose, namely, a model based on the ocular act of 'looking.' According to the 'ocular' cognitive theory, any affective cognition is necessarily epistemically just subjective.

3   My Own Philosophical and Empirical Position on Euthanasia

I concluded chapter 8 by affirming what I take to be Lonergan's position on a set of core philosophical questions, and I defended his stance against some anticipated objections. That section constitutes my own achievement of the first goal of this discussion, which was to explicate and critically assess Lonergan's account of the role of affect in evaluations. In chapter 9 I employed Lonergan's philosophical position on a set of core questions to engage opposing positions on the issue of euthanasia. What remains is for me to articulate my own reply to this question. That is, how would I answer the practical question 'What does all this mean concretely for a medico-ethical issue such as euthanasia?' This section, therefore, completes my achievement of the second goal of the discussion, which was to demon-strate some ramifications of Lonergan's philosophical position for the euthanasia debate.

For the remainder of the discussion, then, I will be advancing my own view about what an adequate answer to the euthanasia question would look like, and specifying what further questions need to be addressed in order to ground a responsible public policy. Although I think this answer is consis-tent with Lonergan's philosophical stance, I take full responsibility for it myself. And although the form of this answer will be distinct from the arguments that both Beauchamp and McCormick have advanced, I wish to avoid controversy by highlighting not deficiencies but rather the positive lessons I take from their stances, lessons I hope to incorporate in my own reply.

3.1 Some Relevant Philosophical and Empirical Questions

The list of questions mentioned at the beginning of the discussion included some core philosophical questions that have to do with cognitional and decisional subjectivity. The central question in the series was, 'What is the role of affect in evaluations?' A distinct set of questions arose from the euthanasia debate itself. A central question in this set was the one posed by the Special Senate Committee on Euthanasia and Assisted Suicide, namely, 'Why do persons request physician-assisted suicide?' I take the first set of

questions to be *philosophical* questions that regard the knowing and deciding subject, and I spelled out an answer to these questions in my exposition
of Lonergan's cognitional theory. I take the second set of questions to be
distinct insofar as they regard not my own performance as a subject, but
what I come to know of objects by means of these acts. For convenience, I
label these questions *empirical.*[4]

   The image I used earlier to capture the distinction between philosophical and empirical categories was that of a pair of scissors. The lower blade of
the scissors represents the a posteriori or empirical data with which I
engage. The upper blade symbolizes the heuristic, merely structural, a
priori, or pre-empirical features of myself as a knowing subject. The coming
together of these two blades results in the action of cutting, which is the
manifold contents of knowledge that result from my cognitional acts actually operating in an authentic manner. With this image in mind, a central
concern of the discussion was to demonstrate that if one is to provide an
adequate reply to any given ethical issue, such as those raised by the
euthanasia debate, it is necessary to have a functioning, two-bladed pair of
scissors – and it also helps if one is clear about the role and limits of each
blade. Although I take answers to the first set of philosophical questions,
which I dealt with first in the discussion, to be most basic and general, I
would also insist that explicit answers to these questions do not provide
sufficient conditions for establishing an adequate stance on this or any
other ethical issue.[5] Nevertheless, I have shown that many of the differences between proponents and opponents of euthanasia actually arise at
the level of what I would call philosophical commitments. This is one
reason why it is important that ethicists be aware of these issues and attend
to them. To summarize the various types of differences that can arise in
these philosophical issues, it is helpful to consider various alternative family
stances that have arisen in the euthanasia debate. Each of these stances
illustrates alternative emphases, and hence more or less truncated viewpoints on what Lonergan would argue is the whole of cognitional and
decisional subjectivity. That is, for Lonergan, a complete account of cognitional and decisional subjectivity would need to include the distinct
and related acts of experiencing, understanding, judging, and evaluating-
deciding-doing/enjoying. He regards this as the philosophical *positional*
stance, and the basic set of philosophical counterpositions are derived from
this set by truncating this account to three or fewer levels of acts.

3.2   Choosing a Philosophical Stance That Is Least Truncated

There were four *family tendencies* that emerged in my analysis of the euthanasia debate, which I now wish to highlight. This is continuous with what I
did in chapter 3 by outlining historical continuities among alternative

families of thinkers (e.g., axiological subjectivists and objectivists). Now, however, I wish to draw attention not only to the fact that each family tends to focus on one or more elements of cognitional and decisional subjectivity, but also that such a focus tends to exclude or diminish the role of other elements. These families represent not distinct cognitional performances, but rather distinct accounts of performances.

The most narrowly focused (and also the most truncated) tendency is best reflected by the family of thinkers who attend exclusively to *sense data* or *sense objects*. This family focuses all its attention on questions regarding sense data. But it does so at the expense of neglecting questions regarding the knowing and deciding subject, which involve attending to *data of consciousness*. Consequently, what this family means by *the real* is simply what is given at the level of sense experience, and hence its account of the real will differ from the accounts offered by other families.

An example of this tendency among the thinkers I have considered is, perhaps, the minority members of the Special Senate Committee. A classic example of someone who belongs to such a family is B.F. Skinner, for whom the only scientifically relevant data are sense data. I suggest that the minority members also exhibit the tendency of this family to exclude attending to the subject's own cognitional processes, which would mean attending to data of consciousness. Moreover, this exclusion plays a crucial role in their endorsement of euthanasia. As I reported this position previously, one has the sense that the evaluating and deciding subject is, for them, an unknowable *black box*. And as I read them, their positive stance on euthanasia is largely a consequence of the presumed philosophical limitations in the ability of individuals to penetrate the *black box* of others, and thereby to understand, judge, and evaluate the cognitive grounds of decisions by others. From this family's perspective, wishes become all important because they are most apparent and evident from what people say. To unpack the cognitive grounds of such wishes is, in principle, an impossible task.[6]

A second family tendency is just the opposite to the tendency of the previous family. Instead of focusing on objects that are given in sense data, this family focuses on the data of consciousness of subjects to the exclusion of objects. Members of this family are very aware of such subjective phenomena as feelings or moods. But for them the distinction between *subject/object* or *self/other* is a fundamental one. Consequently they become stuck on the problem of the bridge, of moving from their own minds through judgment to objects (self and other). Hence, this family's account of the knowing and deciding subject is one in which the content of one's knowledge is never more than *epistemically just subjective*.

An example of someone exemplifying this family tendency among the people I have considered, I suggest, is Sue Rodriguez. This tendency to believe that one's knowledge, and especially one's self-evaluations, are never more than just subjective is most evident from Sue's interchange with Dennis Kaye. Sue expressed publicly her negative self-evaluation when claiming that when her disease progressed to the point where her life was 'a mere biological existence,' life would not be worthwhile. In Dennis's response to her, he said that since his own life is of the quality she refers to as 'merely biological,' her self-evaluation was *relevant* to himself. Dennis also prefaced his own remarks by acknowledging that although he realized that she did not *intend* her self-evaluation to be hurtful to others, such as himself, nevertheless they were. Dennis highlighted for Sue the fact that the content of her knowledge is not just subjective, and his own appreciation of the fact that she had not grasped this herself.[7]

A third family tendency insists most strongly on the objectivity of knowing, including evaluative knowing and deciding. In so doing, members of this family characteristically set aside or repress certain elements of psychological/cognitive subjectivity, such as feelings. This is because they believe them to be *just subjective*, and that they must somehow be transcended in order for one to achieve objective knowledge (this is why, I think, the passive voice is so popular with them). They are not necessarily ill disposed to all elements of psychological/cognitive subjectivity, for they might be quite aware of such conscious acts as those of understanding or judging facts. But, for some reason, affective acts are considered to be too closely aligned with the body, rather than with the mind, and so they are deemed to play a merely psychological function and to have no true cognitive import. Hence, members of this family are open to data of sense, which the first family emphasizes. They are also open to many elements of the data of consciousness, which the second family highlights. They are not open, however, to entertaining affective data as cognitively important, or at least as on a par with other acts, such as those of insight or understanding. Among people with whom I have dealt here, I would suggest that an example of someone belonging to this third family tendency is Richard McCormick. This assessment might not be fair, but it is based on the fact that, at least judging by the way he engages the euthanasia debate, he never once inferred, or made explicit, that affective cognitive acts were important to evaluations.[8]

A fourth family tendency is one that is least truncated in its account of the knowing and deciding subject. This family is open to data of sense (first family), data of consciousness (second family), intellectual cognitive acts (third family), as well as to affective cognitive acts. In the examples I gave, this family was represented by Dennis Kaye, Richard McCormick (probably), the majority members of the Special Senate Committee, and Lonergan.

Interestingly, on each level of the debate, members of this family were consistently opposed to euthanasia. Since I consider the euthanasia question, like any other ethical question, to be one that requires the operation of a two-bladed pair of scissors consisting of a philosophical upper blade and an empirical lower blade, one can critique any position on such an issue on the basis of the kind of scissors they bring to it. A position's upper blade may be overly truncated to begin with. Or its lower blade may have insufficiently engaged the concrete issues. Or, finally, the scissors a position has may function poorly because it tries to cut through these complex issues with only a single blade. It seems to me that at least the opponents of euthanasia have their upper blade in better order. What I would add to their position are some recommendations about lower-blade issues and how they might be ordered by upper-blade considerations.

The critical side of this conclusion is that the proponents of euthanasia have an overly truncated upper blade, and this restricts their attention to lower-blade data. This is, I must admit, a somewhat surprising conclusion. Prominent proponents of euthanasia typically present themselves as closer to the actual experience of persons who are dying than the opponents. Part of the phenomena of this experience they seek to highlight, rightly I think, is affective. They focus on the suffering that people experience, and conclude that society has an urgent duty to respond effectively to this suffering, and propose euthanasia as one part of such an effective response. The way I have sought to engage this position is to affirm the data to which they attend, but to press them to unpack what they mean by *suffering*, and what evaluations lie behind any decision to respond to this suffering.

4   My Own Reply to the Empirical Questions regarding Euthanasia

4.1   An Outline of a Philosophically Sound, Comprehensive Research Program

For what it is worth, my own reply to this difficult euthanasia question would involve taking a stance both on the philosophical questions that regard cognitional and decisional subjectivity, and on the empirical questions that regard the concrete human realities and possibilities from which requests for euthanasia arise. I would locate my own philosophical position as being compatible with Lonergan's. Still, even if Lonergan's philosophical stance is less restricted than the other alternatives I have examined, my commitment to the position he articulates does not settle the empirical questions that arise in the euthanasia debate. The benefit of being clearer about these philosophical issues is that at least then one can approach the empirical questions with an express knowledge of the categories one is employing. My focus on the ramifications of Lonergan's stance on some core questions regarding the role of affect in evaluations for three levels of this debate was, on this view, an empirical exercise. This exercise led me to a number of conclusions regarding the stories of Sue and Dennis, some of which were also relevant to the larger ethical and legislative debates.

Before I offer my own reading of the empirical issues, I would suggest that there are some distinct sets of empirical questions that researchers need to address if they are to make a responsible recommendation regarding a policy on euthanasia. I hope to point out some ramifications not only of Lonergan's stance on the role of affect in evaluations, but, more generally, of an account of human cognitional and decisional subjectivity for answering this public-policy question. Since I consider the public-policy question to be, in the first instance, a decisional issue, I would also relate it to the underlying evaluations, judgments, understandings, and experiences. These connections are perhaps the most important ramifications of Lonergan's position for this debate.

My short reply to the euthanasia question is to highlight what the relevant empirical questions are, how these questions relate to one another, what I take to be the central research questions that need to be addressed, and how such questions might be answered empirically. In other words, my answer is to outline the design for a research program that could address these questions.[9] The end result of such a program would be to reach a shared evaluation about the conditions of persons that would support the view that their lives were 'not worth living.' It would only be in such a context that one might consider collaborating with a request for euthanasia. I take this to be the context of the public-policy questions. I will suggest that this public-policy question is about the concretely functioning human good, a key component of which involves addressing rival notions of justice.

4.2 What Are the Empirical Questions That Need to Be Addressed?

I suggest that there are four interrelated sets of empirical questions that need to be addressed: (1) about the experience, e.g., 'How many persons are requesting euthanasia?' (2) for understanding, e.g., 'Why are persons requesting euthanasia?' 'What alternatives to suicide might be acceptable?' 'What would be the short- and long-term consequences of a new policy on euthanasia for various members of society?' (3) for judging, e.g., 'The ethically relevant concrete possibilities to consider are ...'; and (4) for evaluating, choosing, and acting/enjoying, e.g., 'Would a proposed new policy be truly better, and for whom?' 'Should such a policy be implemented at once or in a step-wise fashion?'

Grasping the distinctions and relations among these empirical questions locates the policy question in Lonergan's scheme as an effort to generalize particular evaluations that are authentic. This general policy question is importantly distinct from, though connected to, the particular evaluations on which I have focused. Lonergan's general cognitional structure provides an outline for a systematic approach to a whole series of questions that need to be addressed in order to make a responsible policy decision on this matter. Since these prior questions are distinct projects, there needs to be some coordination and collaboration among researchers working on distinct questions, similar to what has occurred in the case of the human-genome project.[10]

4.3 Who Might Address the Empirical Questions and How?

Various researchers might address, and indeed have addressed, some of these empirical questions. However, what I want to highlight here is that the most crucial set of questions in this series are those that occur on what Lonergan has named the fourth level, that is, questions for evaluation. Although there might be different reasons for requesting euthanasia, the requests that I think are most important to address are those that follow from the negative self-evaluation 'My life is not worth living.' In the first instance, for Lonergan this evaluation concerns the ontic value of his or her life, in the particular context of debilities, relationships, life histories, and circumstances. Given my (or another's) negative response to this question, the decisional issue becomes whether to do or not do something to end my or another's life. If I am the person making this evaluation, this individual deliberation becomes a public issue if I decide to end my life by enlisting the cooperation and assistance of others. The question these others, and society as a whole, face is whether they affirm my negative self-evaluation and, if so, whether they should choose to allow physicians to cooperate with my plan. The public-policy question that society as a whole is being asked to face is not one of possible fact, such as whether they could ever conceivably affirm my negative self-evaluation. Rather, society's question here is a normative, decisional one, 'Should society's physicians materially cooperate with the suicidal plans of their patients?' On Lonergan's account, to make this decision responsibly, society's legislators need to come to some agreement on the underlying evaluative question, 'Are certain lives truly not worth living (even when the *person in question* says so)?' This question, I think, needs to be faced directly in a comprehensive research program.[11] In my view, it would be irresponsible of society's policymakers to dismiss out of hand this central question simply by appealing to the apparently absolute status of a person's autonomous wishes, or to dismiss it on the basis of a philosophical stance that rejects, in principle, the epistemic objectivity of such evaluations. This is not to say, however, that even if society agrees with a person's negative self-evaluation, that it should necessarily decide to allow physicians to assist such a person in their suicidal plans. There might be other important social values that would make such a decision imprudent, such as the possible negative effects on physician-patient trust. Here again, such concerns need to be demonstrated empirically, not by mere opinion.

However society's policy-makers might answer this question, a central point of the present discussion has been to argue that such an evaluation will inevitably involve the evaluator in some *personal* way. I spelled out the personal, cognitive elements in such an evaluation in terms of the affective dimension of my transcendental intending of value, and in the fact that I grasp particular values by means of my evaluations that result from affective deliberative insights. The point in this issue is that any policy decision that is made will bear some connection to the underlying evaluation. A research program needs to be clear that answers to the prior sets of questions, such as questions for understanding and judgment, though surely important as far as they go, will not answer this central evaluative question. Nor will a particular policy decision *necessarily* or *immediately* follow from a given answer to this evaluative question.[12]

It is important that a number of methodological questions regarding such a research program be addressed. These include questions such as 'Who should do the research?' 'What role should historians, physiologists, psychologists, physicians, sociologists, cultural anthropologists, philosophers, ethicists, theologians, etc., play?' 'Who should be included or excluded as researchers and as subjects?' 'What kind of study, what end-points, duration, control groups should be used?' 'Are qualitative and/or quantitative methods of analysis appropriate?' and 'What level of evidence is reasonable?' Although answering such questions (or even coming up with a complete list) is beyond the scope of the present discussion, I suggest that Lonergan's stance on cognitional and decisional subjectivity will have ramifications for how these questions are answered.[13]

Although I would characterize these research questions as *empirical* questions, they do not presuppose that those who address them adopt a strictly *empiricist* view of reality (i.e., as the 'already out there now' that is known in experience).[14] Nor would I argue that settling strictly philosophical questions, such as those regarding cognitional and decisional subjectivity, by itself, settles any ethical dispute.[15] I suspect that when legislators who have addressed the legal dimension of the euthanasia debate admit their own frustrating lack of competence to deal adequately with the range of questions they cannot avoid, they are not self-deceived. In fact, I suspect that this frustration expresses some awareness on their part of their need to complement the historical evidence of case law and the heuristic or purely structural elements of their knowing with empirical evidence, in order to verify their answers to such questions as 'Is there a difference between killing and allowing to die?' Indeed, the first step in addressing this question is to recognize the type of question it is. If it is an empirical question, legislators would be wise to address it accordingly.[16]

4.4 What Would a Responsible Public Policy on Euthanasia Look Like?

My own sense is that empirical research will provide further evidence of the benefit of palliative-care medicine in meeting the needs of dying patients. It will also verify the suspicion that when certain needs are not met, some persons can be pushed by their illness to the point of suicidal despair.[17] I would also expect research to cast more light on those stories of individuals who are intent on suicide, and for whom no amount of positive *human* response to them would be sufficient to rekindle the flame of hope extinguished in their hearts by life's events.[18] Aware of this reality, I think it is crucially important that our society's words and deeds express an unfaltering and unequivocal support for all persons, most especially for its most vulnerable members who, according to cultural values such as beauty, efficiency, comfort, power, wealth, and so on, might easily be perceived as living lives that are 'not worth living.' This support needs to be underpinned and maintained by society's express affirmation of their moral status, which is not to be thought of as conditional on whatever qualities or attributes happen to be most valued by a culture. The goal of such a policy statement should be nothing less than an expression of the best minds of our day, grounded in a valid philosophy and deliberating on the best empirical evidence available. Only then might the judgments of our day approximate the wisdom of Solomon's decision in the case of disputed maternity. A hallmark of the validity of our own policy decisions would be evidenced, in part, by a broad communal sentiment that our legislators, like Solomon, have a 'wisdom for dispensing justice.'[19]

Since the question of euthanasia arises in the legal and public-policy spheres, I think it is important to recognize it as a question about the human good, which for some can be unpacked in terms of competing notions of justice. Behind the euthanasia debate are concerns, expressed by both proponents and opponents, about violating the demands of justice. In the case of the Special Senate Committee, their concerns were about treating persons equally under the law. Still, there are important differences of opinion about what the demands of justice are, that is, 'who should receive benefits and burdens, good or bad things of many sorts, given that others might receive these things.' In the history of philosophy a variety of criteria have been proposed for ethically just distributions: 'Some think just distributions should be in accordance with contribution, some with effort, some need, some desert, and so on.'[20]

The question regarding legalizing physician-assisted suicide is distinct, I think, from the question that emerges either from the perspectives of individuals who consider this option for themselves or from ethicists who seek to highlight some of the values that might morally constrain such individuals. In the first case, considering this decision is part of a subject's cognitional and decisional response to an illness. In the second case, it is an attempt to make explicit and thematic some of the cognitive activities and achievements that factor into an individual's discernment and might morally constrain their decisions. But the question that arises from the legal or public-policy perspective regards society's response to a suicidal request for assistance. The normative issue from this perspective has to do with legal, rather than moral, constraints and issues of justice.[21]

My request for euthanasia can be an expression of my decision to end my life because I have made the negative self-evaluation that continuing to live would not be worthwhile. This seems to have been one line of thinking and feeling in Sue's story. However, if a legal analysis is unable to explore critically the cognitive grounds of my assessment, the notion that I might be morally constrained from inflicting avoidable harm on myself (and others) could not emerge.

But if one could conclude that I am morally constrained not to do certain acts, and that my life is worthwhile even in the midst of various struggles, how might this change the focus of the debate? If one concludes that I am morally constrained from inflicting self-harm, there is no longer an inconsistency between moral and legal limits. In this way, not only could one reject the view that physician-assisted suicide ought generally to be considered a *benefit*, it might also shift the focus of the debate to attend to how *more genuine benefits*, rather than fewer, could and should be distributed to certain vulnerable individuals. One could make a good argument that justice demands that our communities distribute their benefits in such a way that they give *preferential treatment* to persons who have greater needs. This is a notion of justice that goes beyond mere considerations of equality.[22] Moreover, I would also argue that as a society we must acknowledge unstated benefits of legalizing euthanasia, which include the prospect of economic benefits for healthy members of our society who will be relieved of the burden of responsibly caring for individuals until their natural death.

This side of the issue has been brought to the fore by Jack Kevorkian. If we are to believe him, not only does he benefit suicidal individuals by offering them medical technologies, he is also now demonstrating the benefits of this procedure to a society that has an interest in harvesting human organs. The arguments of the proponents, then, have finally begun to admit to the unstated social benefits of physician-assisted suicide. Any student of the history of the twentieth century might rightly be chilled by the similarities between the current debate and the events of the Second World War that have, according to many thinkers, forever changed the way bioethics can be done.

5   Ramifications of Lonergan's Philosophy for Myself as a Caregiver

One of my goals in bringing Lonergan's philosophy to bear on the euthanasia debate has been to identify, understand, and assess better the affective elements that enter into concrete moral deliberations. I thought that case examples, such as those of Sue Rodriguez and Dennis Kaye, would illustrate some ramifications of Lonergan's normative model of value judging, and provide a way of assessing the contribution his thought can make to bioethics. A more personal way of assessing Lonergan's position would be to reflect on how his contributions have made a difference to my own performance as a physician. Given my affirmation of Lonergan's global philosophical position on the role of feelings in value judgments, I will now attempt to articulate some of the ways in which I have altered my own thinking and clinical performance in light of these broader philosophical commitments. My aim here is to respond to Callahan's challenge that there be some consistency between what moral theorists say and how they actually operate.[23]

5.1   The Intentionality of Knowing, Including Feelings

The first claim that has affected my own thinking and performance is that my knowing, including certain affective cognitive acts, is intentional. As mentioned earlier in the discussion, human knowing, for Lonergan, involves a series of distinct but interconnected intentional cognitive operations that follow a pattern of encountering data, raising questions, and proffering answers. These intentional cognitive operations fit into the broad categories of experiencing, understanding, judging facts, and evaluating. In answer to the epistemological question, 'Why is doing this genuine knowing?' Lonergan responds that one's knowing is authentic to the extent that one follows the transcendental precepts: be attentive, be intelligent, be reasonable, and be responsible. On this basis, he is able to articulate a basic philosophical position on knowing that can be named 'critical realist.' It is a 'realist' position because people can make true fact judgments and evaluations. It is 'critical' because they do so, not by some immediate or intuitive look or feel, but through a series of distinct cognitive operations, each of which can be performed in a more or less authentic manner. It would be hard to overemphasize the importance in ethics of the view that human knowing is intentional, and that persons can actually achieve more than just subjective answers to questions about the good.

As a realist position, Lonergan's value theory falls into the category of 'axiological objectivist' theories. This realist stance is at odds with the views of many contemporary philosophers and ethicists. Still, Lonergan's brand of realism conceives of knowing as a mediated process that culminates in the achievement of knowledge through a judgment. Such a realism is not identical with the empiricist position, commonly presupposed in medicine, which identifies the real with what one experiences. Idealists, by contrast, reject the empiricist account of human knowledge, even though they accept the empiricist view of objective knowing as involving an escape from one's subjectivity. Hence, they conclude that the actually achievable object of human knowledge is not the real, but the ideal. Lonergan moves beyond both empiricism and idealism to a critical realism through the discovery that one's 'intellectual and rational operations involve a transcendence of the operating subject, [and] that the real is what we come to know through a grasp of a certain type of virtually unconditioned.'[24]

Lonergan's analysis of the elements and structure of intentional consciousness has heightened my own awareness of what I am doing when I am knowing facts or values. My reflections on the medical example that I carried through chapters 4 to 7 illustrated my efforts as a physician to appropriate critically my own intentional cognitive processes. This added self-knowledge, though not directly relevant to particular medical judgments, has enabled me to be more precise and critical of my own medical knowing, as well as more critical of the claims that others make. Lonergan's critical realism specifies the elements that come together in an act of judgment. His analysis also brought to light a naive realism that medical thinkers sometimes exhibit in presupposing a model of knowing based on the ocular act of 'looking.' From such a simplistic cognitional model as this there follows a notion of 'objectivity' that entails the suppression of everything that is 'subjective.' This effort to escape one's own subjectivity is presumed necessary in order for one to 'take a good look to see what is truly out there.' With this distrust of subjectivity in the minds of caregivers, there comes, I believe, a suspicion of the relevance of evidently subjective acts, including all affective responses. By rejecting this presupposed cognitional model and the derivative view that all feelings are essentially non-intentional or merely subjective, I believe that I have become more attuned to the legitimate cognitional function of certain affective responses.

5.2   The Cognitive Role of Affect in Evaluations

Coming to accept Lonergan's stance that certain feelings are legitimate and necessary elements of the cognitive enterprise that culminates in evaluations, and indeed that certain affective responses play a crucial cognitive role in one's move from fact claims to value judgments, has been a sort of 'conversion' experience for me. This conversion has had implications for my clinical performance and interests. For instance, Lonergan's theoretical analysis has fostered in me a more genuinely empathic and understanding approach to others, especially to those confused and overwhelmed by their conflicting feelings. A great interest and challenge to me is determining how most effectively to enable persons to distinguish, in their conflicting feelings, their responses to satisfactions and their responses to values. Such an approach and interest stands in sharp contrast to what others have identified as medicine's dominant values of detachment and distance, traces of which I recognize as still present in myself as part of the heritage of my own medical training.[25] Although detachment and distance might be desirable in certain medical settings, educators in fields such as palliative care have found that engaging affectively with patients is the most essential feature of successful performance in caring for people at the end of life.[26] Lonergan's emphasis on feelings as the 'mass and momentum of our lives' offers some counter-balance to the predominantly 'intellectualist' approach to human persons that dominated my own medical education. I am indebted to his analysis of the structure of human knowing for heightening my awareness of my own affective life and, consequently, the importance of attending to the affective lives of others.[27]

Another personal clinical implication that Lonergan's anti-individualistic view of the human person has had on my clinical performance is that I am now more open to the idea of considering medical issues in their social contexts and to the possibility of such things as 'assisted' decision-making. The core issue in these evaluations, in Lonergan's view, is not the locus of a decision (the individual who is making the decision), but the authentic performance of whoever makes the decision. I am likewise inclined to place less emphasis on who decides and more on whether the judgment is authentic or epistemically objective.

Lonergan's analysis has also helped me to understand better, and facilitate responsible medical decisions among, persons by focusing on the cognitive processes and achievements that underpin their decisions. The example of Sue Rodriguez's decision about assisted suicide illustrates the critical moment of applying Lonergan's value theory. This example, however, had the disadvantage of suggesting a lack of sympathy for, and understanding of, Sue's suffering. This was, to some extent, unavoidable, given that my review of Sue's case was necessarily a retrospective one, and thus, in using Lonergan's categories to analyse her decision-making, it may have tended to overemphasize the critical moment. The main thrust of my analysis of Sue's decision-making was that, for various reasons, she was mistaken in her affirmation that physician-assisted suicide was a true value for her. By applying Lonergan's philosophy, I was able to articulate a deficiency in her evaluation, one, I believe, that most other thinkers have overlooked. The legal discussion, in particular, asks virtually no questions about the grounds of decisions such as Sue's. This strikes me as showing insufficient concern about the rightness of such important decisions that might form the basis for a change in public policy. Consequently, Sue's conclusion that physician-assisted suicide is a particular value for her, and the derivative generalization that the legal prohibition of euthanasia should be reformed, become much less convincing. Lonergan's account has helped me to unpack more precisely what the law also seeks to promote and protect, which is a person's ability not only to understand, but also to 'appreciate,' the consequences of his or her medical decisions.

The distinction between intellectual and affective cognitive processes and achievements is well illustrated in individual approaches to counselling by clinical psychologists who employ what they refer to as a 'rational-emotive' approach. For instance, therapists corrected the aggressive behaviour of a young woman with mild mental retardation by helping her to re-interpret, or re-evaluate, the name-calling by her disabled peers who sought to provoke her outbursts of anger. The key point of this case was that the problem was not essentially her angry emotional behaviour. Rather, at its root was her interpretation that the name-calling behaviour expressed their negative evaluation of her, to which she reacted with the anger of someone who had been slighted. By addressing this question of her peer's evaluation of her, her counsellors were able to address her behaviour toward them. [28]

In contrast to these critical implications of Lonergan's analysis, what is more characteristic of my clinical performance in light of Lonergan's philosophy is a more supportive and understanding attitude toward others and their evaluations. It is true that I am less hesitant now to make fact judgments and evaluations than I was before I became familiar with Lonergan's work. Even so, I am now also more critical of my own tendency to evaluate others negatively.

The distinction between evaluating someone's claims and evaluating that person, however, is not always easy to make (and feel) concretely. This is especially true when the claims and consequent behaviour regard moral matters. The risk of conflating these two judgments arises in any review of Sue's case. In this light, one motive for my avoiding any negative judgment

of Sue's decision-making might be to avoid the risk that others will misinterpret me as making a negative judgment about her character or person.
However, my advertence to the historical, psychological, social, cultural,
and personal dimensions of Sue's evaluation of the worth of her own life
helped to underline the communal dimension of her judgments. These
factors surely mitigate to some extent Sue's culpability. Given my tendency
as one trained in philosophy to be critical of the claims I or others make, I
am now more sensitive to the importance of distinguishing clearly between
my negative assessment of the truth of someone's claims or the goodness of
their actions, on the one hand, and my positive regard and respect for the
person making these claims, on the other. For instance, in the case of a
patient, such as Paul, who has an addiction to cocaine, I have become more
aware of the importance of distinguishing clearly my negative affective
response to his behaviour from my positive regard for Paul as a person. This
distinction is often less difficult to make once one becomes more aware of
someone's background, social context, and developmental history.

An important benefit of focusing on the affective elements underpinning evaluations is that it draws one's attention beyond the biological
dimensions of a disease to interpreting the human experience of an illness.
I have found that my ability to understand this process, and to accompany
persons in their efforts to integrate an illness into their life-story, facilitates
the building of genuine solidarity between caregivers and patients. Conversely, failure to attend to the isolating effects of an illness, and to build
some bonds of solidarity with those who are ill, invites the sort of difficulties
that the stories of Sue and Dennis illustrate. Both expressed the devastating
effects wrought by what they interpreted as a lack of empathy for them on
the part of some of their caregivers. Their physicians truthfully communi-
cated to them that there was little hope of a cure for ALS. Still, they failed to
assure them that their future life would not be one of unmitigated evil, and
that they would remain in solidarity with them throughout their illness. Sue
and Dennis interpreted their caregivers' 'professional' responses to them
as indicating indifference toward them. They also thought their caregivers
were conveying their privately held pessimistic views about the value of what
lay ahead for them. In these stories lies a criticism of a traditional mode of
caregiving that fosters an emotionally detached and seemingly distant
attitude. Regrettably, this attitude added to Sue and Dennis's shock in
learning of their situation a sense that their physicians were indifferent to
them as persons and were abandoning them to their biological fates.
Perhaps it was this experience that explains, in part, Sue's ultimate distrust
of physicians and why she pursued other sources of healing among alternative medical practitioners.

In summary, I think that the role of affectivity in value judgments is especially relevant to medical caregivers and to the issue of euthanasia. For attention to the role of affectivity focuses not merely on the grounds for the evaluations patients make, but also on how a caregiver responds to a patient who expresses despair about the value of his or her future life in the context of a terminal illness. The cry of despair that turned into a request for physician-assisted suicide in Sue's case is not adequately understood from an individualistic perspective as being simply *her* response to this illness. More amply, her cry of despair is also shaped by the responses of other persons to her in the context of her illness. The lesson I take from Lonergan's analysis is that I should seek to facilitate a patient's and his or her family's own understanding of the problems they are facing. In so doing, I might encourage them toward those realistic values that they most desire to achieve during this final phase of life. What is crucial is that caregivers be convinced, through their own experiences, that there are important values to be achieved at the end of life. Consequently, they need expressly to commit themselves to providing ongoing support for and solidarity with their patients and their patients' families. In this way, they might conspire with a patient's own efforts to discern and realize important values, even given his or her restricted horizons.[29]

5.3 Distinguishing and Relating Fact Judging, Value Judging, and Choosing

A third claim that Lonergan's global position affirms is that although judging and evaluating are distinct, they are also importantly related. Also, although Lonergan locates value judging and choosing as two acts that are part of the fourth-level evaluative process, these acts are distinct in important ways. Value judging involves the affective cognition of a deliberative insight, the epistemic objectivity of which is prefigured by the affectivity of one's transcendental intending of value. By contrast, the act of choosing ends the ongoing process of deliberation by determining what one will enjoy or do. Such a choice can be positive or privative, and can regard the passive willing of an actual good that is given in the mode of complacency, or the active willing of some concretely possible good that is given in the mode of concern. In the case of a concretely possible good, the fourth-level evaluative process as a whole can only be said to have been 'responsible' if (1) the value judgment was epistemically objective, and not just epistemically subjective, (2) the choice was a positive one, and not just privative, and (3) the possible good was actually executed in some concrete manner. These distinct features seem to capture Lonergan's notion of fourth-level evaluative authenticity.

Before studying Lonergan, my own view, like that of many of my colleagues, was that all clinical judgments were essentially matters of fact. Medical conclusions, I thought, had little, if anything, to do with evaluations. By contrast, I am now more inclined to consider the relations between even the most fact-like activities, such as educating patients about some medical problem, and the values such activities presuppose, express, and promote. Indeed, in Lonergan's analysis, every medical encounter that concludes with a decision to take some course of action or treatment presupposes and is justified by some value judgment. Whether this recommended goal is realistic, that is, a concretely possible good and not just abstractly possible, involves further fact judgments. Attending to these features of evaluative cognitional and decisional processes in my own performance has enabled me to interpret better the differences and sources of problems between, for instance, my own perspective and that of a patient. This has helped me to be more clear-headed about being sympathetic and understanding toward a sufferer, without necessarily agreeing that what the sufferer says is true, or even that what the sufferer wants to do would actually promote the good he or she seeks.[30]

Lonergan's analysis brings clarity to the confusion regarding how one moves from fact to value judgments. One expert medical witness in Sue's court case, for example, drew attention to this distinction in his testimony outlining the facts of ALS. But he went beyond a strictly medical account of the facts of ALS to express his views about what he took to be morally necessary medical responses, as distinct from those that were morally optional and up to the patient to accept or refuse.[31] Lonergan's analysis has helped me to be clearer about the difference and connection between facts and values. It has also convinced me that the connection between fact and value judgments is not to be explained just by considerations drawn from logic. All the decisions about how to respond to someone with ALS follow not only from fact knowledge, but also from the evaluation that a person's life is indeed worthwhile, as is what one has to offer to them.

Finally, being aware of the connection, and also the distinction, between value judging and choosing has helped me to locate more readily the ethical issues that are often presented as strictly matters of personal choosing. For instance, a case was presented to me for comment that involved the decision to provide a severely deformed child with a feeding tube. The prospect of this intervention was met with opposing responses by the parents.[32] The way I circumvented this impasse was to identify the issue as resting fundamentally not on the question of whether the child's life was worthwhile or worth promoting, but on whether the risks of seeking some concretely possible good (i.e., enhanced nutrition) was better than choosing not to intervene in this way. This common point between both parents and physicians was a source of trust, for the parents had already encountered other caregivers whom they perceived as not wanting what was best for their child, that is, who wondered, 'What's the point?'

5.4 Evaluations as Epistemically Objective

A fourth global claim of Lonergan's stance is that even though one grasps values affectively, when they are based on authentic subjectivity, they can achieve epistemic objectivity. Lonergan's analysis has clarified for me the distinction between phenomenological and epistemological cognitional issues. It has also made me more attentive to identifying and distinguishing affective responses from the content of the evaluations themselves. I recall, for instance, my tendency to be dismissive of the affectively based claims of others that I could not personally verify. Indeed, I took both these data and claims to be merely 'subjective,' and hence not available to any critical discernment. I am indebted to Lonergan's account for encouraging me to challenge the predominant medical view of epistemic objectivity that considers such objectivity to be a matter of escaping from one's subjectivity. His analysis has also helped me to be more aware of recurring patterns in my own failures to make correct fact and value judgments, and to address these oversights. In addition, I am less apt to consider value judgments to be merely arbitrary expressions of personal whims.

The epistemic issue concerns not only fact and value judgments, but also decisions. Michael Vertin has added a further nuance to Lonergan's account by distinguishing between two types of decisions. The first type are decisions *to do* or achieve some possible good. These are distinct from a second type, which are decisions *to enjoy* some present good. I recognize that before studying Lonergan's thought I tended to think that I always had to 'do' something in any given circumstance. But this distinction between decisions to do and to enjoy highlights what palliative-care medicine also teaches, namely, that there is still much that I can 'do' for a patient even when I am unable to 'do' anything medically that will reverse the patient's terminal illness. Moreover, it is important sometimes to resist the tendency to 'do' things and decide instead simply to 'enjoy' a person's life and achievements, while allowing some irreversible medical process to unfold.[33]

One paradox I have discovered in moving away from 'doing' things to simply 'being' is that it is in the latter mode that many of the most important events or moments have occurred for me and for my patients. For instance, it is in enjoying a patient, even when he or she might be gravely ill, that we encounter one another on the deepest human level. It has also been my experience that these are the occasions during which the greatest healing can occur, not only for a patient, but also for the patient's caregivers and his or her loved ones. To the extent that Vertin's nuancing of Lonergan's analysis has opened me to the possibility of simply 'being with' others, it has also helped me to undercut the view that the only worthwhile responses to terminally ill patients are ultimately technical acts – including lethal injections.

5.5 A Transcultural Structure of the Human Good

A fifth global claim of Lonergan's position is that not only can we know epistemically objective values or goods that are distinct from mere satisfactions, but also that these values constitute a transcultural structure of the human good. Lonergan's general distinction between transcendental and categorial, and the more specific version of distinct categories of categorial affectivity that Vertin has argued for, have been quite helpful for me clinically. For even if I have had difficulties being persuaded by the particular categorial evaluations a patient has made, at least I have sometimes been able to identify the transcendental notion of value he or she was seeking to express in that concrete evaluation. That is, these categories have heightened my awareness of an inner, prior groaning for some good or fulfilment that underpins all our efforts to achieve some categorial evaluation. It might be that the reader, like myself, remains unconvinced that Sue's categorial response to physician-assisted suicide was actually made in fidelity to the affectivity of her transcendental notion of value. That is, one might interpret her expressions of despair, such as statements like 'I'm already a non-person,' as manifesting a certain incongruity or disharmony between her categorial and transcendental affectivity. Still, behind her decision one can recognize her genuine desire to achieve some good outcome in her situation. One way one might draw out this dimension of her deliberation would be to expand the range of concrete possibilities on which she could have deliberated. In this way, one might also encourage others to discern better the option that most satisfies their fundamental affective orientation to a self-transcending good.

5.6 The Value of Life

Lonergan refers to the value of life not merely as contingent on some qualitative values but as an *ontic* value, that is, the value of being. I end on this issue because, in some sense, it was where I began. This beginning was an 'awakening' on a deep level to what I would now label as the ontic value of being. This awakening originally motivated my move to philosophy and has been an orienting foundation for many of my subsequent decisions. Reflecting on this in light of all that I have read of the euthanasia debate, I cannot help but sense that there are much deeper, personal concerns that people have and express indirectly in this debate. If this is true, then the real issue has little to do with decisions that I hope many will not face personally for many years. Nor does it have to do with extremes of suffering and a desire to have some final means of escaping what is bound to be a lonely time when, as Cardinal Newman says, 'evening comes and the fever of life is over.' What I think this debate is, or perhaps should be, about is the meaning and significance of 'being' and of the 'now' of one's life. As a physician, how I face and respond to these questions will doubtlessly affect the way I deal with others and also how I spend my time. More generally, my sense of human beings as 'terminal' goods (beings that are chosen as valuable), and sometimes also 'originating' goods (i.e., beings capable of responsibly choosing) will surely influence how I answer questions about whether my own or another's life is worth living.

In these reflections, then, I have sought to articulate some personal ramifications of Lonergan's analysis of the role of affect in value judgments for my own performance as a physician. Lonergan's contributions have sharpened my awareness of some of the complexities of reaching reasonable and responsible judgments. They have also convinced me of the important connections between what one thinks, how one feels, what one judges to be worthwhile, and what one decides to do or not do. This foray into philosophy has enabled me to appreciate better some of the wonder and complexity of human intelligence, the remarkable phenomenon of achieving authentic fact judgments and evaluations, and the cognitive role that affect plays in the evaluative process.

In some quarters, not only philosophers and ethicists but also medical practitioners have recognized the deficiencies of a strictly intellectual approach to human persons. In response to the inadequacies of a physician-centred approach to care, for instance, many institutions are tending toward a more 'patient-focused' philosophy of care. Such an approach seeks to be more attentive to the feelings and values that patients express, as part of a broader philosophy of care. It encourages caregivers and ethicists to move beyond the role of merely providing information to patients to one that includes helping them to evaluate their medical options responsibly. I hope that my efforts in this work will help the reader to think about some of the philosophical underpinnings of this shift in emphasis, and to appreciate better its significance, especially for responsibly meeting the needs of those at the end of life.

Afterword

Following this analysis of the cognitional role of affect in knowing the human good, using the euthanasia debate as an illustration, some readers may still be inclined to ask what remains for them the crucially important question: 'So what?' What, if anything, does all this analysis and its application to the euthanasia debate mean or matter? More particularly, what does it mean or matter for those working in the empirical fields of medicine, psychology, and related health-care professions; for those working in the more general or theoretical fields of philosophy, theology, and related disciplines; for those working in fields such as clinical ethics or pastoral care, where part of the goal is to integrate the empirical and more theoretical disciplines? On a more personal level, what, if anything, does this analysis and its application to the euthanasia debate mean or matter for caregivers, or for family members who might be in a situation of caring for a loved one during the final phase of a terminal illness? What does it mean or matter when questions arise about the meaning or worth of a person's life, when that person becomes increasingly restricted by an illness? What does it mean or matter when obstacles and illness, whether terminal or otherwise, cause a person to question seriously, or possibly even reject, the value of his or her life in such a condition? How ought the loved ones of a person in such a condition respond to such conclusions, or to requests for assistance in committing suicide? That is, what does all this analysis mean for those who face the sorts of questions that are at the heart of the euthanasia debate? What significance do the issues posed in this book and the stances taken on these issues mean or matter in the laboratory of real-life experience, when such questions come to the fore? Is all this analysis really relevant to individuals who are confronted by such questions and seek to address them? And is this analysis relevant to other individual and communal or societal questions that currently arise in bioethics, or to those that are likely to arise in the near future?

In this Afterword I shall not attempt a detailed response to such questions. Rather, I shall try, first, to sketch briefly what this analysis and its application to the euthanasia debate has meant for me in the personal context of caring for my late wife during her terminal illness. Then I shall discuss its relevance in my professional life as the director of a bioethics institute.

1   Some Indications of the Relevance of This Work for Caregivers Facing Requests for Euthanasia

Unexpectedly, after writing the present work, the issues connected with terminal illness, suffering, and death touched me in my personal life. Getting married and then accompanying my wife Connie during her final months of life was such a significant event in my life that I decided to honour her by writing a book about her life and her experiences of her illness. The book is entitled *Promise of Mercy: Lessons in Faith and Hope from the Journeys of a Young Woman with Cancer*. In order to illustrate what I have learned in relation to the challenge of euthanasia as a result of this experience, I would like to share a relevant portion of the book:

> Connie's most difficult hour was on May 15th, only a few days before her death. I recorded my own account of this trial in my journal a few days after it had passed:
>
> *On Monday 15/5; Connie was very distressed; angry, anxious and in pain. She was frustrated by a series of issues – back discomfort, for which she was refusing pain medications (because they gave her bad dreams), she was short-of-breath and fatigued from her respiratory efforts and lack of sleep, and she felt like it was time to go (die) and didn't want to wait ('I want to go tonight! Why won't Jesus take me now?'). When I arrived home from work, everyone looked stressed and exhausted. Initially I felt angry toward Connie because she was demanding the impossible ('Do you want us to kill you?'). John [her brother] had tried to talk her out of this mood and to pray with her, but to no avail. It seemed as though she was engulfed in a storm of despair, her tiny ship tossed in the turmoils of the endless dark seas, and she could find no hope or peace while the storm raged and battered her body and soul.*
>
> *The remedy for this was a combination of medical, social and religious interventions. We attended to the things that seemed to be causing discomfort: taped over a leaking nephrostomy tube, removed some rolled up pieces of duoderm on her sacrum, cut the sides of her underwear, which were causing*

some discomfort, adjusted the pressure of her air mattress and obtained a no-slip mat to help prevent her from sliding down the bed … She eventually agreed to take some morphine (at the insistence of her friend Lorraine), and we re-started the fentany-patch (for pain). I also gave her a massage with an aromatic cream and kissed her all the places that hurt (and more) and kept telling her how much I loved her and how sorry I was that I caused her to perceive that I was angry at her.

As for social interventions, we had Lorraine and Susan [Connie's friends and bridesmaids] come over to help console her. They were helpful and supportive of Mrs Heng [Connie's mother] as well. Lorraine said the Rosary with Connie, which helped her. John got Connie talking about the funeral arrangements … This shifted her thinking to more practical and concrete matters that we could actually achieve. Within 24 hours, things were back under control. The urgency and frustration has mostly subsided. Such an experience is likely to unnerve even the most committed to the values of life and of person-centred care. May 17, 2000.

This dark night was perhaps the most challenging one during our journey with Connie. As a result of passing through it we have learned that while faith does not exclude anyone from genuine struggle, it does, however, provide a fundamental commitment from which one can persevere with a loved one through thick and thin. Without an unqualified belief in the inviolability of each human life, it is nearly impossible to avoid the euthanasia option in the face of a loved one's anguish and despair. Our faith in God and love for Connie led us to show mercy to her by drawing closer in loving support as best we could, not by ending her life. This choice always comes at a personal cost (e.g. time, comfort and freedom). Through-out Connie's illness, we had spent innumerable sleepless and difficult nights with her. For some, euthanasia may simply reflect (perhaps without realizing it) an unwillingness to pay this price rather than a genuine desire to show mercy. Despite the cost of caring for Connie during her illness, we had each come to recognize the hidden blessing that our time with her possessed. Earlier in her illness John had written:

It was VERY hard to stir from my half-sleep to fetch water or move Connie's leg a bit or flip her pillow – you know how I like to sleep. It was tough, even tougher for Connie, to accept my washing her underarms, which were sweaty and smelly. But I understand a bit better how service can be prayer and prayer, service. For in serving another, we transcend our self-centredness and this overcomes our principal barrier to our communication with God. God often reminds me that it is WE who 'hang-up' on Him through selfish sin; He always stays on the line waiting our return. What a privilege it is to be able to

> *wait on Jesus on the hospital bed, to be at His disposal, to be on our feet at a*
> *single word from His lips and to do so with a smile of love. This is the*
> *particular way Jesus has chosen to purify us of our past and present self-*
> *indulgence. It is the sure way, the Gospels tell us, of moving Jesus' heart. – In*
> *memoriam, June 11, 2000*

I too had discovered the blessing that Connie had become in her weakness and learned that in loving her I had discovered Love in a new way. Choosing death for Connie in response to her anguish would have robbed her and us of these blessings and the peaceful and holy death that she eventually experienced.

In this brief account of Connie's 'dark night,' it is evident that her cry for euthanasia was more complex than the typical 'rational suicide' that philosophers discuss. Her story illustrates a degree of complexity present in such lived experiences of an illness that one might overlook or not recognize if one goes simply by available interpreted reports. In the experience people have of an illness, particularly at advanced stages, there is likely to be a whole nest of medical, technical, social, psychological, affective, evaluative, and spiritual factors that come interconnected and even intermingled. Such was certainly the case with Connie. Recognizing this helps one to understand better the various situations that may arise and how to act appropriately. On the medical side, for instance, some knowledge of the signs of a delirium, an altered state of cognition during which individuals might say things that are quite inconsistent with their prior and usual non-delirious states, was important in the interpretation of Connie's uncharacteristic behaviour and request 'to go tonight.' Attending to some of the medical reasons for her distress was also an important part of the response to her crisis. Advanced medical technologies place great hope in salvation by technology, and many in our culture deny that meaning and value can be found in the midst of suffering or death. As a result, they often seek technical solutions for human issues. The real challenge is to humanize the dying process in the context of advanced medical technologies.

A person's response to the whole experience of having a terminal illness and suffering is shaped in part by his or her past experiences of loss, by his or her inner resources, and by the outer resources that are offered or withheld. Indeed, some of these inner and outer resources are discovered and developed during the course of a person's illness; and the outer resources can be instrumental in awakening and releasing a person's own inner resources or, unfortunately, if withheld, in preventing such inner resources from being awakened and released. Thus, Connie's responses were shaped by the responses *to her* of her intimate circle of loved ones and by her caregivers. They, in turn, were influenced in their thinking and their responses by various circles of people, circles that extended even to those within our culture who deny there is meaning in the midst of such experiences of illness. I have learned from this experience with Connie that it is the dying who are in the best position to teach others something about the meaning of this time of life. And I have come to understand how much they have to offer those of us who struggle with less-dramatic issues of loss and weakness in the course of our own lives.

Having grasped something about these issues by accompanying Connie through her illness, and especially having learned something of how individuals and families can come out 'on top' in the face of such personal tragedy, and having tried to reflect and say something concrete about this whole process in *Promise of Mercy*, I believe I am now in a much better position to understand in a concrete, personal way the various issues that lie at the heart of the public euthanasia debate. Connie's story is one with an underlying theme of growth in love in the context of her suffering and dying, of acceptance of her dying and death, and of a legacy of family and communal healing. The success of her dying experience was not the result of some technical intervention. Indeed, attention to the human and spiritual dimensions of this experience enabled her and those who accompanied her to humanize her medical care. Such a personal experience undoubtedly places one in a better position to comment on issues such as euthanasia.

I also believe that I am in a much better position now to identify which of Lonergan's philosophical contributions are most helpful to this whole discussion. If I were asked to pick the three most important contributions from Lonergan's work that I found most helpful in grasping some of the issues Connie was dealing with, and by extension anyone facing the experiences and questions that underpin the euthanasia debate, namely, questions about the value or worthwhileness of one's life in the context of a life-threatening illness, they would be (1) apprehensions of value are given in, through, or by means of intentional responses of feelings; (2) judgments of value are simple or comparative, and regard either the ontic value of persons or the qualitative values of beauty, understanding, truth, noble deeds, virtuous acts, or great achievements; and (3) value judgments lead to decisions and actions, and a decision can be either 'to do' some *x* or 'to enjoy' some *x*.

Having had the opportunity in this work, prior to my journey with my wife in her final days of life, to analyse and relate these three elements to one another has provided me with some basis for grasping the complexities of the eye of the human heart that are at the centre of these experiences of terminal illness and of the whole euthanasia debate. The challenge that Connie faced in coming to terms with her illness, and that I and Connie's family and friends faced in responding responsibly to her responses to her illness, throughout its course and during her dark hours, is analogous to the challenge our culture and lawmakers face in articulating policies that will govern such responses for all Canadian families.

In the midst of this personal tragedy, the current law prohibiting euthanasia was for me a compass that I could rely on and trust, even more than I could on my own sometimes disoriented moral compass. I am grateful that this already enormously confusing personal storm was not further complicated by the legal option of ending Connie's life at the point when she seemed to be requesting it. Although such a law may well come about in our country in response to the minority of people who want this legal option, I am convinced that in Connie's situation, if such an option had been in place, it would effectively have been not an option but an obligation, if not on her part to ask for euthanasia (possibly at a much earlier stage in her illness), then upon her family to honour her request, and to do so despite the long-term effects that the knowledge that we had abandoned and killed her in her hour of greatest need would have on our grieving and our lives.

2   Relevance to Collaborative Research in Bioethics

As the founding director of the Canadian Catholic Bioethics Institute (CCBI), which opened in November 2001, I have been challenged to apply concretely the methodology that I sought to elucidate in this book. The most comprehensive attempt at such an application took place in developing the Institute's first think tank on Human Genetics in the Context of Health Care Reform, which took place in June 2002. This think tank was intended to be a first effort to address a pressing set of questions in bioethics of particular interest and concern to Catholics in Canada. The main goals of the think tank were (1) to pose adequately the questions raised by these new technologies and proposed health-care funding reforms, and (2) to identify and address the disputed foundational issues in the opposed positions being taken on these questions. The planning committee envisioned a think tank that would gather a diverse group of specialists: some working in human genetics, health-care economics, and/or particular cognate areas; some more broadly in bioethics; and some even more broadly in philosophy and theology. The aim was to get specialists talking to one another on a common ethical issue, and to publish the results of these collaborative efforts in a multi-authored publication that would incorporate the rich diversity of specialized knowledge from various thinkers and also unify and integrate this knowledge through a shared commitment to a critical-realist stance on the foundational, cognitional issues that are discussed in this book.

In order to save time in identifying these foundational issues and in distinguishing between more or less adequate stances on them, the planning committee expressly opted to employ the work of Bernard Lonergan. Besides the clarity on the foundational nature of cognitional theory that he offers to such a debate, Lonergan also provided us with a heuristic in his articulation of distinct and related functional specialties. On the question of cognitional theory, Lonergan's work was used to identify distinct stances being taken on knowing in general and knowing the human good in particular. For Lonergan, the positional stance on these issues is one that conceives of human knowing as a composite of distinct and related cognitional processes, from experiencing and understanding through to judgments of fact and judgments of value. Less-adequate stances tend to reduce this multi-levelled process to a single act (such as experiencing or choosing). And doing so has the effect, Lonergan argues, of distorting the whole of human knowing and human evaluating.

Related to this four-step process are Lonergan's eight functional specialties. The think tank focused on the functional specialty of *dialectic*, as does this present work. The philosophical task of *dialectic*, for Lonergan, is to relate the opposition between stances on particular issues to more fundamental differences on such general questions as the nature of knowing the human good.

We used both of these key contributions to help coordinate and integrate the labours of the various specialists we commissioned to work on this research project. We called this first think tank *Quodlibet 2002*, and we structured sessions in a manner that sought to integrate the efforts of individuals by (1) exploring the connections between the various academic disciplines; (2) synthesizing discussions of particular and foundational ethical issues; (3) seeking to integrate the claims of faith and the claims of reason; (4) bringing together people who have skills in distinct areas of the research process, from professional librarians to editors and communicators; and (5) tackling the issue of how to proceed from analysis to action in order to engage our culture.

The theme of 'Human Genetics in the Context of Health Care Reform in Canada' provided an arena within which to test these general methodological strategies and commitments and to collaborate across a series of academic disciplines. We divided our time into distinct tasks that would be handled over a four-day period. The goal was to produce an integrated contribution on this issue. The papers, responses, and discussions of the first day, for instance, sought to identify different perspectives on particular bioethical issues arising from genetics and health-care funding. Here the task was mainly to identify the ethical issues and to set forth the range of opposed stances currently being taken on these issues. The papers, responses, and discussions of the second day were aimed at pressing the opposed stances uncovered on the first day to their philosophical and theological *roots* by identifying the different presuppositions that underlie these stances. The third day was spent considering the most appropriate positions on the foundational issues. We used Lonergan's own position on the underlying foundational issues to illustrate what such a stance might look like and what its implications might be for the particular bioethical issues discussed, although it was made clear that this was merely illustrative and not an effort to endorse Lonergan's particular positions. The fourth day was devoted to Lonergan's eighth functional specialty, *communications.* The issue discussed was how one might communicate the results of this collaborative enterprise to various non-specialized audiences in ways that are understandable, interesting, and helpful.

To this end, the results of this first think tank have been made available in a brief summary document of the highlights. In addition, we hope to publish a longer, more detailed work through an academic press.

As important as Lonergan's contributions to understanding the cognitive role of affect might be to the particular issues of euthanasia in this work, and to issues in genetics and health-care reform addressed in the CCBI's first think tank, it is his development of a *method* that one can use to address any particular issue in bioethics that is more important. The crucial issue here is not one of developing more specialized knowledge, but rather of integrating distinct areas of expertise. The model we employed drew explicitly on Lonergan's cognitional theory and his articulation of distinct and related functional specialties, a topic that Michael Vertin has discussed in the foreword to this work.

Lonergan's image of the scissors and its action provides the metaphor employed in this model and suggests the way in which distinct disciplines can come together in an integrated way on topics in advanced studies in bioethics. The lower blade of the scissors involves the empirical disciplines. Their task is to identify the dialectical disputes that arise in their empirical fields (genetics, economics, public policy). The upper blade of the scissors involves the more general philosophical and theological disciplines capable of addressing the foundational issues that underpin the dialectical disputes that arise within the empirical disciplines, one example of which are the opposed views on the role of affect in knowing the human good. Our working thesis is that the lower-blade disputes could only be addressed adequately by engaging the foundational issues at stake, which is the function of those disciplines operating in accordance with the upper blades. Such an inquiry moves forward to the extent that these two blades are brought together successfully. This proposed model is applicable not merely to issues in bioethics, but to any field of human inquiry that seeks to address dialectically opposed positions on claims about the human good. What is crucial is that one first adequately poses the questions that need to be addressed, and second that one addresses these questions in a way that is sufficiently general – which is to say that one identifies and takes a position on dialectically opposed stances on foundational issues having to do with the nature of knowing the human good.

An original part of the approach that Lonergan's philosophy advocates, which this work on the role of affect in the euthanasia debate explicates, and which the CCBI's first think tank attempted to put into practice, is genuine and fruitful interdisciplinary collaboration among a whole range of individuals with specialized knowledge and skills. Lonergan envisages teams of thinkers collaborating on a common task but operating in functionally distinct yet related areas of expertise. In this present work, I as one individual have attempted to integrate elements from the disciplines of medicine, psychology, and philosophy by working mainly from within the functional specialty of *dialectic*. Such a contribution is only possible after many years of training in these disciplines. Following that, several more years are needed for teams of individuals to begin this huge task of integrating the contribution of these various disciplines.

The CCBI's first think tank brought together about forty people with very different areas of expertise in an attempt to make an original, integrated, and fruitful contribution to a very difficult set of questions, and to do so within a short period of time. Yet it was organized by only a few people who understood something of Lonergan's vision. Many of the academics who were part of this process, and who had little if any knowledge of Lonergan's work, were understandably baffled by the whole process; it was something they had never seen happen before. Nevertheless, many of them were energized by the opportunity to discuss these issues with colleagues in other disciplines. One seasoned professor commented in his evaluation of the think tank that this collaborative work was the best experience he had had of what the 'university' (*universitas*) was really meant to be – something that he had never previously experienced in all of his academic life.

Although we certainly recognize the gap between our soaring ambitions for this first collaborative enterprise and our faltering performance, we are hopeful that we are beginning to cultivate a core group of academics who share this vision and whose performance will progress with each successive think tank. If successful, this approach could serve as a model for the roughly thirty other national Catholic bioethics institutes around the world, all of which are grappling with similar questions and with the challenges of approaching these questions in an interdisciplinary manner that adequately poses the range of relevant questions that need to be raised, engages the dialectically opposed stances underpinning different answers to these questions, and formulates responses that are rooted expressly in solid foundations.

Appendix

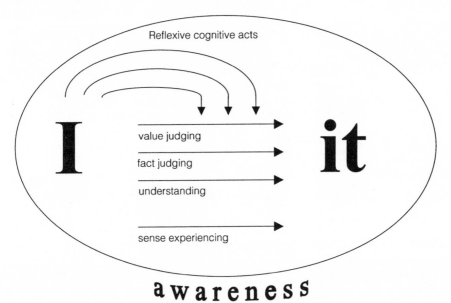

Critical realism (Bernard Lonergan)

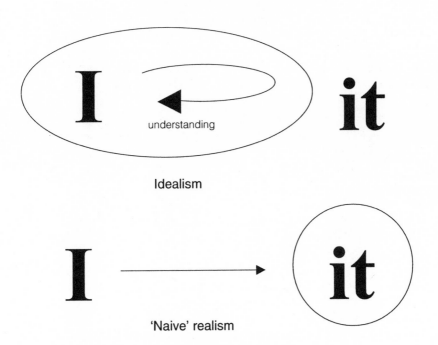

Idealism

'Naive' realism

Figure A.1   Three different accounts of knowing

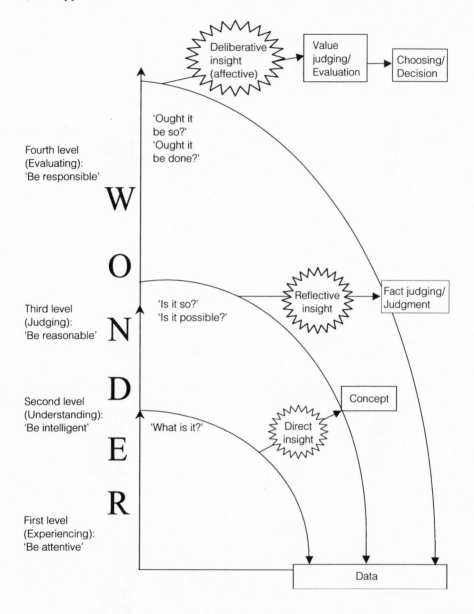

Figure A.2   Cognitional structure according to Bernard Lonergan

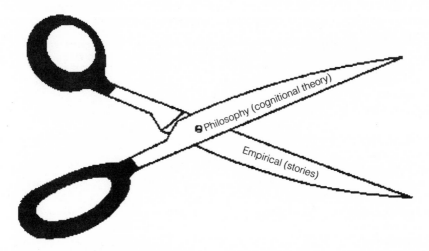

Figure A.3   Ethical reflection on euthanasia involves the 'upper blade' of philosophy and the 'lower blade' of empirical stories.

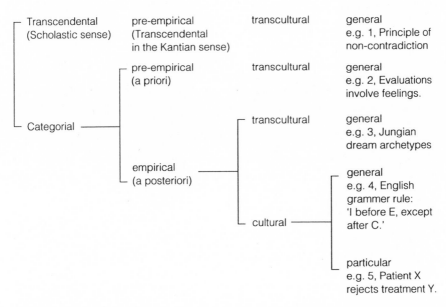

Figure A.4   Particular and general claims, according to Michael Vertin's interpretation of Longeran

Table A.1   Comparing and contrasting core philosophical positions:
Level of stories

	Bernard Lonergan	Sue Rodriguez	Dennis Kaye
Do feelings ever play a cognitive role in my knowing?	Yes	Yes	Yes
If some feelings are cognitive,	Partly	Entirely	Partly
how do they relate to my knowledge?	Necessary, not sufficient	Necessary, and sufficient	Necessary, not sufficient
How are cognitive feelings related to my evaluations?	Mediately	Immediately	Mediately
Do such evaluations ever yield more than just subjective knowledge?	Yes	No	Yes
Is the verbal emphasis on evaluating or choosing?	Evaluating	Choosing	Evaluating
Is there a normative structure of the human	Yes	Yes	Yes
good? If so, how are the individual and social goods related?	Mutually conditioning	Mutually conditioning	Mutually conditioning
Is life a basic good?	Yes	Yes/No	Yes
Is it an absolute good?	No	No	No

Table A.2   Comparing and contrasting core philosophical positions:
Level of ethics

	Bernard Lonergan	Tom Beauchamp	Richard McCormick
Do feelings ever play a cognitive role in my knowing?	Yes	Yes	Yes
If some feelings are cognitive, how do they relate to my knowledge?	Partly	(?) Entirely	Partly
	Necessary, not sufficient	Necessary, and sufficient	Necessary, not sufficient
How are cognitive feelings related to my evaluations?	Mediately	(?) Mediately	Mediately
Do such evaluations ever yield more than just subjective knowledge?	Yes	No	Yes
Is the verbal emphasis on evaluating or choosing?	Evaluating	Choosing	Evaluating
Is there a normative structure of the human good? If so, how are the individual and social goods related?	Yes	Yes	Yes
	Mutually conditioning	(?) Opposed	Mutually conditioning
Is life a basic good?	Yes	Yes/No	Yes
Is it an absolute good?	No	No	No

Table A.3   Comparing and contrasting core philosophical positions:
Level of public policy, Special Senate Committee on Euthanasia and
Assisted Suicide, Canada

	Bernard Lonergan	Minority members	Majority members
Do feelings ever play a cognitive role in my knowing?	Yes	Yes	Yes
If some feelings are cognitive, how do they relate to my knowledge?	Partly	(?) Entirely	Partly
	Necessary, not sufficient	Necessary, and sufficient	Necessary, not sufficient
How are cognitive feelings related to my evaluations?	Mediately	(?) Immediately	Mediately
Do such evaluations ever yield more than just subjective knowledge?	Yes	No	Yes
Is the verbal emphasis on evaluating or choosing?	Evaluating	Choosing	Evaluating
Is there a normative structure of the human good? If so, how are the individual and social goods related?	Yes	Yes	Yes
	Mutually conditioning	Opposed	Opposed
Is life a basic good?	Yes	Yes/No	Yes
Is it an absolute good?	No	No	No

Notes

Foreword

1 Bernard Lonergan, *Method in Theology* (London: Darton, Longman & Todd; New York: Herder and Herder, 1972). See esp. chap. 5, 'Functional Specialties.'

2 In terms that may be familiar to some, Lonergan's distinction between *field specialization* and *subject specialization* is analogous to the scholastic distinction between a discipline's *material object* and its *formal object*.

3 I intend the phrase 'in one way or another' to indicate that although persons may express their stance-taking in technical language, they may also express it in non-technical language, or in deeds, or in non-verbal products. Hence, careful research about the moral value *of euthanasia*, about specifically *moral* value as such, and about *value* as such will take account not only of academic writings but also of autobiographies and biographies and popular histories, of the concrete life-practices of individuals and groups, of novels and paintings and sculptures and music, and so forth.

4 Although the limitations of this foreword do not allow for a detailed account of his findings regarding the role of feelings in valid judgments of value, it is worth making clear that Sullivan, following Lonergan, maintains that certain feelings do indeed have positive cognitive import. More precisely, the constitutive elements of the process of valid value-judging include feelings that are self-transcending responses to values.

5 In the same respect in two parallel examples, he contends that the stance in the writings of ethicist Richard McCormick on euthanasia is superior to that in the writings of ethicist Tom Beauchamp, and that the stance of the majority members in the 1995 report of the Canadian Senate Committee on Euthanasia and Assisted Suicide is superior to that of the minority members.

6 Though he is attracted by Kaye's implicit judgment, Sullivan grants that his relatively sketchy grasp of Kaye's reasons for making it prevent him – Sullivan – from being more firmly approving.

7 More precisely, my contention is not that the book suggests a clear and systematic structure for ethical studies simply or even primarily by way of its *directly asserted claims* on that topic. My contention rather is that the book is helpful on the topic (a) partly by way of its directly asserted claims, (b) partly by way of the *indirectly asserted logical presuppositions* of those claims, and (c) partly by way of the *indirectly asserted methodical presuppositions* of both. In other words, it constitutes a model that is partly *explicit*, partly *implicit conceptually*, and partly *implicit operationally*.

8 For example, 'Choosing irresponsibly is always a moral disvalue.' More broadly, notice three things. First, the ultimate opposite of a categorial MORAL value is a categorial moral *disvalue*, not just a categorial moral *nonvalue*. This terminological nuance reflects the Thomist contention, embraced by Lonergan, that the radical opposite of a moral value is not its *mere* absence but rather its *privative* absence, the absence of what *ought* to be present. Or, more familiarly, a moral evil is the privation of a moral good. Second, and similarly, the ultimate opposite of a categorial NON-MORAL value is a categorial non-moral *disvalue*, not just a categorial non-moral *non-value*. In its own way, a natural evil is the privation of a natural good. Third, however, the ultimate opposite of TRANSCATEGORIAL value is nothing other than transcategorial *nonvalue*. For the Thomist-Lonerganian universe is not dualistic. There is no transcategorial disvalue, no transcategorial evil. Whatever is, insofar as it is, is valuable, good; and disvalue or evil is always parasitic on the valuable, the good.

9 For example, 'Lying (understood as knowingly and freely expressing a falsehood with the aim of deceiving someone who has a right to the truth) is always a moral disvalue'; and 'Murder (understood as knowingly and freely taking an innocent human life) is always a moral disvalue.'

10 What characterizes an investigation as *ethical* is that its distinctive question is about the specific *moral* value of things and properties. (Similarly, what characterizes an investigation as *aesthetical* is that its distinctive question is about the beauty, the specifically *aesthetical* value, of thing and properties.) Note that (a) the endeavour of integral ethical studies stands to (b) bioethics, environmental ethics, business ethics, political ethics, legal ethics, and so forth as (c) *a single distinctive question* and its exhaustive answer stands to (d) the *diverse partial fields of data* to which that distinctive question can be directed and the diverse partial answers to it that emerge.

11 In Lonerganian terms, Sullivan's own labours in specifically ethical studies are limited largely to the special or categorial dimensions of two functional specialties – the fourth, 'Dialectic,' and the fifth, 'Foundations.'

12 Just as for the structure of ethical studies, so also for the structure of trans-categorial valuative studies: I contend that Sullivan's book constitutes a model that is partly explicit, partly implicit conceptually, and partly implicit operationally. (Cf. note 7, above.)

13 For example, 'Whatever totally fails to satisfy the transcendental intention of value is always a transcategorial nonvalue.' (On transcategorial *nonvalue* as the ultimate opposite of transcategorial *value*, recall note 8, above.)

14 For example, 'The ether (understood as the invisible cosmic medium of electromagnetic radiation) is always a transcategorial nonvalue; and schizo-phrenia (understood as a distinctive mental dysfunction whose cause is in no way organic) is always a transcategorial nonvalue.' (The key to these ex-amples is that transcategorial value presupposes reality, such that whatever is unreal is a transcategorial nonvalue. And in the view of many researchers, empirical study of multiple concrete instances seems to support the generali-zations that the ether is always unreal – it never exists – and that schizophre-nia that is in no way organically based is always unreal – it never occurs.)

15 What characterizes an investigation as *transcategorial valuative* is that its distinctive question is about the general *transcategorial* value of things and properties. Note that (a) the endeavour of integral transcategorial valuative studies stands to (b) the endeavours of integral ethical studies and integral aesthetical studies as (c) *a single wider and more gerneral* distinctive question stands to (d) diverse *narrower and more specific* distinctive questions. In other words, the difference between *integral transcategorial valuative studies* and, say, *integral ethical* studies reflects at root the difference between the greater and lesser respective scopes of two distinctive *questions*; whereas the difference between *integral ethical studies* and, say, *bioethics* reflects at root the difference between a single distinctive *question* and one of the diverse partial fields of *data* to which that distinctive question can be directed. (Cf. note 10, above.)

16 In Lonerganian terms, Sullivan's own labours in valuative studies are limited largely to the general or transcategorial dimensions of two functional spe-cialties – the fourth, 'Dialectic,' and the fifth, 'Foundations.' (Cf. note 11, above.)

Chapter 1

1 *Affect* has many senses, and I will attempt to unpack some of these more fully in Chapters 3 to 9. Until then, readers will not be misled if they consider affect to be roughly synonymous with *feeling* or *emotions*. What I will be referring to by these terms are activities that are (1) mental and inward, rather than their physical, outward manifestations; (2) characterized by their distinctive emotional tone, as distinct from an intellectual one; and (3) intentional or cognitive, in the sense that they have objects, unlike non-

cognitive, psychological feelings or moods. *Value judgment* will also be characterized more precisely in chapters 3 to 7.

2 I use *ramifications* to suggest that the relation between Lonergan's philosophy and the euthanasia debate is one in which his philosophy branches out, has outgrowths and consequences for this debate. By the *euthanasia debate* I refer to the debate that primarily concerns voluntary active euthanasia in which a deliberate act is undertaken by one person with the intention of ending the life of another person to relieve that person's suffering, where that act is the cause of death. l engage this debate primarily at the level of concrete stories, and only secondarily at the levels of the ethical and public-policy debates. For the public-policy debate, see Canada, Special Senate Committee Report, *Of Life and Death* (Ministry of Supply and Services Canada, May 1995) 14.

3 Lonergan, *Method* 37.

4 In 1993–4, I had the good fortune to attend a series of seminars on the theme 'Philosophical Perspectives in Bioethics.' This series consisted of 13 contributions from thinkers representing a wide spectrum of views on the nature of bioethics itself as a normative discipline. It was hosted by the Centre for Bioethics and the Department of Philosophy at the University of Toronto. The papers presented in this series have since been published. Daniel Callahan opened the discussion with a plea for 'an ethical theory that would be capable both of being applied to practical problems and of being embodied in the life of the theorist.' He admitted that his own experience in, and reflections on, the professional world of ethics called into question either the usefulness of theories typically devised by moral philosophers or the consistency between what the theorists say and how they actually operate. It is my primary aim to articulate a theory of moral knowing that will satisfy both of Callahan's requirements. See Daniel Callahan, 'Professional Morality: Can an Examined Life Be Lived?' foreword to L.W. Sumner and Joseph Boyle, eds., *Philosophical Perspectives on Bioethics* (Toronto: University of Toronto Press, 1996) 9–17.

5 See the Diagnostic and Statistical Manual of Mental Disorders, 4th ed. (Washington: American Psychiatric Association, 1994), s.v. 'Gillberg's Criteria for Asperger's Disorder.' In addition, the psychological lexicon lists *alexithymia* as a condition that describes an affective and cognitive disturbance in which persons are unable to differentiate or verbalize emotions, often only being able to describe emotions in physiological or behavioural terms (e.g., anger can only be described in terms of physiological sensations such as flushing, or as aggressive behaviour). See H. Krystal, 'Alexithymia and Psychotherapy,' *American Journal of Psychotherapy* 33 (1979) 17–33.

6 Intellectual ability is a quality that is highly regarded in our society. Conversely, persons who are relatively deficient in their intellectual capacity

might be at risk of being undervalued, which might also be reflected in their medical care. For instance, at a Montreal hospital patients are denied heart transplants if they score less than 50 on an IQ test. Although there might be good reasons for such persons not to have a heart transplant (e.g., problems with consent), this policy might also reflect a broader devaluation of persons having cognitive impairment. See Nancy Deutsch, 'Low IQ May Disqualify Patient for Heart Transplant,' *Family Practice*, 4 November 1996, 40.

7 See L.W. Sumner and Joseph Boyle, eds, *Philosophical Perspectives on Bioethics* 7.

8 It is interesting to note inconsistencies between the values that persuade people of the benefit of some public policy and those values that are actually made manifest in the implementation of that policy. For instance, euthanasia in the Netherlands might have gained acceptance on the basis of a persuasive appeal to the personal autonomy of competent, terminally ill individuals. It is difficult to reconcile the value of autonomy that purportedly underpinned this movement with the early claim that as many as 40 per cent of the estimated 3600 cases of euthanasia in the Netherlands were performed either non-voluntarily or involuntarily. See Thomas Gates, 'Euthanasia and Assisted Suicide: A Family Practice Perspective,' *American Family Physician* 55 (1997) 2437–44, at 2440.

9 John Finnis provides an example of such a view. For how he differs, on his understanding, from Lonergan on this issue, see his book *Fundamentals of Ethics* (Washington: Georgetown University Press, 1983) 30–37, 42–45, 48–50, 54.

10 Milton Hunnex outlines a series of examples of such positions in his overview of various value theories, some of which I will explore further in chapter 3. They include theories such as Hume's skepticism ('x has a value' means 'most men prefer x'); Nietzsche's relativism (value judgments serve as *expressions of feelings* and *customs* rather than statements of fact); Ayer's logical positivism (value judgments serve an *expressive function*, giving vent to feelings and, as statements, are emotive or noncognitive, i.e., *factually meaningless*); and Stevenson's logical empiricism (value judgments serve a *persuasive function*: since value judgments are emotive and not subject to error as true or false, persuasion is needed to evoke their acceptance). See Milton Hunnex, 'The Problem of Values,' in *Chronological and Thematic Charts of Philosophies and Philosophers* (Grand Rapids, MI: Zondervan Publishing House, 1986) 22–23.

11 One example of a contemporary philosopher who is sympathetic to the view that human affectivity or emotion plays some cognitive role in knowing and evaluating is Ronald de Souza. In his *The Rationality of Emotion* (Cambridge, MA: MIT Press, 1990), de Souza argues for an objectivist view of emotions where 'the emotion in question apprehends something of the world that exists independently of our reaction to it' (xv).

12 Michael Vertin cites a list of works by Lonergan scholars who offer diverse
    accounts of what he means by 'apprehensions of value,' and distinguishes his
    own account from theirs. See Michael Vertin, 'Judgments of Value for the
    Later Lonergan,' *Method: Journal of Lonergan Studies* 13 (1995) 222 n. 7, in
    which he cites: Patrick Byrne, 'Analogical Knowledge of God and the Value
    of Moral Endeavor,' *Method: Journal of Lonergan Studies* 11 (1993) 103–35;
    Robert Doran, *Theology and the Dialectics of History* (Toronto: University of
    Toronto Press, 1990) 55–58, 86–87; John Finnis, *Fundamentals of Ethics*
    (Washington: Georgetown University Press, 1983) 30–37, 42–45, 48–50, 54;
    Neil Ormerod, 'Lonergan and Finnis on the Human Good,' in William
    Danaher, ed., *Australian Lonergan Workshop* (Lanham, MD: University Press
    of America, 1993) 199–210; and Bernard Tyrell, 'Feelings as Apprehensive-
    Intentional Responses to Values,' in Fred Lawrence, ed., *Lonergan Workshop* 7
    (1988) 331–60.
13 See G.K. Chesterton, 'The Maniac,' in *Orthodoxy* (New York: Image Books,
    1959) 19. For Chesterton 'sane affections' are those affections that work with
    reason and assist it to function in a properly human way.
14 One example of the cognitive and evaluative aspect of certain feelings is
    the feeling of *guilt.* 'Moral guilt' is a state that others might attribute to a
    responsible moral agent who has done some avoidable harm. The feeling or
    sense of guilt is the psychological correlative, in the guilty person, of his or
    her guilty state. The difficulty of focusing exclusively on this feeling is that
    the genuinely guilty person may or may not experience the appropriate
    feeling of guilt and remorse for the avoidable harm he or she caused and
    consequently may or may not have a desire to expiate the wrong done. Con-
    versely, one may not be genuinely guilty of causing some avoidable harm but
    nevertheless may feel guilty. That is, such a feeling may also be excessive or
    unwarranted because one was not responsible, or the harm caused was un-
    avoidable, or there was no real harm caused. The key point here is that the
    feeling of guilt is not merely one of self-reproach: 'it is inseparable from
    awareness of the harm, or neglect, brought about to the others affected by
    one's action or inaction.' Hence, such a feeling has a cognitive, and more
    particularly, an evaluative aspect to it. See Ted Honderich, ed., *The Oxford
    Companion to Philosophy* (Oxford: Oxford University Press, 1995), s.v. 'Guilt,'
    by R.W. Hepburn.
15 By *wisdom* I have in mind 'good judgment about the evaluation of complex
    situations and conceptions of a good life in the light of a reflective under-
    standing of the human condition.' See Honderich, ed., *Oxford Companion to
    Philosophy*, s.v. 'Wisdom,' by John Kekes.
16 Although Lonergan's cognitional theory, epistemology, and metaphysics will
    occupy the core of this discussion, the reader should consider these issues to
    be instrumental to the task of making some creative contribution to the

euthanasia debate. This strategy is consistent with Lonergan's own withdrawal into foundational issues, which, as Frederick Crowe points out, was
preparatory for a thoroughly effective return to deal with a whole range of
practical questions of his day, both moral and technical. In the process of
seeking to apply Lonergan's stance on these global philosophical issues, I
have also discovered the truth of Crowe's further observation that the application of Lonergan's *organon* to questions like those raised by the euthanasia
debate 'is an extremely laborious process requiring further creativity of a
character and magnitude we are just discovering.' See Frederick Crowe,
'Lonergan's "Moral Theology and the Human Sciences": Editor's Introduction,' *Method: Journal of Lonergan Studies* 15 (1997) 2.

17 In order to emphasize that the 'illness' of ALS includes more than merely
biological symptoms of a disease, I will refer to the broader human impact
of a disease as the 'illness experience.' Even though using 'illness' as an
adjective might not be grammatically correct, this expression has become
popular in family medicine where there is an effort to highlight some
human dimensions of an experience of disease, such as the psycho-social-
spiritual challenges of disease.

18 See Ira Brock, *Dying Well: The Prospect of Growth at the End of Life* (New York:
Putnam, 1997).

19 The most significant details of Lonergan's biography are amply outlined in a
variety of sources. The English sources include but are not limited to *The New
Encyclopedia of Philosophy* (1972), *The Fontana Biographical Companion to Modern
Thought* (1983), *The Canadian Encyclopedia* (1988), and *Chambers Biographical
Dictionary* (1996).

20 *The Canadian Encyclopedia* (1988 ed.), s.v. 'Lonergan,' by William Fennell.

21 *Chambers Biographical Dictionary* (1996 ed.), s.v. 'Lonergan,' by Magnus
Magnusson.

22 Sumner and Boyle, eds, *Philosophical Perspectives on Bioethics* 7. I referred to
this seminar series in note 5 above.

23 Ibid. 8.

24 Sumner and Boyle point out that R.M. Hare's position was a conspicuous
exception to the bulk of the presentations because 'his method of supporting his two-level normative theory is neither foundationalist, properly
speaking, nor coherentist.' If, from Lonergan's perspective, one interprets
R.M. Hare's two-level normative theory to be a cognitional theory, his
argument is foundationalist, just as I will argue that Lonergan's position is
foundationalist. For Lonergan, however, the foundations are not, ultimately,
some content, but rather the general structure of one's knowing. In articulating Longeran's position, I will suggest the relevance of these basic categories for expanding the whole particularist/generalist discussion in bioethics. See Sumner and Boyle, eds, *Philosophical Perspectives on Bioethics* 8.

25 Bertrand Russell, *Skeptical Essays* (London: Allen and Unwin, 1977) 127.

26 One of the reasons for exploring Sue Rodriguez's story more closely is the enormous influence it has had in shaping the Canadian euthanasia debate. The possibility that further nuances or twists to her story might come to light even after her book, however, would support rather than undermine my underlying concern. That is, I contend that her story shows that most persons who affirm her conclusion do so with a very limited understanding of why she judged her life to be without value at a certain stage in her decline, and also of what sort of difficulties her decision to die by assisted suicide was intended to address. Further complexities that might subsequently emerge will only strengthen my central claim that affirming Sue's conclusion that assisted suicide was necessary for her to secure a dignified death (as the Canadian Supreme Court judges did) is an opinion based more on larger philosophical issues than on the facts of her particular case.

27 In fact, this is part of my argument against certain proponents of euthanasia. I argue that not only is there a lack of cognitional skill in their assessment of Sue's conclusions (i.e., they are too easily persuaded by her evaluation of the worth of her own life), but also they mistakenly also purport to go beyond her particular case and to draw general policy conclusions from it.

28 Since Tracy Latimer was unable 'voluntarily' to give her father consent to kill her, hers would have been an easier case for me to critique than Sue Rodriguez's. In addition, Tracy's case also argues against relaxing the prohibition on all forms of euthanasia. This is because the substantial outpouring of public sympathy in support of Robert Latimer's actions suggests that the significance of the moral and legal distinction between voluntary and non-voluntary euthanasia has already been lost in the broader public-policy debate. This is a distinction that is very important for proponents of voluntary euthanasia to be able to maintain both in theory and practice. Since most thinkers currently view non-voluntary and involuntary euthanasia to be morally offensive (and rightly so), the fact that this distinction, which rests on the issue of consent, is already blurred in public discussions seriously challenges proponents of euthanasia who think there is a world of moral difference between the case of Sue Rodriguez and that of Tracy Latimer.

29 Although the case of Sue Rodriguez and the issue of euthanasia has captured enormous attention, the discussion of her case has tended to reduce the ethical debate to merely procedural questions, such as who, if anyone, should act on her request of assisted suicide. This tends to distract attention from the more substantive issues, such as the basis for her evaluation that her life was no longer worthwhile. It also obscures the fact that many of the everyday value judgments that caregivers in a family-practice context typically encounter have as much complexity and nuance to them as these more celebrated cases and issues. One benefit of encouraging the dialogue

between philosophers (or lawyers) and medical practitioners is that the former might begin to pay more attention to the particularities of cases, and the latter to more global philosophical issues.

30 In addition, if the laws on euthanasia and assisted suicide are changed, it will be the family physicians, rather than the specialists, who will be most directly affected (as is the case in the Netherlands).

31 There are some important stances on pedagogical issues that underpin my approach, as a philosopher, to a medical audience. I have had the opportunity to try a number of approaches, and the one I will adopt in this discussion seems to avoid better the pitfalls of those approaches that tend to irritate, bore, or be irrelevant to medical persons. The key, I think, is to add a new or expanded perspective on some issue by finding the right combination of what is familiar and of concern with what is philosophically novel and challenging.

Chapter 2

1 The divided public view about the relevance of affectivity or feelings to cognitive acts, such as value judgments or evaluations, corresponds to a similar division that some thinkers claim exists among medical practitioners. One proponent of the view that the modern medical school is divided on this issue is Ian McWhinney, Professor Emeritus of Family Medicine at the University of Western Ontario. (See Ian McWhinney, 'The Importance of Being Different: 1996 William Pickles Lecture,' *British Journal of General Practice* 46 [July 1996] 433–36.) In his address to the Royal College of General Practitioners, McWhinney claimed that one feature that distinguishes general practitioners from their specialist colleagues is their rejection of the dualistic division between body and mind which, he says, 'runs through medicine like a geological fault' (435). According to McWhinney, this fault line 'runs through the affect-denying clinical method which dominates the modern medical school. Not until this is reformed will emotions and relationships have the place in medicine they deserve' (436). My focus on two particular stories in this chapter serves to illustrate how emotions are implicated in evaluations, that is, that they actually play some cognitive role. In so doing, I will be exploring the relation between what McWhinney calls *body* and *mind*, or what I would express as the distinction between human *psychology* and *cognition*.

2 Canada, House of Commons, *Hansard*, 24 Sept. 1991, 2664.

3 This report was the third in a series on physician-assisted suicide requested by the American Medical Association Board of Trustees. See Council on Scientific Affairs, AMA, 'Good Care of the Dying Patient,' *Journal of the American Medical Association* 275 (1996) 474–78.

4 In the age range of 25 to 64 years, the five leading causes of death by number
of deaths per year in the United States are malignant neoplasm, heart disease, motor vehicle accidents, HIV infection, and suicide and homicide.
In the age range of 64 and older, all five leading causes of death are from
chronic diseases: heart disease' malignant neoplasms (lung, colorectal, and
breast), cerebrovascular disease, chronic obstructive pulmonary disease, and
infectious diseases such as pneumonia or influenza. See Paul Frame, Alfred
Berg, and Steve Woolf, 'U.S. Preventive Services Task Force: Highlights of
the 1996 Report,' *American Family Physician* 55 (1997) 567–76, at 570, 571.

5 Robert Buckman suggests that the challenges patients and physicians face in
dealing with death are continuous with the difficulty of giving bad medical
news to patients generally. He speaks of various causes for these difficulties
and distinguishes between causes having to do with specific patients' 'fears of
dying,' and more generally prevailing 'social attitudes to death.' The specific
patient fears he lists echo those previously mentioned, such as physical
symptoms, psychological loss of control, disagreeable treatment side-effects,
and threats to one's family system or social status. But Buckman locates these
concerns within a more general contemporary negative social attitude to the
fact of human mortality. He argues that the problems individuals encounter
when faced with the news of their own impending death reflect contemporary social attitudes, such as: a lack of experience of death as a normal part
of family life; high expectations of health and life; the predominance of
materialist values (such as the value placed on wealth, youth, and health);
and the declining role of religion. See Robert Buckman, *How to Break Bad
News: A Guide for Health Care Professionals* (Toronto: University of Toronto
Press, 1992) 29–33.

6 Frame, Berg, and Woolf, 'U.S. Preventive Services Task Force: Highlights'
569.

7 Council on Scientific Affairs, 'Good Care of the Dying Patient' 475.

8 Harvey Max Chochinov et al., 'Desire for Death in the Terminally Ill,'
American Journal of Psychiatry 152 (1995) 1185–91.

9 Council on Scientific Affairs, 'Good Care of the Dying Patient' 475.

10 Chochinov et al., 'Desire for Death in the Terminally Ill' 1188.

11 James Lavery, Bernard Dickens, Joseph Boyle, and Peter Singer, 'Bioethics
for Clinicians: 11. Euthanasia and Assisted Suicide,' *Canadian Medical
Association Journal* 156 (1997) 1405–1408, at 1407.

12 Canada, Special Senate Committee Report, *Of Life and Death* (Ministry of
Supply and Services Canada, May 1995).

13 Ibid. 24.

14 Ibid. 32.

15 Council on Scientific Affairs, 'Good Care of the Dying Patient' 475.

16 Chochinov et al., 'Desire for Death in the Terminally Ill' 1190.

17 The best source of information on the context of Sue Rodriguez's decision to request physician-assisted suicide is a book she co-authored with Lisa Hobbs Birnie. I follow this report of Sue's story with a parallel report of the story of Dennis Kaye, a peer of Sue's who also wrote about his life with ALS. For more complete accounts of their stories, see Lisa Hobbs Birnie and Sue Rodriguez, *Uncommon Will: The Death and Life of Sue Rodriguez* (Toronto: Macmillan Canada, 1994) and Dennis Kaye, *Laugh, I Thought I'd Die, My Life with ALS* (Toronto: Penguin Books Ltd., 1993).

18 John Keown, ed., *Euthanasia Examined: Ethical, Clinical, and Legal Perspectives,* foreword by Daniel Callahan (Cambridge: Press Syndicate of the University of Cambridge, 1995) 2.

19 Canada, Special Senate Committee, *Of Life and Death* v.

20 In fact, the courts expressly avoided entering the 'existential' dimensions of Sue's decision because they did not wish to presume any authority to address such weighty philosophical questions. Nor did any lawyer subject her to personal criticism or cross-examination. As Hobbs Birnie points out, '[o]nly a lawyer with a death wish would have put her on the stand.' See Hobbs Birnie and Rodriguez, *Uncommon Will* 66.

21 I will organize my comments according to affective themes that Sue and Dennis address in their books. My aim is merely to highlight the affective context of their value judgments and decisions. Although these affective data are also key to a psychological or psychiatric analysis, my aim is to focus on how they might be relevant to value judgments. Hence, I will briefly sample some of the typical categories of a psychiatric assessment, such as a 'history of the present illness,' 'past personal history,' 'social history,' and 'family history.' See Harold Kaplan and Benjamin Sadock, *Synopsis of Psychiatry: Behavioral Sciences, Clinical Psychiatry,* 6th ed. (Baltimore: Williams & Wilkins, 1991) 193–205.

22 Sack Goldblatt Mitchell, 'The Sue Rodriguez Case: A Legal Perspective,' *Ontario Medical Review* 60 (1993) 79. Note that this 'medical description' also suggests a normative stance on what patients with ALS 'require' as a medical response to this disease.

23 Sue Rodriguez, 'To Die with Dignity,' letter to the *Vancouver Star,* republished in the *Toronto Star,* 4 March 1993, 1(B).

24 Deborah Wilson and Donn Downey, 'Obituary,' *Globe and Mail,* 14 February 1994, 4(A). This legal statement seems to concede the key claim that Sue's death would be dignified only on the condition that physician-assisted suicide was allowed. One ultimate aim of addressing this issue is to challenge this rather arbitrary view of the conditions of Sue's dignity. I will attempt to do this in chapter 9.

25 The end that Sue sought was a declaration by the courts that would permit a physician to connect her to a mixture of intravenous fluids containing a

lethal agent at the time of her own choosing. She could trigger the device to deliver this lethal agent herself. Sue's lawyers argued that the legal grounds for such a declaration are given in section 7 of the Canadian Charter of Rights and Freedoms. This section of the Charter guarantees her the right to control what happens to her body while she is still living, and the liberty to make fundamental decisions concerning her life. They maintained that this should be interpreted as including her choice of the timing, method, and circumstances of her death, without interference from the state. See Sack Goldblatt Mitchell, 'The Sue Rodriguez Case' 80.

26 I will focus, as much as possible, on understanding Sue's emotional life. Although Sue spoke critically of those who did not 'respect the truths of others,' or who 'want to impose their own value system on me,' my first aim is to highlight what her truths and values were, insofar as they can be gleaned from what she and Hobbs Birnie say in her biography. See Hobbs Birnie and Rodriguez, *Uncommon Will* 69, 116.

27 Ibid. 137–38.

28 Ibid. 138.

29 In other words, she received no 'anticipatory counseling' prior to being told about her diagnosis. Such counselling has become part of the routine practice in other cases of giving 'bad news,' such as prior to testing someone for an HIV infection.

30 Hobbs Birnie and Rodriguez, *Uncommon Will* 3.

31 Ibid. 2–5.

32 Ibid. 6.

33 Ibid. 24.

34 Ibid. 20.

35 Although Sue was only briefly exposed to the Baptist faith of her parents when she was a child, she could identify with the Puritan work ethic her family motto expresses. This work ethic links material achievement and productivity with one's moral justification. See Anne Mullens, 'Just Getting Through the Day Was the Hardest Part,' *Toronto Star*, 14 February 1994, 19(A).

36 Hobbs Birnie and Rodriguez, *Uncommon Will* 20.

37 Ibid. 21.

38 Ibid. 21.

39 Ibid. 23.

40 Ibid. 23.

41 See ibid. 22. My own interpretation of this incident is that Sue's behaviour was motivated by her need to be included and accepted by her friends. The controlling, disciplinary response of the new coalition of her parents and grandparents alienated Sue from her family and friends. Consequently, at this time in her life she had no real supports whatever. In this light, it is not

surprising that in her later life Sue was bitter toward her family and controlling of others, for fear that they would use their power once more to betray
or control her.

42 Ibid. 25.

43 Daniel Wood, 'Death Wish,' *Chatelaine* 66 (1993) 26.

44 Hobbs Birnie and Rodriguez, *Uncommon Will* 26–27.

45 Ibid. 23.

46 Ibid. 135–36.

47 Given Sue's personal background, it is less surprising that the focal issues at
the end of her life had to do with control (whose life is it anyway?) and
boundary issues (challenging the medical profession to extend its role of
healer to include acts of killing).

48 Surprisingly, physical pain was never an important worry for Sue. That is, the
source of her suffering was not merely one of pain. See Hobbs Birnie and
Rodriguez, *Uncommon Will* 27.

49 In fact, it was not Sue's loss of her speech, but relational losses, that finally
prompted her decision to kill herself.

50 Mullens, 'Just Getting Through the Day.'

51 Hobbs Birnie and Rodriguez, *Uncommon Will* 36–37.

52 Ibid. 63. In the minds of many members of the public, these biological
issues, including pain, seem to be the most persuasive grounds for arguing in
favour of physician-assisted suicide. Given what Sue has said elsewhere, her
own emphasis of these issues might have had more to do with a courtroom
strategy than with her with personal concerns about losing control or of not
mattering to anyone as her condition progressed.

53 Ibid. 90.

54 Rodriguez, 'To Die with Dignity.'

55 Ibid.

56 Ibid.

57 Hobbs Birnie and Rodriguez, *Uncommon Will* 152.

58 Ibid. 162. Doe later reported to Hobbs Birnie that she did not speak to Sue
on the phone that day because by that time she could not understand a word
Sue said. Doe said that it was painful to try to understand, and she thought
that there really wasn't any point in just saying hello.

59 Ibid. 128–9.

60 Ibid. 163. All of these events need to be interpreted in light of Sue's open
wish to kill herself. It seems that her threat of suicide had negative implications for many of her relationships. In her husband's case, it was a source
of guilt. Henry had the feeling that, had he cared for her better, he might
have helped her to avoid the decision to commit suicide. For Sue's mother
Doe, Sue's decision was a foregone conclusion, so she didn't think there
was any point in talking to her. As for Sue's friend, she might have been

reluctant to become involved with Sue for fear of being implicated in her suicide plans.

61 Ibid. 164.

62 Ibid. 37. Sue seems to have based this view of what would be best for her son on her own negative images of her father's dying.

63 Ibid. 74, 132.

64 Ibid. 129.

65 Ibid. 129.

66 Ibid. 130.

67 Ibid. 136.

68 Dennis was diagnosed with ALS at age 30 and died at age 41. By contrast, Sue was diagnosed at age 42 and died at age 44.

69 Kaye, *Laugh, I Thought I'd Die* xi.

70 Ibid. 203. I will draw primarily on Dennis's own account of his affective life with ALS in order to contrast it with Sue Rodriguez's.

71 Ibid. 207–208, 233 (item 14).

72 Hobbs Birnie and Rodriguez, *Uncommon Will* 122.

73 Kaye, *Laugh, I Thought I'd Die* 106.

74 Ibid. 101.

75 Ibid. 163.

76 Ibid. 164. Although the issue of control was also important to Dennis, the control he sought was not external, as in Sue's case, but internal and emotional. That is, he directed his efforts toward his own response to his illness experience.

77 Ibid. 164.

78 Ibid. 64.

79 Ibid. 65. Grasping the humour of a situation illustrates the close link between cognitive and affective acts, of which I will have more to say in chapters 4 through 7.

80 Ibid. 98.

81 Ibid. 100.

82 Ibid. 100.

83 Although I think that substituting *Our* for *My* in the title of Dennis's book would more accurately underline a key theme of this work, I note that the original subtitle was 'From Diagnosis to Rigor Mortis.' This original title highlights the 'times' of Dennis's illness (i.e., from diagnosis to death). The title he later chose for his book helpfully focuses our attention on the story of his 'life,' appreciated from the vantage point of those times near its end. The title I am suggesting would further emphasize the role that others played in this life story. For while Dennis's book is certainly about his life with ALS, it is also the story of the responses of his wife, daughters, parents, friends (even strangers) to his life with ALS. Even what we might properly call

Dennis's response to his illness cannot be understood apart from the responses of others to him. Nor did his own response to this illness end with himself. Rather, his 'laugh' had a contagious quality about it that even infected radio audiences. Dennis acknowledged that his life had been especially blessed because it had been part of the life of a family and community. We, along with his family, might well reach a similar conclusion about how our lives have been blessed by him when we reflect upon his gifts to us (including that of taking ourselves – even our decline and death – less seriously). See Wood, 'Death Wish' 29.

84 Kaye, *Laugh, I Thought I'd Die* 96.

85 Ibid. 200.

86 Ibid. 85.

87 According to Tom Beauchamp, the traditional debates about suicide centred on whether suicide violates one or more of three types of obligations: to oneself, to others, or to God. See Ted Honderich, ed., *The Oxford Companion to Philosophy* (Oxford: Oxford University Press, 1995), s.v. 'Suicide,' by Tom Beauchamp.

88 This was essentially David Hume's famous argument for the permissibility of autonomous suicide. In this argument, Hume responds to the traditional obligations to oneself and others, but not to God. See Honderich, ed., *Oxford Companion to Philosophy*, s.v. 'Suicide.'

89 Another way of expressing this evaluative issue is to focus on the 'intentions' behind various decisions and actions. The purported ethical significance of 'intentions' has been used to highlight the controverted ethical distinction between euthanasia and assisted suicide, on the one hand, and decisions to forgo life-sustaining treatments, on the other. Decisions to perform euthanasia or assisted suicide follow from the evaluation that a life is not worth living. Consequently, the death of the patient is the intention behind whatever means is employed to bring about this death. By contrast, death is said to be a predictable, though non-intended, consequence of the morally justified withdrawal of life-sustaining treatments. Such withdrawal is thought to be morally justified only in cases where there is a fatal underlying condition. It is that condition, not the action of withdrawing treatment, that causes death. I would argue that the issue of intention highlights the connection between the fundamental question of whether a life is worth living and subsequent questions that are raised in light of this evaluation and that lead to decisions and actions. It also locates the key ethical issue to be an evaluative, rather than a decisional, one. The key difference in stances on this evaluative issue, I think, is between proponents of euthanasia who view human moral status as developmental, and opponents who view it as non-developmental. See Lavery et al. 'Bioethics for Clinicians.'

90 Richard Norman points out that the moral importance of this notion of

autonomy has prompted attempts to express more precisely what it is. He suggests that '[o]ur idea of the autonomous person seems to involve more than just the capacity to act on particular desires and choices. It suggests a more general capacity to be self-determining, to be in control of one's life ... The autonomous person is one who is able to assess his or her own first-order desires, to reject or modify some of them and to endorse others, and to act upon these second-order preferences.' Such a view suggests that there are more or less 'authentic' expressions of personal autonomy. This notion of authenticity is one that I will explore. See Honderich, ed., *Oxford Companion to Philosophy*, s.v. 'Autonomy in Applied Ethics,' by Richard Norman.

91 This identification of the problem is consistent with the view of the main arguments and beliefs for euthanasia that predominate in the literature according to John Williams, Fred Lowy, and Douglas Sawyer. In a five-part series of articles published in the *Canadian Medical Association Journal*, these authors distinguished between the main patient and physician beliefs about and arguments for euthanasia. For patients, the two main arguments for euthanasia are relief of suffering (based on the belief that suffering is worse than death), and the exercise of personal control (based on the belief that autonomy is paramount). For physicians, the two main arguments for euthanasia parallel patients' arguments. The first is respect for a patient's choice based on the belief that patient self-determination must be respected, and the second argument is one of 'compassion' based on the belief that suffering must be relieved. Interestingly, the authors begin this article by stating that '[s]ome arguments are based on equally strong feelings or beliefs, which unlike arguments are often not susceptible to rational deliberation.' See Williams, Lowy, and Sawyer, 'Canadian Physicians and Euthanasia: 3. Arguments and Beliefs,' *Canadian Medical Association Journal* 148 (1993) 1699–1702.

92 Daniel Callahan, 'Foreword' to Keown, ed., *Euthanasia Examined* xiii–xv.

93 An opinion poll conducted by the Harvard School of Public Health in 1991 reported that 64 per cent of Americans favour physician-assisted suicide or euthanasia for terminally ill patients who request it. This number was as high as 79 per cent among adults under 35 years of age. See R. Knox, 'Poll: Americans Favor Mercy Killing,' *Boston Globe*, 3 November 1991, 1(A).

94 Callahan, *Euthanasia Examined* xv.

95 Ibid.

96 Leon Kass, a prominent medical ethicist from Chicago, agrees with Callahan's analysis. He contends that proponents of euthanasia typically cite two main reasons in support of their position: (1) whether a debilitated life is worth living, and (2) whether euthanasia is an expression of freedom and personal autonomy. But of the two reasons, Kass also suggests that the former plays the greater role. That is, '[i]t is not his or her autonomy but

rather the pitiable condition of the body or mind that justifies doing the patient in.' Accordingly, in my discussion I will focus on the grounds for this underlying evaluation that seems to be at the heart of this debate. See Leon Kass, '"I Will Give No Deadly Drug," Why Doctors Must Not Kill,' *Bulletin, American College of Surgeons* 77 (1992) 6–17, at 8.

97 Tom Beauchamp, 'Refusals of Treatment and Requests for Death,' *Kennedy Institute of Ethics Journal* 6 (1996) 371–74, at 371.

98 This question is even more restricted than the one Hume raised more than two centuries earlier in his rebuttal of the traditional views on suicide. The key question for Hume was whether more value is produced for the individual or for society than would be produced by not performing the act of taking one's life. The question now concerns only the individual, although there is evidently some social interest in containing the costs of caring for persons at this stage of life. See Honderich, ed., *Oxford Companion to Philosophy*, s.v. 'Suicide,' by Tom Beauchamp.

99 Beauchamp, 'Refusals of Treatment and Requests for Death' 374.

100 Philip Hébert is an example of a Canadian ethicist who argues in a style that is similar to Beauchamp's. As a medical ethicist and physician, he maintains that the key reasons to support physician-assisted death are consistent with the training and intuition of many doctors to focus on the particularities of individuals, rather than on broader public considerations. These reasons include putting the needs of a particular patient ahead of other third-party interests (e.g., such as the risks this practice holds for other vulnerable patients, for family members, or for the integrity of physicians). Hébert understands such decisions to be an instance of 'individualized decision making' that is part of what physicians do best. Just as we trust physicians with all sorts of responsibilities, Hébert argues that we should also trust them with this one. He concludes that 'if such decisions can be made properly they should be decisions of conscience, such as ones regarding elective terminations of pregnancy.' Philip Hébert, *Doing Right: A Practical Guide to Ethics for Physicians and Medical Trainees* (Toronto: Oxford University Press, 1996) 191–92.

101 Richard McCormick, 'Killing and Allowing to Die,' *America* 177 (6 December 1977) 6–12.

102 Ibid. The other cultural biases that McCormick addressed was the tendency to make autonomy absolute and the tendency to what he called 'technological monism.' The latter is the view that every death is preventable by technology. As a result of this view, there is a sense of failure and culpability when, for instance, a 93-year-old person dies in an intensive care unit.

103 Philip Hébert adds that withdrawal of life supports was a contentious moral and legal issue only 20 years ago. Although it is now considered to be 'humane medical care,' he interprets it to be still against the provisions of

the Criminal Code of Canada. Hébert and Schafer were cited as two Canadian experts in medical ethics commenting on the case of a Halifax intensive care physician, Dr. Morrison, who was charged with first-degree murder of a patient under her care whom she removed from life-support systems. See Leslie Scrivener, 'MD's Often Give Drugs That Speed Up Dying,' *Toronto Star*, 10 May 1997, 29(A).

104 Canada, Special Senate Committee, *Of Life and Death* 1.
105 Ibid. 1–2.
106 This minority view corresponded to the minority opinion of the Supreme Court of Canada that ruled on Sue Rodriguez's case.
107 Canada, Special Senate Committee, *Of Life and Death* 88.
108 Ibid. 87.
109 Ibid. 72.
110 Ibid. x.

Chapter 3

1 It is interesting to note the universality of the symbol of the heart, a symbol that extends beyond the Western traditions. This symbol represents something at the core of a person, and in some cultures is explicitly linked to cognitive abilities. The Chinese character for insight, for instance, is the symbol of the heart under the symbol for field (i.e., wisdom for the Chinese involves 'cultivating the heart'). Among biblical writers, the anatomical locus of various emotions is differentiated further than the mind/heart distinction. For instance, the author of Luke/Acts localizes compassion to the 'bowels.'

2 See Cheshire Calhoun and Robert Solomon's 'Introduction,' in Calhoun and Solomon, eds, *What Is an Emotion? Classic Readings in Philosophy and Psychology* (Oxford: Oxford University Press, 1984) 3–40.

3 Simon Blackburn, *The Oxford Dictionary of Philosophy* (Oxford: Oxford University Press, 1994); and Ted Honderich, ed., *The Oxford Companion to Philosophy* (Oxford: Oxford University Press, 1995). My choice of the Oxford works over other equally legitimate options, such as the *Cambridge Dictionary of Philosophy*, is merely to simplify the discussion.

4 Note that, on this division, this first family of positions includes members who express both 'axiological subjectivist' and 'axiological objectivist' value theories according to Milton Hunnex's classification system. (See Hunnex, *Chronological and Thematic Charts of Philosophies and Philosophers* [Grand Rapids, MI: Zondervan Publishing House, 1986] 22–29.) Besides this distinction, I will also distinguish thinkers on the basis of whether they consider emotions to play any cognitive role in value judgments, what I will later refer to as a phenomenological, rather an epistemological, issue.

5 The definition of 'cognition' is itself controversial. The traditional view, which is presupposed by most of the thinkers I will survey, understands human cognition to be the domain of thought and inference. By contrast, the non-cognitive domain includes perceptual experiences, sensations, feelings, and other mental phenomena that, it seems, are not specifically human. Those mental elements that humans share in common with animals are thought to provide input into thinking and reasoning, but are not themselves thoughts or cognitions. More recently, cognition has been defined as 'the representational states and processes studied by cognitive psychology' (see Honderich, ed., *Oxford Companion to Philosophy*, s.v. 'Cognition,' by Barry Smith). This new definition includes some aspects of sensory perception as cognitive, such as representations of a spatial world and intelligent processing of this sensory input. It also prescinds from the concern to distinguish between animals and humans on the basis of their mental capacities. For my purpose, I will follow the traditional understanding of the term 'cognitive,' but will later nuance this understanding by appealing to intentionality analysis rather than to faculty psychology.

6 Calhoun and Solomon, *What Is an Emotion?* v.

7 Honderich, ed., *Oxford Companion to Philosophy*, s.v. 'History of Moral Philosophy,' by Richard Norman.

8 Calhoun and Solomon, *What Is an Emotion?* 3.

9 Ibid. 6.

10 Ibid. 9.

11 Ibid. 10.

12 Ibid. 20.

13 Ibid. 18.

14 Ibid. 9.

15 Honderich, ed., *Oxford Companion to Philosophy*, s.v. 'History of Moral Philosophy' 588.

16 Ibid. 588. Note that although both Hobbes and Hume maintain that emotions play a role in knowing the good, for Hume one can at best know the 'apparent' good; on the other hand, for Hobbes, one can at best know the 'genuine' good. In this sense, Hobbes represents a thinker outside of the Aristotelian tradition for whom emotions are relevant to knowing epistemically objective values.

17 Ibid. 589.

18 Calhoun and Solomon, *What Is an Emotion?* 17.

19 See Frederick Copleston, *A History of Philosophy* 5: *Hobbes to Hume* (New York: Doubleday, 1985) 332.

20 Calhoun and Solomon, *What Is an Emotion?* 18.

21 Honderich, ed., *Oxford Companion to Philosophy*, s.v. 'Immanuel Kant,' by Henry Allison.

22 Calhoun and Solomon, *What Is an Emotion?* 32.

23 Honderich, ed., *Oxford Companion to Philosophy*, s.v. 'History of Moral Philosophy' 590.

24 Calhoun and Solomon, *What Is an Emotion?* 33.

25 See Copleston, *History of Philosophy* 6: *Wolff to Kant* 319.

26 Immanuel Kant, *Foundations of the Metaphysics of Morals*, trans. Lewis White Beck, 23rd ed. (Indianapolis: Bobbs-Merrill Educational Publishing, 1983) 43.

27 Interpreting Kant's claims from the perspective of the *Second Critique*, this knowledge is, nevertheless, merely of *appearances* rather than of *noumena* or 'things in themselves.' Still, other thinkers, such as John Finnis, who follow Kant's view that emotions are irrelevant to knowing values maintain that such knowledge is genuine and not merely theoretical.

28 See Blackburn, *Oxford Dictionary of Philosophy*, s.v. 'Rationalism,' and Honderich, ed., *Oxford Companion to Philosophy*, s.v. 'Kantian ethics,' by R.S. Downie.

29 Honderich, ed., *Oxford Companion to Philosophy*, s.v. 'History of Moral Philosophy' 578.

30 See W. Fortenbaugh, *Aristotle on Emotion: A Contribution to Philosophical Psychology, Rhetoric, Poetics, and Ethics* (Worcester and London: Harper & Row Publishers, 1975) 12.

31 See ibid. 31 n. 3.

32 Calhoun and Solomon, *What Is an Emotion?* 43.

33 Honderich, ed., *Oxford Companion to Philosophy*, s.v. 'History of Moral Philosophy' 587.

34 Aristotle, *Nicomachean Ethics*, trans. Terence Irwin (Indianapolis, IN: Hackett Publishing Co., 1985), II, 4, 1105b 6–12, p. 40.

35 Ibid. II, 2, 1103b 21–25, p. 35.

36 W.S. Hett translates this as 'the thinking faculty thinks the forms in mental images.' See Aristotle, *On the Soul*, trans. W.S. Hett (Cambridge, MA: Harvard University Press, 1936; repr. 1986), iii, 7, 431b 2–5, p. 177.

37 Lonergan interprets Aristotle to mean that understanding (the faculty) actually understands. For him, the Aristotelian and Thomist program arrives at this conclusion through 'a process of introspection that discovers the act of insight into phantasm and the definition as an expression of the insight.' Hence, understanding involves both acts of 'grasping' some unity in a diversity and of abstracting this intelligibility to express it in a definition. See Lonergan, *Verbum*, CWL 2:88.

38 Aristotle, *On the Soul*, III, 7, 431a 1–5, p. 175.

39 Honderich, ed., *Oxford Companion to Philosophy*, s.v. 'Virtues,' by Michael Slote, 900–901.

40 See Terence Irwin's 'glossary' in Aristotle, *Nicomachean Ethics*, s.v. 'Virtue' 431.

41 Some thinkers, such as Kenneth Melchin, make this same argument independently of these Platonic presuppositions. For him, the moral consequences of certain acts on one's virtuous disposition would be important considerations for ethical reflections generally. See Kenneth Melchin, 'Revisionists, Deontologists, and the Structure of Moral Understanding,' *Theological Studies* 51 (1990) 389–416.

42 See Honderich, *Oxford Companion to Philosophy*, s.v. 'History of Moral Philosophy' 586–91 passim.

43 Recall that for Kant the fact that the virtuous person's good acts are in keeping with his or her personal inclinations detracts from the moral worth of those acts. See Kant, *Foundations of the Metaphysics of Morals* 43.

44 Honderich, ed., *Oxford Companion to Philosophy*, s.v. 'Virtues.'

45 Ibid., s.v. 'History of Moral Philosophy' 587.

46 Ibid.

47 Copleston, *A History of Philosophy* 2: *Augustine to Scotus* 411.

48 Ibid.

49 Eric D'Arcy discusses some of the difficulties in rendering an English translation of Aquinas's *passiones animae*. He considers a variety of options, such as *affect*, *sentiment*, and *feeling*. He settles on the term *emotion* and restricts the use of the term *passion* to those occasions in which he wishes to emphasize the passive quality of certain emotions. See Eric D'Arcy's 'Introduction,' in Thomas Aquinas, *Summa Theologiae* 19 (London and New York: Blackfriars in conjunction with Eyre & Spottiswoode and McGraw-Hill Book Co., 1967) xxvi–xxix.

50 John P. Reid, 'Introduction,' in Thomas Aquinas, *Summa Theologiae* 21: xx.

51 Fathers of the English Dominican Province, trans., *Summa Theologica of St. Thomas Aquinas* 2 (Westminster, MD: Christian Classics, 1981) q. 26, a. 2, p. 704.

52 Ibid. 2: 689–789 passim.

53 Mark Drost, 'Intentionality in Aquinas' Theory of Emotions,' *International Philosophical Quarterly* 31 (1991) 451.

54 Fathers of the English Dominican Province, trans., *Summa Theologica* 2, q. 1, a. 2, p. 584, and q. 24, a. 3, p. 699.

55 Ibid. 2, q. 24, a. 1, p. 697.

56 Mark Drost, 'In the Realm of the Senses: Saint Thomas Aquinas on Sensory Love, Desire, and Delight,' *The Thomist* 59 (1995) 58.

57 Fathers of the English Dominican Province, trans., *Summa Theologica* 2, q. 78, a. 2, p. 942.

58 Ibid. 2, q. 58, a. 5, p. 837.

59 See Calhoun and Solomon, *What Is an Emotion?* 215.

60 See Honderich, ed., *Oxford Companion to Philosophy*, s.v. 'Max Scheler,' by M.J. Inwood.

61 Manfred Frings, 'Foreword,' in Max Scheler, *Formalism in Ethics and Non-Formal Ethics of Values*, trans. M. Frings and Roger Fung (Evanston, IL: Northwestern University Press, 1973) xiv.

62 Lonergan, *Method* 30–31 n. 2.

63 Frings, *Formalism in Ethics* xxiii.

64 Calhoun and Solomon, *What Is an Emotion?* 217.

65 Ibid. 217–18.

66 See Honderich, ed., *Oxford Companion to Philosophy*, s.v. 'Max Scheler.'

67 Ibid.

68 Edith Stein, 'On the Problem of Empathy,' in *The Collected Works of Edith Stein* 3, trans. W. Stein (Washington: ICS Publications, 1989).

69 Ibid. 10.

70 Ibid. 11.

71 Ibid. 116.

72 Ibid. 108.

73 Frings, *Formalism in Ethics* xxiii.

74 See Honderich, ed., *Oxford Companion to Philosophy*, s.v. 'Passion,' by Robert Solomon.

75 Lonergan, *Method* 39.

76 Ibid. 37.

77 Ibid. 30–31.

78 Admittedly, this is a very preliminary and sketchy definition of 'affect.' I will later specify which affects are important, and precisely how they enter into evaluations for Lonergan. It is important also to point out that many contemporary philosophers would accept the view that moral responses and moral judgments have an emotional dimension. As R.W. Hepburn remarks, this connection 'can hardly be reasonably denied by any philosopher.' Still, it is helpful to distinguish clearly my use of the term *affect* from its use in rival non-cognitivist theories, such as emotivism. These theories hinge on a presupposed dichotomy of reason-feeling or belief-desire, a dichotomy that I will argue Lonergan rejects. A central task of this discussion is to point out some of the consequences for the euthanasia debate of rejecting this dichotomy. See Honderich, ed., *Oxford Companion to Philosophy*, s.v. 'Emotive theory of ethics,' by R.W. Hepburn.

79 *The Oxford English Dictionary*, unabridged version (1971), s.v. 'Affect.'

80 Blackburn, *Oxford Dictionary of Philosophy*, s.v. 'Affective.'

81 By contrast, Lonergan understands certain feelings to be not merely states, but cognitive acts. See Blackburn, *Oxford Dictionary of Philosophy*, s.v. 'Emotion.'

82 The distinction between one's intellectual and emotional nature corresponds to the traditional distinction between *head* and *heart*. But in the *OED*, even the term 'heart' has several senses that are relevant to Lonergan's

discussion. In the 9th sense, for instance, 'heart' is 'the seat of the emotions generally,' as distinct from 'head,' the seat of one's intellectual nature. In the 10th sense, it is the seat of love or affection. In the 13th sense, 'heart' is a term used for one's moral sense or conscience. See *Oxford English Dictionary* (1971), s.v. 'Heart.'

83 Blackburn, *Oxford Dictionary of Philosophy*, s.v. 'Emotion' 117.

84 That is, the feeling is cognitive in the sense that it is directed to some object (i.e., it apprehends a quality of some thing or object). But it is also cognitive in as far as it plays a specifically evaluative role. See *Oxford English Dictionary* (1971), s.v. 'Feeling.'

85 James Drever, *A Dictionary of Psychology* (Middlesex: Penguin Books, 1955), s.v. 'Fear.'

86 Harold Kaplan and Benjamin Sadock, *Comprehensive Glossary of Psychiatry and Psychology* (Baltimore: Williams & Wilkins, 1991), s.v. 'Fear' and 'Anxiety.'

87 On the distinction between feelings that are non-intentional and feelings that are intentional responses, see Lonergan, *Method* 30–31.

88 Ibid. 34.

89 Note that *value*, in the transcendental intending of 'value,' is always singular. By contrast, one's categorial intending regards particular *values*, in the plural. That is, the contrast is between intending transcendental 'value' and categorial 'values,' which is parallel to the contrast between intending transcendental 'intelligibility' or 'reality,' on the one hand, and intending categorial 'intelligibilities' or 'realities' (facts) on the other. I will return to this crucial distinction for Lonergan in chapters 4 to 7.

90 In this account I have summarized what Lonergan has said in *Method*, 34–41, and also qualified some of his expressions, which I will attempt to justify in chapter 7.

91 Hunnex, *Chronological and Thematic Charts of Philosophies and Philosophers* 22.

92 Honderich, ed., *Oxford Companion to Philosophy*, s.v. 'Epistemic,' by Leslie Stevenson.

93 Ibid., s.v. 'Objectivism and subjectivism, ethical,' by R.W. Hepburn. Note that although I think the adjective 'epistemic' surely brings out what Lonergan means, Lonergan himself may never have used this terminology. I will address this issue in detail in chapters 5 and 7.

94 Canada, Special Senate Committee, *Of Life and Death*, 13–15.

95 The definition of euthanasia adopted by the Senate committee fails to specify certain conditions that Tom Beauchamp cites as necessary. For Beauchamp, euthanasia occurs if and only if three conditions hold: (1) the death must be intended by at least one other person who is either the cause of death or a causally relevant condition of the death (i.e., this could include not only 'active' means, but also 'passive' means, such as certain omissions to act with the intent to cause death); (2) the person killed is either acutely

336 Notes to pages 83–91

suffering or irreversibly comatose (or soon will be) and this alone is the primary reason for intending the person's death; and (3) the means chosen to produce the death must be as painless as possible, or there must be a sufficient moral justification for a more painful method. Since I will be challenging Beauchamp's position on this question later (particularly on his first condition), I will refrain from explicitly adopting his definition at this point. See Honderich, ed., *Oxford Companion to Philosophy*, s.v. 'Euthanasia,' by Tom Beauchamp.

96 Calhoun and Solomon, *What Is an Emotion?* 22.

97 In figure A.1 of the appendix, I depict three distinct models of knowing. In light of these models, the key distinction that I have sought to draw in this chapter is between (1) a *critical realism* and (2) the alternatives of *naive realism* and *idealism*. Despite the many differences between these alternative accounts of knowing, what they hold in common, as I will argue later, is the view that the subject/object distinction is fundamental. Hence, for these accounts the philosophical 'problem of the bridge' between subject and object, or more generally the mind/body problem, is fundamental. So if feelings are inevitably connected to 'body,' on these alternative views, they are inherently problematic for knowing 'objective' values.

98 Calhoun and Solomon, *What Is an Emotion?* 3.

Chapter 4

1 *The Canadian Encyclopedia*, 1988 ed., s.v. 'Lonergan,' by William Fennell.

2 See Frederick Crowe, 'Lonergan's New Notion of Value,' in Michael Vertin, ed., *Appropriating the Lonergan Idea* (Washington: Catholic University of America Press, 1989) 52–55; cf. 5–12, 55–70, 98–105, 345–55; cf. Vertin's 'Review: *Collection*: Vol. 4 of *Collected Works of Bernard Lonergan*,' *Toronto Journal of Theology* 6 (1990) 145.

3 Lonergan sometimes refers to third-level *fact judging*, in contrast to fourth-level *value judging*. For the sake of consistency of expression, I will use *judging* to refer to third-level fact judging, in contrast to fourth-level *evaluating*, unless I qualify judging as *value* judging.

4 Lonergan, 'The Original Preface of *Insight*,' *Method: Journal of Lonergan Studies* 3 (1985) 4.

5 This is Lonergan's definition of the notion of structure. See his 'Critical Realism and the Integration of the Sciences,' transcript of six lectures given at University College, Dublin, Ireland, May 1962 (Toronto: Archives, Lonergan Research Institute, University of Toronto, File 253) 17.

6 Lonergan, 'Original Preface of *Insight*' 6. See Lonergan, 'Questionnaire on Philosophy,' *Method: Journal of Lonergan Studies* 2 (1984) 25–27; repr. in *Philosophical and Theological Papers 1965–1980*, vol. 17 of Collected Works, ed.

Robert C. Croken and Robert M. Doran (Toronto: University of Toronto Press, 2004).

7 In this and the next chapter I will restrict the discussion to direct and reflective insights. In chapter 6 I will focus on what Lonergan calls 'apprehensions of values,' which Michael Vertin refers to as 'deliberative insights.' See Vertin, 'Judgments of Value for the Later Lonergan,' *Method: Journal of Lonergan Studies* 13 (1995) 235–36.

8 Lonergan, *Method* 6.

9 Ibid. 7.

10 Lonergan, 'The Original Preface of *Insight*' 4.

11 For a diagrammatic representation of the distinction between (1) consciousness, which is the non-reflexive self-presence of one's cognitional acts, and (2) self-knowledge, which is (in its understanding and judging), the reflexive self-objectification of one's cognitional acts, see figure A.1 of the appendix.

12 See J. Doud, 'Use-effectiveness of the Creighton Model of NFP,' *International Review of Natural Family Planning* 9 (1985) 54.

13 Note the three distinct perspectives in such an analysis. The patient experiences dysmenorrhoea and mood swings (i.e., data of sense and consciousness). The physician normally helps her to grasp and verify a relationship between these experiences (understanding and judging). Finally, the philosopher brings expressly to light the activities of experiencing, understanding, and judging in which both patient and physician engage. I would take the second and the third steps here to be self-knowledge, though only the third step involves the self-knowledge of oneself as a knower.

14 See Lonergan's discussion of three senses of 'presence' in *Understanding and Being*, CWL 5:15–17.

15 For the sake of clarity, I will take *level*, in its strict sense, to refer to one of four sets of cognitional activities, rather than the three sets to which the early Lonergan refers. Hence, I will maintain with the later Lonergan the subdistinction within the level of judging between fact and value judgments. For an account of the difference between the strict and wide sense of *level* in Lonergan, see Michael Vertin, 'Lonergan on Consciousness: Is There a Fifth Level?' *Method: Journal of Lonergan Studies* 12 (1994) 21–23; cf. n. 52.

16 I present here only a summary of Lonergan's general ideas. The process of (a) coming to some self-awareness of one's cognitional operations and (b) moving from this awareness to knowledge of one's own knowing, is something that Lonergan refers to as self-appropriation. This development 'occurs only slowly, and, usually, only through a struggle with some such book as *Insight*'; *Method* 7 n. 2; cf. 6–25. For other helpful discussions of self-appropriation by Lonergan see *Insight*, CWL 3: 558–60; *Understanding and Being*, CWL 5:16–17; and 'Cognitional Structure,' *Collection*, CWL 4:205–21.

17 Lonergan refers to this contradiction as occurring 'between what explicitly I

say and what implicitly I am.' I will later point out how this type of operational inconsistency can also obtain even in my negative evaluation of a
theory about evaluating. See *Understanding and Being*, CWL 5:141.

18 Lonergan, 'The Original Preface of *Insight*' 4.

19 See Lonergan, 'Critical Realism' 4–5.

20 This is especially true if that philosopher *is also* the patient.

21 See Lonergan, *Verbum*, CWL 2:104–105, 148–51, 186–90. Since I will be
drawing primarily on Vertin's interpretive exposition of Lonergan's *Verbum*
articles, I also refer the reader to his helpful article 'Judgments of Value'
221–48.

22 Another reason for introducing the reader to the early Lonergan is that
the later Lonergan says very little about affect. Hence, one must rely on the
categories that he sets out clearly in his early writings to interpret best the
little he does say about the role of affect in value judgments.

23 Although I will be drawing on Vertin's interpretation of Lonergan's position
as he articulates it in his 'Judgments of Value,' I will not also be arguing that
his interpretation is correct or superior to rival ones. In this article, Vertin
himself distinguishes his own interpretation of Lonergan from rival accounts
and provides textual evidence supporting his reading, some of which I will
also be referring to. Since I take Vertin's interpretation to be well founded
in Lonergan's own writings and correct in its main lines, I will engage in
those interpretive disputes only secondarily and when I judge the discussion
among Lonergan scholars to be helpful in elucidating Lonergan's stance.

24 Lonergan, *Understanding and Being*, CWL 5:333.

25 Lonergan, '*Insight:* Preface to a Discussion,' *Collection*, CWL 4:152.

26 Lonergan, *Insight*, CWL 3:205.

27 In contending that experiencing is a cognitional process, Lonergan is using
the term 'cognition' in a sense that is consistent with modern philosophical
usage where 'cognitive processes are those responsible for knowledge and
awareness.' Note that sensation is a cognitive process because it *results* in an
awareness of data. That is, sensing is the *act* of experiencing. See Simon
Blackburn, *Oxford Dictionary of Philosophy*, s.v. 'Cognition.'

28 Michael Vertin, *The New Dictionary of Catholic Spirituality* (Collegeville, MN:
Liturgical Press, 1993), s.v. 'Intention, Intentionality.'

29 For Lonergan, to be conscious is to be *present* to oneself. But this *presence* is
not given in perception by looking, even if this is looking at myself. For I am
not an object, but a subject. Moreover, not only am I a subject who is present
to myself empirically, that is, empirically conscious at the level of sense
experience, I am also intellectually, rationally, and deliberatively conscious.
Hence, the cognitional self that I come to know is constituted by the
different acts in which I engage. See Lonergan, *Understanding and Being*, CWL
5:16–17, 20–21; and Vertin, 'Judgments of Value' 224.

30 Eventually, I will expand this discussion to include not only sense acts, but all cognitional acts, wherein I will make the same threefold distinction among the (a) contents of cognitional acts, (b) acts themselves, and (c) cognitional subject who is constituted by these acts.

31 That is, I am present to myself through these acts. Moreover, this self-presence can be heightened and differentiated. For instance, I am more self-present at the deliberative level than at any prior level, which, as I will argue later, is why attention to my affective responses is so crucial at this level.

32 Lonergan, *Insight*, CWL 3:299. See figure A.1 of the appendix for a diagram of Lonergan's distinction between direct and reflexive modes of the cognitional process.

33 Ibid. 3:138. To illustrate the distinction between receptive and productive acts, consider my sensing Paul's heart sounds. Besides achieving some awareness of these data, I also form an image of them. This image might be auditory, visual (e.g., a sonagram), or tactile (e.g., a palpable precordial heave). By means of an apprehensive act of imaging, I am able to construe these sense data in suggestive ways. These images are also linked closely to my second-level cognitive acts because they facilitate my subsequent grasp of some intelligible pattern in these data.

34 That is, the distinction between first-level sensing and what I will later describe as fourth-level affective responses.

35 It would seem that refuting the assumption that human knowing can be helpfully understood by comparing it to looking, and working out the implications of this refutation, are central contributions that Lonergan offers to contemporary philosophy. See, for instance, Lonergan's discussion of knowing conceived of as looking versus knowledge conceived of as an ontological perfection of the subject in *Understanding and Being*, CWL 5:159–60.

36 Lonergan notes that animals, no less than humans (even philosophers) *know* things (e.g., their masters, bones, other dogs). Such knowledge involves, however, the 'sensitive integration of sensible data,' which I will later distinguish from 'knowledge,' taken in the strict sense, as proper human knowledge of the real, known through the act of judgment. See Lonergan, *Verbum*, CWL 2:20.

37 See Lonergan's discussion of 'Patterns of Experience,' in *Insight*, CWL 3:204–12.

38 In this context, introspection 'is a matter not of inward inspection but of inquiry, enlarged interest, discernment, comparison, distinction, identification, naming.' See Lonergan, *Method* 15.

39 Lonergan, 'Cognitional Structure,' *Collection*, CWL 4:206.

40 Later, I will contrast these second-level 'aha' experiences of direct insight with those 'aha' experiences on the third level called 'reflective insights' and, on fourth level, 'deliberative insights.' Vertin has described these insights as

pivotal cognitive events by means of which I grasp a unity in some diversity. They are the cognitional grounds for achieving some content of knowledge. Besides the intellectual character of this cognitive grasping, which is the most prominent feature of a direct insight, there is also an affective aspect, such as the satisfaction of the insight. I will later argue that on the fourth level the affective component is also cognitive. See Vertin, 'Judgments of Value,' 227–30.

41 On Lonergan's insistence that knowledge is *discovered* rather than *created*, see Vertin, 'Judgments of Value' 226. Later I will refer to the advantage of my awareness of the various causes of chest pain over those who have no such prior knowledge.

42 I will later contrast the *simple* mental words of concepts and *complex* mental words of judgments. One difference, for instance, is that simple mental words issue from direct insights as compared to complex mental words, which issue from reflective insights.

43 Considered in this light, one can better understand why physicians are sometimes frustrated when talking to patients who are unable to give a coherent 'medical' account of their sense experience. When describing a patient's ability to report the quality of his or her chest pain, physicians are apt to characterize him or her as a 'good' or 'vague' historian. By this qualification medical persons seek to distinguish the patient who is able to abstract relevant medical data of his or her sense experience from the one who is unable to provide a concise, descriptive interpretation of his or her experience.

44 Lonergan, *Insight*, CWL 3:313. I will return to this discussion of the grounds and limits of generalizing concepts when I later explore the role of principles in ethics.

45 In fact, this 'scientific' description differs from an 'ordinary' one because 'the scientist selects the relations of things to us that lead more directly to knowledge of the relations between things themselves.' See ibid. 3:317.

46 See Lonergan's distinction between nominal and explanatory definitions, ibid. 3:35–36, 37.

47 Ibid. 3:316. I will later return to these fundamentally different manners of envisioning things when I contrast person-centred and person-neutral approaches to ethics.

48 Later, I will argue for a similar functional distinction between the academic and clinical ethicist. The academic is more concerned with the 'bottom-up' approach, which I will label 'conceiving.' The applied ethicist brings the results of academic ethics to bear on clinical cases, in what is often referred to as a 'top-down' approach, here labelled 'verifying.'

49 Lonergan, *Method* 10–11. For Lonergan, all our cognitional acts are both intentional and conscious. They are intentional in that they include a

content of awareness distinct from the act itself. They are conscious since they include a content of awareness identical with the act itself. Just as different operations yield qualitatively different modes of being conscious, they also yield qualitatively different modes of intending. But the most fundamental difference in modes of intending is not between these various categorial, cognitional acts on levels one through four but between the mode of categorial intending and that of wonder or transcendental intending. See also Vertin, 'Judgments of Value' 224.

50 Aristotle, *Metaphysics, Books I–IX,* trans. Hugh Trendennick (Cambridge, MA: Harvard University Press, 1933; repr. 1980), I, 980a 22, p. 3.

51 Later, I will introduce further differentiations of 'wonder,' such as the transcendental notions of reality, on the third level, and of value, on the fourth level.

52 Art collector Dr Albert Barnes expressed this desire to find meaning by saying, '[W]e ask of a work of Art that it reveal to us what is profound.' As a viewer of part of his collection, one experiences a desire to find some intelligibility especially, for example, when confronting a work like Rousseau's 'Unpleasant Surprise.' Indeed, referring to the dream-like images of this painting by Rousseau, his contemporary Pierre-Auguste Renoir asks, 'Is it necessary to understand what it means?' It seems that if there is any necessity, it is in our asking questions, in the human desire to understand. This painting effectively frustrates and exasperates this desire. Perhaps the fact that we do not always fulfil this desire by achieving satisfactory understanding, while initially unpleasant, motivates one to conceive of various interpretations, which I find to be a key part of the pleasure and stimulation of such works. See Michael Hogg's essay on Rousseau's 'Unpleasant Surprise,' in *Great French Paintings from the Barnes Foundation: Impressionist, Post-impressionist, and Early Modern* (New York: Alfred A. Knopf, in association with Lincoln University Press, 1993) 184.

53 See Lonergan, *Method* 73.

54 See ibid. 12.

55 For these notional and terminological clarifications of Lonergan's position, see Vertin, 'Judgments of Value' 227.

56 I will later argue that a similar meaning of the preposition 'in' obtains in the case of the apprehensive act of grasping values 'in' affect. For Lonergan, the relation between the imagined object and the object as understood is the critical point in philosophy. He maintains that, for the Aristotelian, by contrast with the materialist, idealist, and Platonist, both the terms that imagination presents and the intelligible relations or unities that insight grasps are objective. See his *Verbum,* CWL 2:189 n. 199.

57 Although all cognitive acts, for Lonergan, are both intentional and conscious, he describes the intending of our senses as an attending, which is

normally selective but not creative. See Lonergan, *Method* 10 and Vertin, 'Judgments of Value' 224, 226.

58 On the second and higher levels, my knowing is *mediated* by the agency of my own intellectual wonder, traditionally referred to as 'agent intellect.' Not only does there result a procession of a mental word in me, but as the result of this procession I can speak of a perfection of myself as a knower. By contrast, the achievements of my first-level sensing are *unmediated* by my wonder. But by raising the level-two question 'What is it?' I become more attentive in my sensing. This is an example of the influence of a subsequent level on an earlier one. See Lonergan, *Verbum*, CWL 2:188 and Vertin, 'Judgments of Value' 231 n. 34.

59 'Critical Realism and the Integration of the Sciences' (Lectures at University College, Dublin) 18a. Lonergan provides here a schematic representation of his 'Structural Analysis' (fig. 4) and the correlative 'Ontological Analysis' (fig. 5). In the structural analysis, he indicates that the 'state of wonder' promotes the whole process from sense to judgment. Moreover, he remarks that this *state of wonder* in his 'structural analysis' corresponds to the *agent intellect* of a Thomist 'ontological analysis.'

60 Lonergan illustrates the distinction between the content of an insight and of conception using the definition of a circle. My insight grasps a relation between what I imagine to be equal radii and the roundness of *this* curve. I subsequently abstract what is essential for this insight by omitting the 'empirical residue' of this circle that is incidental to defining any circle as 'a locus of coplanar points equidistant from a centre.' Lonergan, *Understanding and Being*, CWL 5:40–43.

61 Lonergan, *Method* 10–11.

62 Lonergan, 'Cognitional Structure,' *Collection*, CWL 4:206–207.

63 Note that by trying to include the most medically serious or life-threatening cause of a symptom in my differential diagnosis, I am indicating an ulterior concern to treat patients responsibly by being sure that I do not overlook the worst possibilities, which I might be able to avoid.

64 The sort of factors that would put Paul into a higher risk group include such data as middle or higher age group, male sex, previous AMI, family history of premature coronary artery disease, personal history of smoking, high blood pressure, elevated cholesterol, diabetes, or sedentary life style. See Allan Goroll, Lawrence May, and Albert Mulley, *Primary Care Medicine*, 3rd ed. (Philadelphia: J.B. Lippincott Co., 1995) 143, table 27-5.

65 The sort of description one would seek is that of a retrosternal squeezing or heavy sensation that radiates into the neck or down the left arm, is associated with sweating or nausea, builds up gradually, lasts for more than ten minutes and improves with nitroglycerine. See David Cline et al., *Emergency Medicine: A Comprehensive Study Guide*, 4th ed. (New York: McGraw-Hill, 1996) 71–73.

66 For instance, are his physical signs indicative of cardiac compromise, such as forward cardiac failure with low blood pressure or cardiogenic shock, or backward congestive heart failure, with an elevated jugular venous pressure and/or abnormal breath sounds from pulmonary edema? Or do Paul's physical signs support an alternative diagnosis, such as a musculoskeletal problem with tenderness on palpating his chest wall, or some gastrointestinal problem suggested by tenderness in the area of his epigastrium? See Cline et al., *Emergency Medicine* 73, table 6-1; 75.

67 See Vertin, 'Judgments of Value' 230. The issue of 'sufficient evidence' pertains to all such judgments. In this example, as in the clinical setting, I will focus on evidence that is available at the time treatment decisions need to be made (which will exclude later, even post-mortem, evidence). Note that evidence can support contrary conclusions, each admitting various degrees of probability. For instance, I might conclude that (a) Paul is (or is probably) having an AMI, or (b) Paul is not (or is probably not) having an AMI. For the sake of simplicity of expression, I will limit this discussion to case (a), and will omit indicating judgments of probable facts, deferring this issue to a later discussion.

68 More specifically, Lonergan speaks of the *direct borrowed content* that is found in the question to which one answers yes or no. See *Insight*, CWL 3:300–301.

69 In chapter 10 of *Insight*, Lonergan gives a series of instances of judgments to illustrate the act of a reflective insight. But he also believes that 'any instance in which we grasp the sufficiency of the evidence qua sufficient can be formulated in terms of the virtually unconditioned' and expressed in the form of a syllogism. See Lonergan's 'Critical Realism' 22–23.

70 For Lonergan, 'the function of the syllogism is to present the conclusion B as a virtually unconditioned; something that has conditions, A, which however are fulfilled and so B becomes a virtually unconditioned ... [I]f you think of the syllogism as an expression of the virtually unconditioned then the whole attention centres on B.' See Lonergan, 'Critical Realism' 21.

71 See Lonergan, *Insight*, CWL 3:305–306.

72 For common symptoms, especially an important one such as chest pain, most physicians would be able to produce a list of possible causes that they would consider, and they would have a good idea what each of these possible causes meant. In practice, as previously stated, the main task is not one of conceiving of possible explanations but of verifying which of these is actually occurring in a given patient.

73 This merely reiterates Lonergan's opposition to views that puff up a part of human knowing to the status of the whole. For instance, even among nuanced medical thinkers there is a tendency to express their own knowing as a matter of taking a good look at some chest X-ray, or cardiogram; one will have the diagnosis if one can see the pattern. For Lonergan, the move

from the X-ray or cardiogram to diagnosis, when philosophically analysed, involves a *mediated* process, not an *immediate* one. Moreover, this whole process goes forward when one is perplexed, that is, in a state of wonder that gives rise to questions, insights, and hypotheses. For Lonergan, the whole problem in cognitional analysis is to discover that there is something else there besides sense. For him, not only is intellect nothing like sensation, but the real that one might affirm need not be limited to what can be imagined (e.g., the wave/particle theories of quantum physics). See Lonergan, 'Critical Realism' 19.

74 This fact judgment, though based in part on a reflective insight, purports to transcend my own cognitive processes to achieve knowledge of the real. Later, I will highlight the parallel between third-level intellectual insights and fourth-level affective insights. Regarding fact judgments, it is interesting to note that high-school students commonly qualify fact claims by prefacing their remarks with 'I feel ...,' instead of 'I think ...' This has the effect of emphasizing the self-constitutive grounds of even judgments of fact. It also seems to express their hesitation to affirm that some immanently (i.e., self-) generated fact claim might actually transcend their cognitive activities and achieve not merely experiential knowledge of themselves, but also knowledge of some fact.

75 See Lonergan, *Insight*, CWL 3:728–39 and 'Belief: Today's Issue,' *A Second Collection* 87–100. I will highlight the same contrast between knowing and believing in end-of-life decisions, where the caregiver is more likely to be in a position of believing than in the case of medical fact judgments.

76 It might seem obvious that there is an important difference between my judgment that Paul is having an AMI and the actual reality of the matter, which I purport to grasp through my fact judgment in diagnosing Paul. But when I speak not about medical judgments, but about philosophical judgments regarding my knowing, I am apt to become confused and substitute the concept for the conceived, the explanation for the explained, or the judgment for the judged. To avoid this 'psychological fallacy,' Lonergan spends the first 10 chapters of *Insight* acquainting the reader with knowing through experiencing his own acts of understanding and judging. Lonergan's strategy is to encourage the reader to interpret what he says according to his or her own experience of what understanding is, and not by some definition or explanation of it. See Lonergan, 'Critical Realism' 33–34.

77 Lonergan, '*Insight,* Preface to a Discussion,' *Collection,* CWL 4:150.

78 Lonergan, 'Cognitional Structure,' *Collection,* CWL 4:207.

79 This is one reason why evidence-based medicine is so important to providing responsible medical care. For instance, despite the expense there is a general consensus in medical circles that hyperbaric-oxygen therapy is a good treatment for patients with carbon-monoxide poisoning. A recent

review article, however, challenges conventional wisdom by concluding that '[n]o randomized, controlled, blinded clinical trial demonstrated a clear advantage of HBO [*hyper*baric oxygen] over NBO [*normo*baric oxygen therapy] in reducing morbidity and mortality in carbon monoxide poisoning.' If this is true, then this would be an example of a medical consensus favouring some treatment that is based either on unverified fact judgments or on some other, possibly arbitrary, grounds. See Patrick Tibbles and Peter Perrotta, 'Treatment of Carbon Monoxide Poisoning: A Critical Review of Human Outcome Studies Comparing Normobaric Oxygen with Hyperbaric Oxygen,' *Annals of Emergency Medicine* 24 (1994) 269–76.

80 Lonergan, *Collection*, CWL 4:214.

81 Lonergan, *Method* 18.

82 Speaking of moral judgments, Lonergan writes that 'one can do too much in formulating true moral judgments. It is something that has all sorts of facets to it; trying to put it into syllogisms is more or less evacuating it.' Lonergan, 'What Are Judgments of Value?' typescript by N. Graham of lectures given at the Massachusetts Institute of Technology, May 1972 (Toronto: Archives, Lonergan Research Institute, University of Toronto, 1985), file 695, 26. His point here can also serve to alert one to the danger of mistaking analysis of the first three levels for the dynamic flow of thought.

83 Lonergan, 'Critical Realism' 17.

84 Lonergan, *Collection*, CWL 4:206.

85 Joseph Flanagan expresses the notion of the unity of this knowing cycle as 'a dynamic, relational whole, structured by three phases of operation [omitting deciding], each of which provides the term and direction for the other two.' See Flanagan, 'The Self-Causing Subject: Intrinsic and Extrinsic Knowing,' *Lonergan Workshop* 3 (1982) 34.

86 For Lonergan, what one desires to know is not only intelligibility, nor reality, but above all value. As I will explain later, this desire is not just to *know* value but also to *enjoy or produce* it.

87 Lonergan, *Method* 73; see also 11–12, 23–24, 36, 74, and 282.

88 This is Lonergan's answer to the Platonic problematic of how one achieves knowledge if one begins in a state of ignorance. It seemed to Plato that if I begin in complete ignorance, I could never break out of my ignorance because I would not even be able to recognize a correct answer. The fact that a person occasionally moves from ignorance to knowledge suggested to Plato that a person must possess some innate knowledge, which he expressed in his theory of recollection. Lonergan agrees with Plato's premise that we do not begin in a state of ignorance, but concludes instead that the world we en-counter empirically is not innately known but rather is a 'known-unknown.' That is, we already have some clue about what would count as an adequate answer even as we pose our questions. See Lonergan, *Method* 77.

89 Michael Vertin, 'The Doctrine of Infallibility and the Demands of Epistemology: A Review Article,' *The Thomist* 43 (1979) 643–44.

90 The act of *sublation* is key to Lonergan's intentionality analysis. For him, sublation is a matter of incorporating or integrating the incremental achievements of prior cognitional levels in those acts proper to the subsequent level. By sublating the achievements of the prior level, one not only adds some further increment of knowledge to that achievement, but also shifts these achievements into a new context. According to Lonergan, 'each successive level sublates previous levels by going beyond them, by setting up a higher principle, by introducing new operations, and by preserving the integrity of previous levels, while extending enormously their range and their significance.' Lonergan, *Method* 340.

91 Ibid. 28. I can express this same point in terms of a principle of movement and of rest. As a principle of movement, the transcendental intentions are the source of my questions that relate me immediately to being. Like Aristotle, Lonergan considers the beginning of all science and philosophy to be *wonder*, the eros of our spirit ('Critical Realism' 19). In Lonergan, this wonder is contained in the transcendental intentions, which function as the principles of movement for the whole of my intentional consciousness. But my transcendental intentions also supply the principles of rest for the whole process. My striving to answer a particular question ends when I achieve some knowledge that satisfies the eros of my transcendental intending. Beyond this, for the later Lonergan, the embodied-intending-that-I-am, and the ultimate eros that my answers seek, is not satisfied merely by intellectual knowledge of facts. Such ultimate satisfaction is affective, as I will elucidate later, and involves not only knowing, but also producing or enjoying values.

92 Lonergan, *Method* 25.

93 Ibid. 265.

94 Ibid. 37.

95 Beyond understanding his position is the further question of judging its truth and value for oneself.

96 Vertin, 'The Doctrine of Infallibility' 642.

Chapter 5

1 On the three basic questions, see Lonergan, *Second Collection* 37, 86; cf. *Method* 20–21, 25, 83, 238–40, 261, 297, 316.

2 For a diagrammatic depiction of 'the problem of the bridge,' see 'Idealism,' figure A.1 of the appendix.

3 Lonergan, *Method* 265.

4 Lonergan suggests that Einstein himself was aware of the difference between one's successful and confident knowing and one's subsequent ability to

articulate accurately the operational features of knowing and the basis of this confidence. To the person who asked Einstein how a theorist of knowledge ought best learn from physicists, Einstein answered: 'Pay no attention to what they say, watch what they do.' My goal here is to learn from physicians by reflecting philosophically upon what they (myself included) do when making medical judgments. See Lonergan, *Understanding and Being*, CWL 5:81.

5 This type of critical reflection on the performance of physicians is typical of the publications of medical insurance companies, such as the Canadian Medical Protective Association. It also constitutes a valuable part of medical literature. From Lonergan's perspective, this literature serves the role of enhancing the 'self-correcting process of learning.' My goal here is to draw attention to the types of misjudgments to which physicians might already be quite attuned. This will highlight the move from methodology to *successful* methodology. See, for instance, the regularly appearing column entitled 'Avoidable Errors in Emergency Practice,' in *Emergency Medicine, Acute Medicine for the Primary Care Physician* 8 (1988) 41–45.

6 A notorious way that students fail their clinical patient examinations is by missing such rather obvious findings as amputated legs or a glass eye. But the distinction I am making between skills of physical examination among clinicians also applies to patients. Most patients are able to distinguish cardiac chest pain from indigestion. Still, only exceptional patients are able to provide, even with prompting, a precise account of their experience of pain, such as its location, quality, quantity, duration, radiation, and associated relieving and aggravating factors. Despite the fact that 1.5 million people in the United States suffer from an AMI each year, about 5% of these patients are erroneously discharged from Emergency Departments by their attending physicians. Consequently, about 20% of malpractice insurance claims by emergency physicians in the United States involve errors in the diagnosis and treatment of chest pain. See Michael Albrich, 'Acute Myocardial Infarction: Comprehensive Guidelines for Diagnosis, Stabilization, and Mortality Reduction,' *Emergency Medicine Reports* 6 (1994) 51.

7 Although the story of chest pain that began after an injury adds probability to the hypothesis that Paul's pain is not from his heart, peers reviewing my performance have the advantage of knowing that Paul was, in fact, having an AMI. With this knowledge, they seek to determine whether I am culpable for my misdiagnosis (or delayed diagnosis). This example illustrates the importance of a proper understanding of statistical probabilities in interpreting data and making fact judgments.

8 I have encountered both of these diagnostic dilemmas in practice, as well as other clinically important examples of a double diagnosis, such as a middle-ear infection and meningitis, or gastroenteritis and appendicitis. One learns,

by reflecting on such cases, the difference between the prior probability of a diagnosis and the judgmental grounds for verifying a particular diagnosis. I suspect that it was on the basis of a collective review of such misdiagnosed cases (and the tragic consequences of these errors) that certain rules came about in medicine, such as 'If you think of meningitis, do a lumbar puncture' or 'Better safe than sorry.'

9 Concretely, this decision is complicated by a number of factors. These drugs have life-threatening risks associated with their use (e.g., allergic reactions, internal bleeding, strokes, etc.); some are expensive; and their potential for benefiting someone having an AMI depends upon how soon they are given. So before exposing a patient to the risks and expense of these drugs, I would want to be fairly certain he or she was having an AMI. On the other hand, I would also want to start these drugs as soon as I made the judgment that he or she was *probably* having an AMI in order to increase their possible benefit. The emphasis here is on the prior cognitional issues involving judgments that underpin subsequent evaluations and decisions, which I will address in chapter 6.

10 The American Heart Association has developed a course called 'Advanced Cardiac Life Support' (ACLS). For students taking this course, a key procedural point is to base all treatment decisions upon correct fact judgments. For instance, the course emphasizes that only after one has correctly interpreted a pattern on the electrocardiogram should one proceed with the treatment specified in the relevant algorithm. This course seems to be a practical way of teaching caregivers to avoid overly rash or hesitant judgments. See American Heart Association, *Textbook of Advanced Cardiac Life Support*, 2nd ed. (Dallas, TX: AHA), 1990.

11 Lonergan, *Insight*, CWL 3:400.

12 Lonergan, *Method* 263.

13 Note that these are not Lonergan's own labels. As I will argue, however, these labels highlight various senses of objectivity to which he does refer.

14 My focus in this chapter is on Lonergan's various meanings of 'epistemic objectivity.' Table 5.1 highlights his distinction between the various meanings of epistemic objectivity, on the one hand, and phenomenal and metaphysical objectivity, on the other hand. For the sake of simplicity of expression, when I refer to 'objectivity' in an unqualified sense I mean 'epistemic objectivity.' I will also speak of partial notions of objectivity as a criterion, such as the *criterion* of genuine experiencing, and partial notions taken together as criteria, such as the *criteria* of genuine knowing.

15 Although there is some unity in sense data already at the level of perceptual experience, which is the sensitive integration of sense data, much of my attentiveness is directed by higher-level questions. For instance, when I listen to Paul's heart sounds I systematically place my stethoscope not over any or

all body parts, but only over those areas of the chest where these data are relevant to my questions for understanding whether there is a problem with the functioning of his heart. Moreover, I attend not to any or all sounds, but rather I deliberately attend to very specific auditory frequencies and patterns by filtering out certain other sense data, such as background noise.

16 Lonergan, *Critical Realism* 24.

17 Lonergan, *Understanding and Being*, CWL 5:173–74.

18 Lonergan, *Insight*, CWL 3:399.

19 On the one hand, it is unreasonable to make a judgment without sufficient evidence. On the other hand, it is also unreasonable to fail to make a judgment given sufficient evidence to support the diagnosis of a probable AMI and to delay treatment further by insisting on additional, time-consuming investigations. But whether my judgment in this particular case might have been overly rash or hesitant is a determination that my peers seek to make. Moreover, they might also judge me incompetent generally in the practice of medicine because of a habitual pattern of overly rash or hesitant judgments.

20 Lonergan, *Understanding and Being*, CWL 5:172–73.

21 Frederick Crowe, 'The Galilean World-view and Its Modern Echoes,' *Lonergan Review: A Multidisciplinary Journal* 3 (1994) 141. For the moment, I will defer speaking about the fourth-level precept of responsibility.

22 See Vertin, '"Knowing," "Objectivity," and "Reality": Insight and Beyond,' *Lonergan Workshop* 8 (1990) 256.

23 Ibid. Here Vertin is referring to 'objectivity' in Lonergan's book *Insight*, CWL 3, chap. 13.

24 By 'non-self' here I would include other 'selves' as well as objects that are not also 'selves,' such as stones.

25 Lonergan, *Understanding and Being*, CWL 5:173.

26 Ibid. 171.

27 Ibid. 172.

28 Lonergan, *Insight*, CWL 3:377; cf. 375–76.

29 I have sought to highlight this basic philosophical point by deliberately using the first person and the active voice. This stylistic commitment is opposed to conventions, especially those entrenched in the modes of expression used by writers in the sciences, in particular, those who use the indefinite 'one' and the passive voice. Both of these techniques obscure the issue of authorship for the claims being made. I suggest that this is, in part, to satisfy certain supposed norms of objectivity in expression. The larger point I hope to make by this stylistic commitment is that genuine knowing is not guaranteed merely by overlooking the obvious and inevitable fact that each of us is the origin of his or her own claims. On the contrary, the key to objectivity is to make this fact explicit and to develop an accurate and nuanced understand-

ing of the recurring features of our own successful cognitive processes that underpin whatever apparent knowledge we might claim to have discovered. Although the claims I make about the structure of my own cognitive performance are, in the first instance, accounts of my own subjectivity, they can subsequently be generalized to other subjects who verify, in their own objectifications of themselves, the structural similarity between this account and their own findings.

30 Lonergan, 'Critical Realism' 30.

31 I have already discussed this sense of the subject-object distinction in chapter 4 where I followed Lonergan's early use of scholastic terminology in his *Verbum* articles. There he used metaphysical labels to discuss both phenomenally subjective conscious-intentional acts and phenomenally objective achievements of those acts in terms of distinct 'objects': 'We spoke of the moving object, agent object, such as the external sensible object; we spoke of terminal object, the immanently produced image, concept, judgment; we spoke of final object, what you know through the image, what is imagined, what is conceived, the "what is" reached through judgment' (*Understanding and Being*, CWL 5:170–71). According to the clarifications just made, Lonergan's terminology is now more understandable. To speak of agent, terminal, and final objects of cognition is to supply metaphysical categories for phenomenally objective contents of conscious-intentional acts. All of these 'objects' are distinct from my phenomenally subjective receptive or productive apprehensive acts (e.g., sensing, imagining, direct understanding, formulating, reflective understanding, and judging). Moreover, the self versus non-self distinction that is behind the principal notion of objectivity is a distinction between different types of final objects.

32 These reflections on the various meanings of objectivity in medicine are based on my own impressions of what medical persons typically have meant by this term and the role that this notion has played in my medical judgments. In fact, a key personal source of motivation to studying philosophy was my discontent with the dominant view in medicine that all evaluations are epistemically just subjective judgments. In chapter 7 I will return to these opposed views of objectivity when discussing the crucial issue of evaluative objectivity.

33 Later, in my criticism of ethics conceived of as a strictly empirical enterprise I will take up this view of objective knowing as it applies to evaluations.

34 This 'SOAP' format is commonly used by physicians in family medicine, as well as allied health-care workers in fields such as nursing, occupational therapy, and physiotherapy.

35 I will later suggest that this notion of 'objectivity' also emerges in ethics and seems to discredit first-person moral judgments in favour of a 'person-neutral' ethical perspective.

36 Labelling the descriptive mode 'subjective' and the explanatory mode 'objective' suggests that the explanatory mode better captures what medical persons presuppose genuine knowing to be. This has the unfortunate effect of creating the impression that an important criterion of epistemically objective knowing is that the subject himself cannot achieve genuine knowledge of his own experiences.

37 Both of these notions of objectivity also have implications for evaluations. For instance, if I grasp some value myself that has to do with myself, such as 'My chest pain is bad,' this evaluation would fail to meet the perspectival and explanatory criteria of epistemic objectivity presupposed by the medical uses of this term. On this basis, the notion that evaluations can be based on feelings, which could never meet either medical criterion for objectivity since they are necessarily first person in perspective and are essentially related to myself, could easily be dismissed since such a notion would yield irredeemably 'subjective' evaluations.

38 For instance, the perspective of my peer group might have been helpful in revealing to me my own feelings as a source of individual bias. Such a bias might predispose me to refuse certain insights, or to fail to question my hastily drawn conclusions made within moments of encountering a patient.

39 Lonergan, *Insight*, CWL 3:8. Of interest to me in chapter 7 will be the criticism of a group bias in the scientific community against the role of feelings in value judgments.

Chapter 6

1 A central part of my effort will be to specify what Lonergan means by the term *feeling* or *affective response*. It would not be helpful to appeal to a standard definition here since, as Bernard Tyrrell notes, 'there is no consensus among psychologists and philosophers regarding the technical meaning of the words feeling, passion, affect, and emotion.' Bernard Tyrrell, 'Feelings as Apprehensive-Intentional Responses to Values,' in Fred Lawrence, ed., *Lonergan Workshop* 7 (1988) 331–60, at 348. As in the cases of other cognitive events, Lonergan ultimately pins down the meaning of these terms phenomenally. This will enable me to contrast Lonergan's understanding of these terms with those of other prominent figures in the history of psychology and philosophy.

2 As Lonergan points out: 'Moral feelings and moral judgments are occurring all the time – there is nothing recondite or rare about them. "What a brute he is!" Or "What a nice person!" Most of human conversation is praising or blaming somebody or something.' Lonergan, 'Milltown Park Lectures on *Method in Theology*' (1971) 26, Q. 9.

3 In an article entitled 'Judgments of Value, for the Later Lonergan,' Vertin

first notes how this set of issues has been understood in various ways by various Lonergan scholars and then proceeds to advance his own interpretation of Lonergan's later position regarding where feelings enter into evaluations. In this chapter, I will elaborate an interpretation of Lonergan that seeks to be consistent with Vertin's understanding of Lonergan's mature views. Since the dialectical issue concerning evaluations in a medical context is a focal contribution of the present discussion, rather than exploring the diverse interpretations among Lonergan scholars, I will attend only briefly, and in the footnotes, to how this interpretation of Lonergan differs from those offered by other Lonergan scholars. For a fuller account of such diverse interpretations, see Vertin, 'Judgments of Value,' *Method, Journal of Lonergan Studies* 13 (1995) 221–48.

4 Lonergan, *Method* 30.

5 Lonergan, 'Lecture on *Method in Theology*' 45, Q. 13.

6 John Finnis, for instance, distinguishes his own rationalist position that rejects any properly philosophical role of feelings in evaluations from Lonergan's stance. Neil Ormerod and Michael Vertin are two Lonergan scholars who defend Lonergan against Finnis's interpretation that Lonergan's position is a 'refined but unequivocal empiricism.' For this discussion, see John Finnis, *Fundamentals of Ethics* (Washington: Georgetown University Press, 1983) 30–37, 42–45, 48–50, 54; Neil Ormerod, 'Lonergan and Finnis on the Human Good,' in William Danaher, ed., *Australian Lonergan Workshop* (Lanham, MD: University Press of America, 1993) 199–210; and Vertin, 'Judgments of Value' 221–48.

7 Lonergan's position on these issues, which is consistent with neither the empiricist nor the rationalist stance, is continuous with John Henry Newman's view as interpreted by Jamie Ferreira. On Ferreira's reading, Newman, who links heart with imagination, rejects 'the rationalist denigration of imagination and the sentimentalist romanticization of the imagination.' Newman viewed the imagination as having a double-edged capacity, which is akin to Lonergan's view of the ambiguity of certain feelings. For Newman, the imagination was 'a wonderful faculty in the cause of truth, but it also subserves the purposes of error.' See M. Jamie Ferreira, 'The Grammar of the Heart: Newman on Faith and Imagination,' in Gerard Magill, ed., *Discourse and Context: An Interdisciplinary Study of John Henry Newman* (Carbondale: Southern Illinois University Press, 1993) 129–43, at 131.

8 See Antonio R. Damasio, 'Descartes' Error and the Future of Human Life,' *Scientific American* 4 (1994) 144.

9 Frederick Crowe provides a helpful contribution to what he calls 'the tired old is-ought question.' On his interpretation of Lonergan, the *is* refers to knowledge achieved through fact judgments and the *ought* to knowledge achieved through evaluations. Although Crowe fully accepts the assertion

that one cannot logically derive an *ought* from an *is*, he nevertheless rejects
what he refers to as 'the tyranny some logicians would impose on cognitional
operations.' On this interpretation, the move from is to ought questions 'is
simply a natural unfolding of conscience,' and if there is any struggle, 'it
would be a struggle not to respond to the emergent "ought," and, if "ought"
keeps rearing its head, to suppress it – which is exactly what happens in the
rationalizations of bad conscience.' See Crowe, 'Rethinking Moral Judgments: Categories from Lonergan,' *Science et Esprit* 40 (1988) 137–52, at
141–42.

10 The medical therapy involves the use of some drug, such as streptokinase, to
dissolve the offending blood clot that is presumably obstructing blood flow
to the heart muscle. Surgical options involve using a catheter with an inflat-
able balloon in its tip, which is advanced into the narrow portion of the
coronary artery, and the narrowing is mechanically relieved by inflating the
balloon. Alternatively, the narrowed portion of the artery can be bypassed
using a grafted blood vessel. Of course, each of these options carry their own
costs, risks, and benefits.

11 According to the 'Guidelines for Mortality Reduction in AMI,' these are but
two of twelve risk factors listed among the exclusionary criteria for thrombolysis. See Michael Albrich, *Emergency Medicine Reports* 6 (1994) 56.

12 This is not meant to imply that physicians tend to prefer more aggressive
treatment options than do their patients. Indeed, palliative care units, for
instance, often have rather restricted admission criteria that tend to exclude
patients who prefer more active medical interventions such as intravenous
fluids, or even antibiotic treatment.

13 Decision-making in a medical context tends to be most effective when there
is some collaboration between the physician and patient, rather than either
the physician or the patient making these decisions in isolation. In this
sense, the role of the physician is like that of the mediator or ethicist who
facilitates the whole process of coming to a decision. On this issue see Moira
Steward, 'Effective Physician-Patient Communication and Health Outcomes:
A Review,' *Canadian Medical Association Journal* 9 (1995) 1423–33.

14 For an account of an application of Lonergan's approach toward a phenom-
enology of the feelings of anxiety and gratitude, see Elizabeth A. Morelli,
Anxiety: A Study of the Affectivity of Moral Consciousness (Lanham, MD: University
Press of America, 1985) and Tyrrell, 'Feelings' 347–53.

15 These are some of the symptoms that constitute the syndrome psychiatrists
refer to as a *major depressive episode*. See Mark J. Berber, 'Helping Patients
Overcome Major Depression,' *Canadian Journal of Diagnosis* 5 (1995) 32–49.

16 David B. Posen, 'Stress Management for Patient and Physician,' *Canadian
Journal of Continuing Medical Education* 4 (1995) 43–58.

17 There seems to be a consensus, at least in North American legal and medical

circles, that in order to be capable of making decisions one needs 'knowledge, intelligence, and voluntariness.' Still, there is little guidance as to the degree to which these are needed or how each of these relates to the others. In addition, some persons deemed capable of consent apparently grant it with relatively little information, and with a very limited ability to weigh risks and benefits. The voluntary aspect of their decision might be compromised by a variety of procedures that influence them to 'make the choice desired by the treatment provider.' My aim is not only to clarify the relations between intelligence, fact knowledge, and the voluntariness of decisions using Lonergan's categories, but also to show how feelings enter into the evaluative process of weighing and choosing. Such an understanding is needed to facilitate this process better, especially in persons with cognitive disabilities. See C. Morris, J. Niederbuhl, and J. Mahr, 'Determining the Capability of Individuals with Mental Retardation to Give Informed Consent,' *American Journal on Mental Retardation* 2 (1993) 263–72, at 264.

18 See Philip McShane, 'An Interview with Fr. Bernard Lonergan, s.j.,' *Second Collection* 220–21.

19 Lonergan, *Topics in Education*, CWL 10:214.

20 Ibid. 228. Footnote 51 has 'Time of the music, virtual movements of music, isomorphic with the life of feeling of the subject – an objectification in which the subject can see how to live.'

21 Lonergan, 'Questionnaire on Philosophy,' *Method, Journal of Lonergan Studies* 2 (1984) 12.

22 Lonergan, *Method* 30–31.

23 Ibid. 37.

24 Lonergan used labels other than the ones I will be using to refer to the operations of the fourth level. For example, in 1976 he referred to the fourth-level sequence of operations as those of 'deliberation, evaluation, decision and praxis.' (See Lonergan, 'Questionnaire on Philosophy' [1984] 7.) For the most part, I will be following Michael Vertin's suggestions. I referred already to the second level as the level of *understanding*, consisting in the acts of direct insight and conceiving, and to the third level as the level of fact judgment or simply *judging*, consisting in the acts of reflective insight and fact judging. To highlight the continuity and parallels between these prior levels and the fourth level, I will be referring to the fourth level as the level of *evaluating* and *deciding*, consisting in the act of deliberative insight, rather than Lonergan's apprehending values, value judging, deciding and executing. See Vertin, 'Judgments of Value' 228.

25 On this account, then, deliberative insights are more akin to reflective insights than to direct insights. In the case of fact knowledge, Lonergan expresses the cognitional content of my 'grasping' the unity between a conditioned and its conditions as 'a grasp of a virtually unconditioned, of an

unconditioned that has conditions which, however, in fact are fulfilled.'
Thus the question 'Does it exist?' presents the prospective judgment as a
conditioned. Reflective understanding grasps the conditions and their
fulfilment. From that grasp there proceeds rationally the judgment 'It does
exist.' What he rejects is the view that 'it is through knowledge of existence
that we reach true judgment.' Hence, knowing culminates in affirming, but
what is given in the *grasping* of a virtually unconditioned is not some pre-
affirmational 'knowledge of existence' through which I reach true judgment.
Rather, it is the cognitive grounds that justify my asserting the judgment, in
and through which I come to knowledge of the real. See Lonergan, '*Insight*:
Preface to a Discussion,' *Collection*, CWL 4:150–52.

26 Lonergan, '*Insight* Revisited,' *A Second Collection* 277.
27 McShane, 'An Interview' 221–22. See *Insight*, CWL 3:754 n. 1.
28 Ibid. 223.
29 Vertin, 'Judgments of Value' 227.
30 'Not only do the transcendental notions promote the subject to full consciousness and direct him to his goals. They also provide the criteria that
reveal whether the goals are being reached.' Lonergan, *Method* 35.
31 Ibid. 73–74.
32 Note that as one advances to address questions for deliberation there is a
heightening of self-involvement, a heightening of one's self-presence.
33 Or the intending of transcendental value, reality, intelligibility, as distinct
from categorial values, realities, and intelligibilities.
34 I will return to this issue of affective fulfilment in my discussion of complacency in chapter 7.
35 Vertin, 'Judgments of Value' 236.
36 On Vertin's reading of Lonergan, the cognitional processes on levels two
through four are similar insofar as each involves three main steps: questioning, having an insight, and producing a mental word. Here I am highlighting
how each insight comprises my grasping a 'concrete supra-experienceable
unity in the diversity I have questioned.' See Vertin, 'Judgments of Value'
227–28. This grasping, however, is not some pre-affirmational knowing, but
rather an element in the overall process wherein I come to know only *in* and
through a judgment. As Lonergan puts it when speaking of judgments, 'it is
only through the actuality of truth that we know the actuality of being; and
truth is reached, not by intuiting actual, concrete existence, but by a reflective grasp of the unconditioned.' See Lonergan, '*Insight*: Preface to a Discussion' 152.
37 See Vertin, 'Judgments of Value' 236 n. 50; Patrick Byrne, 'Analogical
Knowledge of God and the Value of the Moral Endeavor,' *Method, Journal of
Lonergan Studies* 11 (1993) 124; and Bernard Tyrrell, 'Feelings as Apprehensive-Intentional Responses to Values,' *Lonergan Workshop* 7 (1988) 335.

38 By 'all hanging together,' I mean not merely the link 'If A then B,' but rather grasping the truth as the fulfilment of those sufficient conditions specified by the link, that is, 'But A.'

39 Vertin provides a more expansive contrast between all four levels by speaking of both the intentional objects that evoke feelings, a subset of what he contends Lonergan names agent objects in *Verbum*, and the intentional responses to these objects. On the first level there is a *datum of sense* (the agent object) and 'the act of sensing' (intentional response). Correspondingly, on the second level there is the *potentially intelligible* unity in the diversity of data of sense or consciousness and (at best) 'an intelligent grasp of that potentially graspable unity.' On the third level, there is the *reflectively graspable* unity in the diversity of a prospective fact judgment, its link to conditions sufficient for its rational assertion, and the fulfilment of those conditions; the intentional response to which is (at best) 'a rational grasp of that reflectively graspable unity.' Finally, on the fourth level there is the *deliberatively graspable* unity of a prospective value judgment, its link to conditions sufficient for its responsible assertion, and the fulfilment of those conditions; the intentional response to which is (at best) 'a responsible grasp of that deliberatively graspable unity.' Vertin, 'Judgments of Value' 232–33.

40 For instance, the inconvenience, my fatigue, the heat, rain, insects, and so forth, versus the fitness benefits, opportunities to share this experience with friends, the inspiring wonder and beauty of nature, and so on.

41 In a taped discussion of this point, which Vertin had with Lonergan in 1975, Lonergan refers to J.A. Stewart's *Myths of Plato*. In his introduction to the book, Stewart suggests that these myths are about transcendental feeling. Lonergan relates Stewart's interpretation of this non-argumentative side of Plato to his own understanding of where feelings enter into evaluations in his comment 'In other words, values apprehended through feeling, I'd say. That's the sort of thing, you see, that's prior to everything else.' More broadly, from Lonergan's perspective, one might interpret Plato's cave metaphor as an allusion to what Lonergan labels as the transcendental/categorial distinction, where what is prior to everything else are the transcendental, a priori, merely structural features of conscious intentionality. Quoted in Vertin, 'Judgments of Value' 235 n. 46.

42 This diversity is more primitive and basic in the sense that 'we perform acts of reflective understanding, we know that we have grasped the sufficiency of the evidence for a judgment on which we have been deliberating, but without prolonged efforts at introspective analysis we could not say just what occurs in reflective insight.' In the case of our medical example, the diversity of the contents in which I grasp a rational or responsible unity are also far more complex than their syllogistic representation might suggest. For instance, the conditions represented as A might be a series of conditions that

can only be fulfilled with some degree of probability. See Lonergan, *Insight*, CWL 3:304.

43 Ibid. 306.

44 Lonergan, *Method* 37.

45 Because feelings are not centrally important to the 'restless mind' nor to acts of direct and reflective insight, the little importance that feelings play in *Insight*, except as a likely source of bias, remains legitimate even from the perspective of the later Lonergan. But, as Bernard Tyrrell suggests, by the time of *Method*, Lonergan was leaning more toward the Augustinian 'restless heart,' and his new understanding of certain feelings as intentional responses to values provides a basis for revising the earlier view of a possible ethics Lonergan provides in *Insight*. See Tyrrell, 'Feelings' 331–32.

46 See ibid. 336–38.

47 On Vertin's reading of Lonergan, to say that values are apprehended 'in feelings' means that values are apprehended by means of feelings that are self-transcendent, not within feelings, as within data. Such feelings are to be distinguished from feelings as satisfactions. Like acts of direct and reflective insight, these feelings are intentional responses, not intentional objects. They constitute part of my 'cognitional access to, not the content of, particular values.' See Vertin, 'Judgments of Value' 235.

48 Admittedly, Lonergan's view is at odds with David Hume's position, as outlined in chapter 3. For instance, Lonergan does not think, as Hume did, 'the human mind to be a matter of impressions linked together by custom.' Moreover, Lonergan points out the performative inconsistency between Hume's own mind, which Lonergan thinks was quite original, and Hume's philosophical account of what he considered the human mind to be, which was something without any possibility of originality. See Lonergan, *Method* 21.

49 It is important to emphasize that, as intentional responses to known contents, deliberative insights presuppose fact knowledge. Although the fourth-level process is not *merely rational*, as is the third level, it nevertheless sublates the third level. Hence, it would be a misinterpretation to object that the fourth level is irrational.

50 It would seem that more complex than the absolute value judgment I have previously outlined is a further 'relative' value judgment (e.g., thrombolysis is better than a coronary angioplasty). On the distinction between simple and relative value judgments, see Lonergan, *Method* 263.

51 Ibid. 30.

52 Vertin, 'Judgments of Value' 231.

53 My interpretations of these feelings (as experienced) and judgments regarding these interpretations could be confirmed by the changes they undergo when I address their presumed causes or goals. If a feeling that I

358 Notes to pages 159–62

provisionally label as fatigue is relieved by rest, or another feeling that I presumptively label as hunger is satisfied by ingesting food, then I have further grounds for labelling these experienced feelings as I did. By such a process of attending to and naming my affective states and trends, I develop a heightened awareness of the non-intentional feelings that are part of my data of consciousness. But these feelings are not to be confused with 'feelings' as data of sense. When speaking of the feeling of anxiety, then, I refer primarily to a datum of consciousness, which might or might not also be manifest in sensible bodily changes, for example, increases in breathing rate, heart rate, or gland secretion.

54 Lonergan, *Method* 30–1.

55 I have already noted that modern psychologists distinguish between the intentional, affective responses of anxiety and fear on the basis of whether the object to which I affectively respond is realistic (fear) or not (anxiety). Based upon this interpretation of Lonergan, what is called *fear* might be thought of as a proper fourth-level affective response to some real, actual, or possible object known through a third-level judgment. Although anxiety is an intentional response to some cognitional object (i.e., an affect linked to some image), it is distinct from fear in as much as the object is unrealistic. Hence, the problem of anxiety on this reading is not in my fourth-level affective response, but rather in my third-level intellectual judgment. By contrast, an *adjustment disorder* suggests a fourth-level affective problem. This is a psychiatric diagnosis defined as 'the development of emotional or behavioural symptoms in response to an identifiable stressor(s).' Here, the distress provoked by some stressor 'is in excess of what would be expected from exposure to the stressor.' One might interpret the psychological problem as a distinctively fourth-level one of an excessively negative affective response to some fact. Alternatively, the problem might not be that of an excessive affective response, but of my correct interpretation of the source of this emotional response. See the American Psychiatric Association, 'Adjustment Disorders,' in *The Diagnostic and Statistical Manual of Mental Disorders*, 4th ed. (Washington: APA, 1994).

56 Lonergan, *Method* 31.

57 Vertin, 'Judgments of Value' 231–32.

58 Lonergan, *Method* 243.

59 Ibid. 37.

60 For instance, in Sue Rodriguez's case, a key issue was not so much her valuing control and autonomy in decisions effecting her care. Rather, the real issue was that she concluded that certain values, such as having certain capacities like speech, were relatively more important than the value of her life. Understanding this issue as one of differing rankings of values is an important contribution to the debate.

61 This is a notion that I will explore further in chapter 7. The term itself derives from the Latin word 'complacentia' and is used here in a technical sense. Accordingly, many of the current connotations of the word 'complacency' in English are irrelevant to what is meant here.

62 Lonergan, *Method* 115.

63 Ibid. 36.

64 Ibid. 38

65 Although, in the case of self-inflicted harm, the agent and the patient would be identical.

66 Lonergan, *Method* 38

67 Ibid. 37.

68 Lonergan, 'Natural Right and Historical Mindedness,' *A Third Collection: Papers by Bernard Lonergan, S.J.*, ed. Frederick Crowe (New York: Paulist Press; London: Geoffery Chapman, 1985) 173.

69 Lonergan, *Phenomenology and Logic*, CWL 18:238.

70 In distinguishing between patterns of complacency and concern, I am expanding beyond what Lonergan has said by drawing upon a series of articles by Frederick Crowe titled 'Complacency and Concern in the Thought of St Thomas,' *Theological Studies* 20 (1959) 1–39, 198–230, 343–95; reprinted in Frederick E. Crowe, *Three Thomist Studies*, ed. Michael Vertin (Boston: Lonergan Institute of Boston College, 2000) 71–203.

71 Lonergan, *Method* 31.

72 It is important to emphasize that acts of deciding or choosing follow from acts of knowing or, more specifically, evaluating. Deliberation reveals an actuality or a limited range of possibilities. This process is brought to a close by deciding to enjoy the actual good or to bring about one of the possible goods.

73 Elisabeth Kübler-Ross set forth a stage-based model for understanding the process of coping with dying in her 1969 classic *On Death and Dying*. In addition, she also remarked that hope was possible throughout this entire process. I would suggest that the sequence of stages she articulates (i.e., denial, anger, bargaining, depression, and acceptance) can be understood as cognitive and decisional advances that persons facing death tend to achieve. See Charles A. Corr, 'Coping with Dying: Lessons That We Should and Should Not Learn from the Work of Elisabeth Kübler-Ross,' *Death Studies* 17 (1993) 69–83.

74 On this analysis, I recognize that the bulk of my medical practice proceeds in the mode of concern. A practical difficulty is to learn to be comfortable with persons who are sick. This is important so that my concern to help them does not truncate or shortcut my cognitional processes of discovering what I ought to do. Nor should my cognitional concern undermine the decisional and effective processes of choosing and doing, in a careful manner, what I

recognize I ought to do. In addition, it is important to learn to enjoy persons who also happen to be my patients, throughout the whole range of these cognitional and decisional processes. Many difficulties that arise in the physician–patient relationship stem from poor communication, that is, from communication that results in misinformation, or gives patients the message that their physician is not concerned about them. Perhaps greater clarity on the affective elements of evaluations could enhance this process of communication by helping physicians to distinguish more clearly their cognitive and decisional concerns from their positive regard for their patients.

Chapter 7

1 Reflecting on more than twenty years of discussions with undergraduate and graduate philosophy students on the possibility of knowing values 'objectively,' Michael Vertin concludes that most of the disputes about this matter 'have little to do with the specific issue of knowing values, and much to do with the prior and more general issue of knowing anything at all.' For this reason, I have addressed Lonergan's epistemology of knowing *simpliciter* prior to his epistemology of evaluative knowing. See Vertin, 'Judgments of Value for the Later Lonergan,' *Method, Journal of Lonergan Studies* 13 (1995) 241–42.

2 Lonergan, *Method* 265; cf. 16–17.

3 As in the previous chapter, I will be drawing primarily upon Michael Vertin's recent interpretation of Lonergan on the epistemic objectivity of value judgments, as argued for in his 'Judgments of Value' 221–48, esp. 241–45.

4 I will use *authentic* in reference to the subject's cognitive activities, and *genuine* in reference to the validity of the knowledge reached on the basis of authentic cognitive activities.

5 In a 12-month period in 1994–95, for instance, the Canadian Bureau of Drug Surveillance disciplined 49 Canadian physicians for inappropriately prescribing narcotics. Dr Russell Portenoy is the editor-in-chief of the *Journal of Pain and Symptom Management* and a leading authority on the role of opioids (e.g., morphine) in the management of chronic non-malignant pain. He argues against the strong societal and political views that reject chronic opioid therapy for all conditions except the control of pain from cancer. But even his position, and that expressed in the Canadian Guidelines for Managing Chronic Non-malignant Pain, accepts society's negative view of addictions and addictive behaviour, while suggesting that not all opioid treatment leads to such behaviour. See Craig Sumi, '49 Doctors Disciplined for Abuse in Prescribing,' *Toronto Star,* 15 January 1996, A3; Neil Gagen et al., 'Guidelines for Managing Chronic Non-malignant Pain,' *Canadian Family Physician* 41 (1995) 49–53.

6 As a practising physician, I sometimes interpret my role as that of a 'peer reviewer' mediating good decision-making among patients who seek my advice. Although much of the literature on mediation recommends that the mediator be neutral regarding normative issues and outcomes, I have found that patients who deny a value that I accept often raise morally problematic issues for me. This seems to be because I perceive myself to be morally implicated in what I judge to be their mistaken evaluations and subsequent decisions and actions. Indeed, in this hypothetical case, I became subject to the censure of my peers precisely because of my involvement with a patient with whom I was unable to negotiate a more responsible treatment plan, for example, a plan to admit him to hospital and, subsequently, to arrange a referral to a facility that specializes in treating addictive behaviours.

7 That is, does one not risk being perceived as insensitive or uncaring if, as a physician, one is critical of a patient's evaluation? And does such a physician not also risk being perceived as abusing one's power, on the basis of some *paternalistic* justification, by denying a patient access to the medical means to what they judge to be their good (e.g., morphine)? This issue is important to address in this case since it also emerges in the context of requests for euthanasia, to which I will return in chapter 9.

8 For instance, decisions by Paul's family or caregivers not to challenge his decision itself implies their own evaluations. If I decide to help Paul execute his decision, even though I judge him to be mistaken, there may be significantly different accounts of this response. One view might be that I am presupposing that my *functionary* service to him is my sole role, and it is not my job to question or help him to discern what he should do. Indeed, there may be practical reasons, such as *time and trouble*, that provide a disincentive for me to extend my institutional role. Lonergan discusses these issues under the heading 'The Structure of the Human Good,' to be discussed in chapter 8.

9 Paul seeks medical attention in order to obtain some terminal value, in this case, the treatment of his chest pain. The proximate ground of the evaluation that it would be good to seek medical attention is, on this account, an affective response to the disagreeable experience of this pain, or the possibility that it might signify a life-threatening emergency.

10 Lonergan, *Method* 31.

11 Ibid. 31.

12 Ibid. 31.

13 Ibid. 35.

14 Ibid. 35.

15 Although most persons who are free of drug addictions would readily agree that a life oriented to the euphoric effects produced by narcotics falls short of an adequate ideal of human flourishing, such an evaluation might also be agreed to by the drug addict whose habits are alien to his will. The distinc-

tion here is, in psychological terms, between a person with narrowed interests who might never have reflected critically on the objects or effects of these interests (e.g., a contented drug addict) and someone who engages in the same behaviour but is discontent and critical of it, and hence wishes to change (e.g., someone whose drug addiction manifests an obsessive-compulsive disorder).

16   Responses to what is agreeable, however, might be a sufficient criterion for other fourth-level evaluations, such as *aesthetic* evaluations. But I would argue that even such evaluations will have an ethical or moral flavour if they involve persons. One example of this is the surgeon who sought to express an aesthetic evaluation by incorporating coloured beads into the sutures of a native Canadian patient on whom he was operating. His claim to the court that this act was merely a matter of aesthetics proved to be unconvincing.

17   Walter Conn, 'The Desire for Authenticity: Conscience and Moral Conversion,' in Vernon Gregson, ed., *The Desires of the Human Heart: An Introduction to the Theology of Bernard Lonergan* (Mahwah, NJ: Paulist Press, 1988) 41.

18   It is on some such reading of human nature that one might argue that no morally degenerate person is beyond reform.

19   Lonergan, *Method* 240. This contrast corresponds to one that characterizes a person of integrity. According to R. Hepburn, for such a person 'the fundamental question whether to conduct life on the plane of self-concern or of moral seriousness has been decisively resolved.' In this sense, Lonergan's account of the person whose life is oriented to satisfactions seems to correspond to what others refer to as the person who conducts his or her life on the plane of self-concern. See Ted Honderich, ed., *The Oxford Companion to Philosophy*, s.v. 'Integrity,' by R. Hepburn.

20   Lonergan, *Insight* 254. Lonergan suggests that this resistance to raise further relevant questions is characteristic of the egoist. I will have more to say on this later when discussing the topic of bias and its various kinds.

21   From this perspective, one might consider the Kantian imperative that 'I should never act in such a way that I could not also will that my maxim should be a universal law' to be a procedural check that ensures that my evaluations are not based on feelings that respond merely to what is satisfying to myself. Kant expresses the altruistic character of the good by insisting that 'the sublimity and intrinsic worth of the command is the better shown in a duty the fewer subjective causes there are for it and the more there are against it.' See Immanuel Kant, *Foundations of the Metaphysics of Morals*, trans. L.W. Beck (Indianapolis, IN: Bobbs-Merrill, 1959) 18, 43.

22   Although the label *Epicureanism* is commonly used in this way, as I noted in chapter 3, Epicurus himself (341–270 BC) advocated only the pursuit of those pleasures that can be controlled and enjoyed in moderation. See Simon Blackburn, *The Oxford Dictionary of Philosophy*, s.v. 'Epicurus.'

23 See John Finnis, *Fundamentals of Ethics* (Washington: Georgetown University Press, 1983) 42–45.

24 I am happy to report that Germain Grisez, one of John Finnis's colleagues, has recently taken up this issue of moral psychology and the role of feelings in moral judgments. It strikes me that the attention this topic is receiving by such thinkers provides evidence that this is an important issue for all thinkers who are concerned about the human phenomena of evaluating. Still, for Grisez, '[s]ince emotional motivation pertains to sentient nature, it is fairly well proportioned to sentient goods and bads. But for the same reason, feelings are not naturally adequate to motivate us to act for intelligible goods and to avoid intelligible bads.' Grisez proceeds to list four natural limitations of emotional motivation, and bases this critique on his interpretation of the role such emotions play in *non-human animal* behaviour. This position illustrates what I would take to be an intellectualist account of human moral knowing. By contrast with Lonergan's account, for Grisez it is always the case that, 'feelings need to expand so that they can work in harmony with practical reason.' In this analysis, there appears to be little, if any room, for what Pascal has called *the heart's reasons, which reason knows not.* Both Lonergan and Pascal would admit the possibility that certain affective responses might actually expand Grisez's practical reason. See Germain Grisez, 'Appendix 1,' in *The Way of the Lord Jesus, Volume 3: Difficult Moral Questions* (Quincy, IN: Franciscan Press, 1997) 863–65.

25 Lonergan, *Method* 31–32.

26 Conn, 'The Desire for Authenticity' 41.

27 Lonergan, *Method* 50–51.

28 Vertin, 'Judgments of Value' 221–48.

29 Conn, 'The Desire for Authenticity' 38.

30 Lonergan, *Method* 34.

31 Ibid. 35.

32 An example of this felt incongruity is, perhaps, the experience of guilt.

33 Lonergan, *Method* 39.

34 Ibid. 32.

35 Ibid. 32–33.

36 Ibid. 33–34.

37 For instance, 'objectivity is simply the consequence of authentic subjectivity, of genuine attention, genuine intelligence, genuine reasonableness, genuine responsibility.' In another place, he writes that '[g]enuine objectivity is the fruit of authentic subjectivity. It is to be attained only by attaining authentic subjectivity. To seek and employ some alternative prop or crutch invariably leads to some measure of reductionism.' See ibid. 265, 292.

38 Ibid. 233.

39 Ibid. 292.

40 Vertin, 'Judgments of Value' 245 n. 63.

41 Indeed, this is precisely his argument regarding how I know facts; that is, my judgments are based on reflective insights, which are intellectual cognitions rather than affective ones.

42 If one interpret's Kant's position on the objectivity of knowledge claims in the framework of the *Second Critique,* however, what he means is a merely practical epistemic objectivity, rather than a genuine or speculative objectivity as thinkers such as John Finnis would mean by objectivity.

43 Lonergan, *Method* 37.

44 This is assuming that Paul has the freedom to choose otherwise.

45 Vertin suggests that the main ways one can fail at cognitional and decisional self-transcendence on the fourth level can be illustrated with precision by the main ways one can fail at deductive inference. For a more detailed account of these different possibilities, see his 'Judgments of Value' 243–44 n. 61.

46 Lonergan, *Method* 231; cf. *Insight* 214–31, 269.

47 Lonergan, *Insight* 622–23.

48 Lonergan, *Method* 40.

49 Ibid. 240.

50 Ibid. 54.

51 Ibid. 54.

52 Ibid. 53.

53 Ibid. 40.

54 Ibid. 40.

55 Ibid. 54.

56 Ibid. 55.

57 Lonergan, *Insight* 622.

58 For Lonergan, value judging, deciding to do or enjoy, and doing or enjoying are all part of the fourth level. Still, I can know what I ought to do and not do it. That is, the fourth level involves both cognitional and decisional issues.

59 In Sue Rodriguez's case, for instance, many of her concerns were based upon future possible events. To the extent that these events were merely 'possible' eventualities, all of her plans were also contingent.

60 Lonergan, *Method* 30.

61 Ibid. 31.

62 Ibid. 241.

63 I would argue, with Lonergan, that the allegedly requisite escape is impossible. One sign of this effort to escape subjectivity is to express oneself in the passive voice, thereby avoiding the apparent subjectivism of first-person claims. In this discussion, I have deliberately tried to avoid doing this. Passive-voice thinking and expressing puts physicians, qua scientists, at a disadvantage when it comes to dealing with the feelings a patient might have and express, either verbally or in their behaviour. For not only are physicians

apt to have little to say about the affective dimension of an experience of an illness, the medical training that has prepared them to be scientists may also have encouraged in them a bias against attending to and raising questions about feelings or other 'subjective' data of consciousness. Without a prior self-awareness and self-knowledge of their own cognitive and decisional subjectivity, physicians and other caregivers may be of little help to those patients who are in need of this type of human understanding and compassion. For instance, only a minority of elderly persons with cognitive impairment who are examined by Emergency physicians are correctly diagnosed as having a problem with their thinking. One interpretation of this fact is that Emergency physicians are disinclined to attend to the non-physical symptoms of their patients, which would involve a formal assessment of their mental functioning. See Arthur Sanders, 'Recognition of Cognitive Problems in Older Adults by Emergency Medicine Personnel,' *Annals of Emergency Medicine* 21 (1992) 831–33.

64 These same reflections also hold true in the story of Dennis Kaye. I regard his story as providing a counter-balance to Sue's because he also had ALS, but responded differently to it. One aim of this analysis is to identify some of the elements of their stories that might account for their different conclusions. In the interest of space, therefore, I will contrast the stories of Sue and Dennis only when this seems helpful for highlighting differences between them.

65 Lonergan, 'Milltown Park Lectures on Method in Theology,' transcript by N. Graham of lectures delivered at Milltown, Dublin, Ireland (Toronto: Lonergan Research Institute, file 641), q. 14, p. 30.

66 Lonergan, *Method* 38–39.

67 In the euthanasia debate, some thinkers invoke the concept of moral autonomy to support voluntary euthanasia. Thus, Norman points out, the wrongness of killing, which rests, in part, on the fact that such an act normally violates someone's autonomy by depriving them of life, does not apply in a case where someone requests that their life be ended. In such a case, respect for autonomy would require one to comply with that person's wishes. In his own name, Norman argues for a more precise account of autonomy that involves some deliberation about possible choices. See Richard Norman, *The Oxford Companion to Philosophy*, s.v. 'Autonomy in Applied Ethics' 70.

68 Heil points out that the divorce of philosophy and psychology occurred relatively recently when, in the mid-nineteenth century, psychologists came to regard themselves as engaged in 'a fully-fledged science emancipated from its empirically feeble predecessors.' Heil concludes that many philosophers now concede it to be a mistake to assume that philosophical inquiry could be altogether insulated from empirical findings in psychology.

Lonergan's position on the relevance of the findings of child psychologists to moral philosophy supports this view. See J. Heil, *The Oxford Companion to Philosophy*, s.v. 'Psychology' 728–29.

69 Norman Care suggests that one way to assess the adequacy of an ethical theory is to attend to the underlying conception of the individual it presupposes. For him, a key difference between individualistic and anti-individualistic theories is the importance of social connections to an adequate understanding of individuals. From this perspective, Lonergan's account of the human person is evidently anti–individualistic. See N. Care, *The Oxford Companion to Philosophy*, s.v. 'Individualism' 404–405.

70 I refer the reader to Lonergan's own more detailed explanation of this chart. My aim here is merely to situate the value judgments grasped through feelings, here labelled terminal values, within Lonergan's understanding of the structure of the human good. See Lonergan, *Method* 47–52.

71 Lonergan, *Topics in Education*, CWL 10:33–34.

72 Lonergan, *Method* 48.

73 Lonergan, *Topics in Education*, CWL 10:34.

74 Lonergan, *Method* 49–50.

75 Lonergan distinguishes three kinds of habits: cognitional habits, volitional habits, and skills. He speaks of such habits as conditions of coordinated human operations. Such habits are the conditions of not having to learn, not having to be persuaded, and not having to acquire a skill every time something has to be done. See Lonergan, *Topics in Education*, CWL 10:35.

76 For a good and concrete summary of Lonergan's account of the human good, see Conn, 'The Desire for Authenticity' 43.

77 Lonergan, *Method*, 50.

78 Lonergan speaks in *Topics in Education* of ethical value as a quality of a subject who does things, and develops the idea that things are to be done because they are right. In so doing, one becomes 'a centre of initiative, free and yet good.' He points out that in our upbringing we are apt to develop the false notion that being good and being unfree or constrained go together. But the proper good of humans, for Lonergan, is doing what is right because one is free. Conversely, one's freedom is to realize the good. See Lonergan, *Topics in Education*, CWL 10:38.

79 Lonergan, *Method* 51.

80 Ibid. 55.

81 Lonergan, *Topics in Education*, CWL 10:39.

82 Ibid. 39–40.

83 Lonergan points out that during various historical periods, certain aspects of the good were emphasized. Positivistic and pragmatic consciousness, for instance, emphasizes the particular good. Idealistic consciousness is primarily concerned with the intelligible good or the good of order. Realist

consciousness insists on the good of value. See Lonergan, *Topics in Education,* CWL 10:41, 106 n. 76.

84 Lonergan, *Method* 38.

85 Note that the distinction between transcendental intending and categorial knowledge is indicated by the singular and plural uses of the term 'value.' Transcendental intending is an a priori orientation toward *value* or genuine goodness. Categorial evaluations grasp particular *values,* categorial goods. See Lonergan, *Method* 36. Note also that I use the term 'evaluation' as synonymous with 'value judgment,' although it is actually broader. To be precise, evaluation refers to the whole fourth level, one element of which is a value judgment. Moreover, not all evaluations involve value or moral judgments; they could also be aesthetic judgments.

86 Ibid. 55.

Chapter 8

1 Lonergan, *Method* 37.

2 As mentioned before, by using the term *phenomenal* I seek to highlight the apparent features of the cognitional process, those features that are sought in answer to Lonergan's first basic question, 'What am I doing when I am knowing.' This sense of 'phenomena' or 'phenomenology' is in contrast to the 'epistemic' status of my cognitive achievements, or what is sought in answer to Lonergan's second basic question, 'Why is doing this genuine knowing?', where *this* is given in answer to his first basic question. In other words, 'phenomenal' here does not mean 'merely' phenomenal, which is equivalent to 'merely subjective.' For this use of terminology, I am following Vertin, 'Judgments of Value,' *Method, Journal of Lonergan Studies* 13 (1995) 233 n. 10.

3 Note that throughout this discussion I have flagged the affective dimension of Lonergan's distinction between the transcendental and the categorial by using the term 'feeling' in its singular and plural forms. 'Transcendental affectivity' corresponds to the singular 'feeling,' in contrast to the particular categorial affective responses to satisfactions or values, which I have designated by using the plural 'feelings.' This distinction is important because one's transcendental 'feeling' is the underlying 'mass and momentum' of one's living, and one's categorial 'feelings' are responses to particular contents that emerge in the context of one's encounters with data. One's intending of transcendental value has an important affective dimension that makes it distinct from one's intending of transcendental intelligibility or reality. This intending of value (singular), is not the sum of particular categorial intendings of values. Rather, it is what opens one to a horizon of value. See Vertin, 'Judgments of Value' 246–47.

4 Ibid. 233.

5 Lonergan, *Method* 231.

6 Ibid. 36.

7 Ibid. 38.

8 Ibid. 31.

9 Lonergan, *Topics in Education*, CWL 10:33–43.

10 The main point here is that for Lonergan, goods/values are ultimately always concrete. Although his scale of preferences among values provides a general or heuristic ranking of values, it should not be interpreted as specifying fairly clear substantive values prior to considering any concrete set of circumstances. Lonergan, *Method* 38.

11 For some Lonerganian distinctions regarding the types of general metaphysical claims that follow from this analysis, see figure A.4 of the appendix.

12 Lonergan, *Method* 37.

13 Ibid. 115.

14 In his own name, Vertin contrasts various other thinkers with Lonergan on the basis of what each takes to be the most basic evidence in support of his or her position. Although this sort of contrast is beyond the scope of the present discussion, it is helpful to note Vertin's conclusions regarding the type of evidence to which Lonergan appeals, and the epistemic status of this evidence. On Vertin's interpretation, the most fundamental evidence to which Lonergan appeals is 'the normative structure of myself in my cognitional enterprise.' Vertin also affirms that this evidence is the most basic type of evidence to which one might appeal and, in addition, that the content of this evidence is operationally incontrovertible: 'I can argue against it however I will; but if I attend carefully to my own performance in elaborating and asserting my objections, I will discover that operationally I invariably invoke what verbally I would reject.' See Vertin, 'Judgments of Value' 242.

15 Lonergan, *Understanding and Being*, CWL 5:187; cf. *Method* 20–21.

16 See Graham Bird, *The Oxford Companion to Philosophy*, s.v. 'Hume' 379–80, and 'Kantianism,' 439–40.

17 Lonergan, *Insight*, CWL 3:364.

18 See figure A.2 of the appendix for a diagrammatic depiction of these different accounts of knowing.

19 I will restrict myself to addressing Lonergan's answers to the first five questions, and defer his answer to the metaphysical questions to chapter 9.

20 Again, as figure A.2 of the appendix indicates, a key difference between Lonergan's account of knowing and the main alternative accounts regards whether the subject/object distinction is taken to be a fundamental one. For Lonergan, one's field of awareness (large circle) includes all being (there is nothing outside of being). Hence, the distinction between self and non-self

is a subdistinction made within the field of being; but first I arrive in the field of being through judgment.

21 As I noted previously, the discipline of psychology has been distinct from philosophy for little more than a century. Still, diverse positions on this global philosophical issue shape the way in which psychologists conceive of their discipline. For instance, behaviourists deliberately prescind from attending to data of consciousness as a basis for understanding emotions. They focus instead on the observable emotional behaviour of their fellows, rather than on their private, i.e., subjective, experiences. This preference, I think, is fuelled by the presupposition that 'private' experience is merely epistemically subjective. See Cheshire Calhoun and Robert Solomon, eds, *What Is an Emotion?* (Oxford: Oxford University Press, 1984) 11.

22 Lonergan, *Method* 11.

23 As I discussed in chapter 3, Aristotle thought that in posing a question one was already partway to the answer. To this early allusion to intentional consciousness, Aquinas adds the notion of judgment and the transcendentals. Subsequent thinkers, such as Scheler, shift the emphasis from faculty psychology to intentionality analysis. Lonergan, on my reading, integrates a number of these insights into his cognitional theory.

24 Michael Shevell has published a series of articles that examine the moral collaboration of the German medical profession with the Nazi regime during the Second World War. These articles raise the question of what sort of conditioning occurred that allowed these medical people to continue to function, if indeed they did so. They are based upon the eye-witness testimony of Dr Leo Alexander, an American army neurologist who prepared medical reports on the Third Reich's army, its mental institutions, and its prison camps immediately after the end of the war in 1945. Although he was also a witness at the Nuremberg war crimes trials, the United States military classified his original reports as 'restricted,' and they have only recently been declassified and made publicly available. Of relevance to the role of fourth-level affectivity is Alexander's interpretation that one of the reasons that German physicians lost their moral sense was the disregard of feeling that was encouraged in their professional training. As he contended, 'Scientific objectivity bred detachment and distance from the object of study. This distance minimized any perceived intrinsic humanity or dignity for the victims, robbing them of the respect they deserved.' See Michael Shevell, 'Racial Hygiene, Active Euthanasia, and Julius Hallervorden,' *Neurology* 11 (1992) 2214–19, at 2217.

25 Lonergan, *Method* 265.

26 On Vertin's interpretation, both fact and value judgments can manifest actualities as well as possibilities. In the case of a value judgment that

manifests an actual value, this process occurs in what Vertin labels the pattern of *complacency*, and this process properly terminates in a decision to enjoy the value. A value judgment that manifests a merely possible value belongs to the conscious intentional process in the mode of *concern*, and this process properly terminates in a decision to attempt actualization of the possible value. See Vertin, 'Judgments of Value' 239 n. 55.

27 As Vertin puts it, '[T]he cognitional criterion of every self-transcending value apprehension, and thus the ultimate cognitional criterion of every epistemically-objective value judgment, is the transcendental notion of value – and, more precisely, the transcendental affectivity of the transcendental notion of value.' Ibid. 244.

28 These are not uncommon feelings among homeless girls I have encountered in inner-city Metropolitan Toronto. Some statistics indicate that in this population, 70 per cent of these youths were sexually and/or physically abused in their family homes. Also, there are about 200 pregnancies each year among these youths (out of a total population of 4000 to 12,000). As one 14-year-old girl put it, 'I want to be a mother so I can do a better job than my mother did with me.' See Michael Valpy, 'The Streets Where They Live,' *Globe and Mail*, 17 Feb. 1994.

29 Lonergan acknowledges that he draws on Dietrich von Hildebrand for this distinction. See Lonergan, *Method* 30, 31 n. 2. In order to avoid confusing the much broader notion of *feelings*, which include first-level sensations, with the fourth-level intentional, affective responses that Lonergan flags, I have referred to the latter as *affects*.

30 Frederick Crowe, 'Dialectic and the Ignatian *Spiritual Exercises*,' in Michael Vertin, ed., *Appropriating the Lonergan Idea* (Washington: Catholic University of America Press, 1989) 249. This limitation, however, does not exclude a report of an actual past example of an evaluation, which is what I have tried to do in chapters 4 to 7.

31 Even if non-intentional feelings are not negatively biasing a particular value judgment, it seems that at least a certain general sense of well-being is an important condition for properly functioning intentional responses to values (e.g., calm deliberation).

32 In defence of Lonergan's position, I would also admit that to the extent that these decisions were mainly based on personality traits and non-intentional feelings, they were not fully personal or authentic, in the sense of an 'existential discovery.' See Lonergan, *Method* 38.

33 Lonergan speaks of *egoism* as 'an interference of spontaneity with the development of intelligence.' See Lonergan, *Insight*, CWL 3:245.

34 Robert Doran expands Lonergan's position in this area. He underlines the importance of non- or pre-intentional feelings. Doran also illustrates that such an expansion of Lonergan's basic position in this area need not under-

mine the latter's central claims concerning the cognitive role of intentional feelings in value judgments. Indeed, the intrusive effects of non-intentional feelings (such as anxiety or depression) in undermining the cognitive processes or the well-being of persons is an issue to which psychologists and psychiatrists frequently address themselves. Difficulties in one's early-life attachments to parents, for instance, can condition one's relationships in later life. Doran acknowledges the important positive and negative role of such non-intentional feelings. He also suggests that one may effect 'psychic conversion' by intentional consciousness operating on non-intentional feelings, as can occur in psychotherapy. See, for instance, the chapters on psychic conversion in Doran, *Theology and the Dialectics of History* (Toronto: University of Toronto Press, 1990) 42–63.

35 Lonergan, *Method* 31.

36 See Lonergan, *Topics in Education*, CWL 10:228 n. 51.

37 This suggestion that some readers' own self-awareness may not be as invulnerable as they initially think ought not be too shocking, given that physicians frequently have difficulties in this area. Having recognized this, some groups specializing in communication skills in health care have designed courses to help physicians become more aware of their own feelings that may arise during an interview with a 'difficult' patient. This initial awareness is a first crucial step. For without it, one never explicitly addresses one's affective responses. Once one is aware of one's own feelings of frustration or irritability toward a patient or circumstance, one can begin to sort out these feelings. At the end of this process, one might decide that they are one's own problem (i.e., the patient reminds one of a difficult relation with a family member), the patient's problem (e.g., certain responses can be helpful in diagnosing some patients, such as someone with a personality disorder), the illness, or all three. See the Bayer Institute for Health Care Communication, *'Difficult' Physician-Patient Relationships: Workbook* (West Haven, CT: Bayer Institute for Health Care Communication, 1995) 61.

38 This point distinguishes Lonergan's position from that of the hedonist and the puritan. For both, the ultimate criterion for the goodness of some entity concerns whether or not it is satisfying. For Lonergan, by contrast, the ultimate criterion is one's intending of transcendental value, which places one within the horizon of value (i.e., beyond any particular value, or even the sum total of particular values).

39 In the case of the last two classes, it would seem that the degree of satisfaction or dissatisfaction might influence one's assessment of the object's value.

40 Lonergan, *Method* 48.

41 Lonergan, *Insight*, CWL 3: 622.

42 Lonergan, Insight Seminar' (St Mary's University, Halifax, 1958, Lecture 8,

Slide I, Discussion), cited by Bernard Tyrrell, *Bernard Lonergan's Philosophy of God* (South Bend, IN: Notre Dame Press, 1974) 194–5.

43 Whether or not they are, in fact, overlooking some aspect of their conscious data, the point is that this is the issue. Moreover, it is not one that can be settled by mere speculative arguments. It can only be settled by readers returning to the laboratory of their own evaluations. As I have done in my own name regarding my medical evaluations, so also readers must determine whether Lonergan's account does justice to their own experience of making true and false judgments and evaluations.

44 Bernard Lonergan, *Collection*, CWL 4:210–11.

45 This is a key claim in my support of Lonergan's whole emphasis on cognitional theory. It is also a claim that my experience as a medical knower, and my insights into my own performance in the medical sphere, allows me to substantiate. The most serious objection to this project, then, would come from a person who is not only successful in some practical endeavour such as diagnosing accurately myocardial infarctions, but who is also able to provide a nuanced account of his or her own performance that differs radically from the one Lonergan provides, and which I accept.

Chapter 9

1 In chapter 1, I suggested that Lonergan's metaphor of the *pair of scissors* neatly captures the relation between particular cases (lower blade) and more general considerations (upper blade). On this issue, I acknowledge the validity of the question L.W. Sumner and Joseph Boyle pose in the introduction to *Philosophical Perspectives on Bioethics* (Toronto: University of Toronto Press, 1996), namely, 'whether the generalist/particularist distinction is any longer a useful analytical device for identifying basic methodological differences' (7). In answer to this question, I hope to demonstrate not only that it is not helpful, but also that, inevitably, imbalanced results occur when persons focus exclusively on either particular cases or general considerations in an effort to address an issue as complex as euthanasia. To press the metaphor, a single-bladed scissors does not cut very well.

2 I have been referring to the latter category as *affects*, rather than the more generic *feelings* or *emotions*. See my characterization of these terms in section 4.1 of chapter 3, and Ted Honderich, ed., *The Oxford Companion to Philosophy*, s.v. 'Passion,' by Robert Solomon.

3 See, for instance, Hunnex's discussion of the 'axiological objectivist' family of thinkers who purport to know true values but deny that feelings play a cognitive role in this knowledge. Milton Hunnex, 'The Problem of Values,' in *Chronological and Thematic Charts of Philosophies and Philosophers* (Grand Rapids, MI: Zondervan Publishing House, 1986) 2. As mentioned previously,

John Finnis is someone who regards all feelings as of just psychological im-portance; see Finnis, *Fundamentals of Ethics* (Washington: Georgetown University Press, 1983) 30–37, 42–45, 48–50, 54.

4 Of course, neither Sue nor Dennis was a philosopher. They did not, to my knowledge, verbally express their answers to this question, nor to any of the others that I will be posing in relation to the available information regarding their stories. For this reason, it would be unfair of me to expect them to give a precise account of what sort of feelings they regard as relevant and which ones not. Nor do I expect them to be able to give a nuanced account – in the scholarly, reflective way that could fairly be expected of philosophers – of the point at which these feelings enter into their cognitive processes. Even so, if one is attentive to their stories, one can glean the answer to these questions that, I think, would fairly represent their positions.

5 Lisa Hobbs Birnie and Sue Rodriguez, *Uncommon Will* (Toronto: Macmillan Canada, 1994) 69. Similarly, Dennis is dismissive of the validity of claims made by persons without this personal experience, even by apparent 'experts' who presume to understand and pass judgment on Sue's experience and concerns. He points out that these individuals might not personally face similar issues for another thirty or forty years. Without access to this personal side of the issues, Dennis insists, 'I don't care if they have masters degrees in forensic pathology, their opinions are inherently invalid.' See Dennis Kaye, *Laugh, I Thought I'd Die* (Toronto: Penguin Books, 1993) 204–205.

6 In chapter 2 I mentioned the disparity between the majority view on euthanasia among ethicists, on the one hand, and the general public, on the other. I wonder whether one reason for this disparity might be poor communication. The fault might lie, in part, with the experts, who tend to address these issues in a strictly intellectual or logical fashion, as is the case when the discussion focuses almost exclusively on the distinction between killing and allowing to die. Even if readers are unconvinced by the end of this discussion that human affect plays a positive cognitive role in evaluations, perhaps they can still learn a lesson from the reactions of Dennis and Sue to the 'experts.' Their stories are replete with instances of poor physician–patient communication. Even if physicians insist that all feelings have no cognitive merit, this should not absolve them from learning to be empathic when communicating with patients. At least such responses acknowledge feelings as worthy of attending to and labelling. On empathic responses in medicine, see Robert Buckman, *How to Break Bad News: A Guide for Health Care Professionals* (Toronto: University of Toronto Press, 1992) 29–33.

7 One example of this is provided by Sue's own account of how she decided that she would die by physician-assisted suicide, which I related in chapter 2. The night following her first meeting with a local ALS Society, Sue decided to commit suicide. As Hobbs Birnie relates the story, 'Sue made this decision

without fuss, hesitation or moral argument. The idea came and she accepted it. It felt right.' See Hobbs Birnie and Rodriguez, *Uncommon Will* 36–37.

8 Some of Dennis's most descriptive accounts of such a deficiency are directed at members of the medical community. He titles his chapter 4 'Doctors and Other Deities,' and it begins with the quip 'It's been said that the primary difference between doctors and God is that God doesn't think he's a doctor' (47). Recalling the manner in which he was told that he had ALS, he describes this specialist as 'Mr. Personality,' and says he had 'all the bedside manner of an impeccably dressed mannequin.' Note that this deficiency is at the human, affective level. For Dennis, there is no conflict between such a criticism and acknowledging that this specialist was also highly respected within his field. This view raises the further question of the relation between moral and intellectual development. Lonergan's short answer is that moral conversion precedes intellectual conversion. See Kaye, *Laugh, I Thought I'd Die* 46, 47, 49.

9 Hobbs Birnie and Rodriguez, *Uncommon Will* 67–69.

10 A positive feature of Lonergan's position that certain feelings are necessary but not sufficient grounds for certain knowledge claims is that it highlights both personal and communal features of the process of knowing. On the personal side, his position argues for the necessity of one's feelings, and the importance of integrating intellectual and affective acts in evaluations. Put negatively, his position acknowledges the insufficiency of one's affective responses in the totality of this process. There is also the insufficiency of one's *individual*, as distinct from communal, cognitive efforts to know values. This is a limitation that is important to acknowledge. Given the fact that, as an individual, my knowing facts or values is limited, how should I respond to others who challenge my claims? Far from being defensive, a fitting acknowledgment of the corrective influence of the wisdom of a community is for me to welcome challenges with gratitude. For they are important contributions to my own faltering efforts to achieve evaluative authenticity.

11 What I mean by immediate, by contrast with mediate, is that there is some presupposed *identity* between the cognitive act of feeling and the content grasped in this act. I take this to be Hume's position, as I described it in chapter 3. What I do not wish to deny is that mediate knowing can occur in a temporally rapid manner, as in 'love at first sight.' The fact that the stories of both Sue and Dennis can be characterized as documentaries of personal growth suggests to me that feelings are part of a discernment process, one that can even take years. In other words, mediate knowing involves a process that is far more complex than an initial reaction to some object or possibility.

12 In my view, differences among thinkers on this and other ethical issues can be most sharply located by their differing answers to this third question.

13 Kaye, *Laugh, I Thought I'd Die* 208.

14 Another incident in which the devaluation of another ALS sufferer had interpersonal implications for Dennis was the story of Aleza, which I related in chapter 2. She was hospitalized with ALS near the end of her life and was mistreated by the staff, who all assumed that she was mentally handicapped rather than merely physically handicapped. There is no question in Dennis's mind that the 'raw personal nerve' this story touched in him was compatible with his evaluation that treating Aleza more appropriately would really have 'made a world of difference' to her and her husband. That is, Dennis's view opposes the stance that *personal* or first-person involvement in an issue necessarily is a disadvantage, or makes one's judgments or evaluations suspect. Because of his empathy for Aleza, and his feelings of indignation that her story aroused in him, it seems that he was even more convinced in his negative evaluation about how she was treated. The 'personal raw nerve' her story touched in him motivated him to add a further chapter to his book, which was expressly on the facts of ALS, and implicitly, I think, on the value of treating those afflicted by this condition with the respect that is their due.

15 Hobbs Birnie and Rodriguez, *Uncommon Will* 116.

16 In the debate about the ethics of euthanasia, this question also lies behind Beauchamp's concerns about the possibility of others genuinely knowing whether someone else's evaluation that his or her life is not worth living is true or not. I will explore this issue further in section 9.4.

17 Note that there might be some equivocation in Sue's thinking about 'constraints.' One can be legally at liberty but morally constrained to act or not to act (e.g., rescue a drowning child if this could be done without grave risk to oneself). Her stance seems to be that she is morally at liberty to kill herself, but legally constrained. This begs the question.

18 More specifically, some X is choiceworthy because it is deemed to be not a just possible good, but a concretely possible good, rather than a just abstractly possible good. And just as one's knowing the good can be authentic or inauthentic, one's choosing the good that is known can be positive or privative. To 'operate responsibly,' then, means not only to make an authentic value judgment but also to choose positively and execute this choice, if pertinent. For instance, I judged that treating Paul's AMI with streptokinase would bring about a concretely possible good. A positive or privative choice regarding whether to recommend this option to Paul and, if he agreed, to carry it out would characterize my fourth-level operation as either responsible or irresponsible. For these terminological precisions, see Michael Vertin, 'Lonergan's Metaphysics of Value and Love: Some Proposed Clarifications and Implications,' *Lonergan Workshop* 13 (1997) 189–219; esp. n. 20.

19 On relating Frederick Crowe's discussion of complacency and concern to passive and active willing, see Vertin, 'Lonergan's Metaphysics' n. 20.

20 A counter-argument might be that Sue's legal right to physician-assisted

suicide would actually impose a duty on people who are dying to choose physician-assisted suicide.

21 If this deliberative syllogism adequately expresses the content of Sue's value judgment, her position becomes much less convincing than when it is expressed in terms of a philosophical position regarding the freedom to choose what one deems to be good. But this emphasis on the act of choosing merely obscures the key evaluative issues. Although the value judgment that her life was 'not worth living' was perhaps a persuasive argument for suicide, it was clearly not Sue's only argument, nor can one be sure that it actually articulates what she felt. For instance, she also speaks about this decision as being forced upon her by the fear of dying *in extremis* from ALS, concerns about the negative effects of 'lingering on in life' on her son, and the burden and pain that her lingering is causing others. Although the media and ethicists frequently cite the first reason in justifying euthanasia, namely, 'If life is not worth living, then one can ethically choose to kill oneself,' in Sue's case this account did not seem to do justice to what she actually thought and felt.

22 Lonergan's view is that the key element on the fourth level is the deliberative insight, which issues first in the evaluation or value judgment, and second, at best, in the act of choosing. That is, the deliberative insight is the ground of both, but first the evaluation, and second the choice. One might analyse the elements of a deliberative insight by distinguishing the responsible unity that Dennis grasped in some diversity. In its bare logical form, there are three elements: (a) the possible value judgment, (b) the link of that possible value judgment to its responsible conditions, and (c) the concretely possible fulfilment of those conditions. For example, 'If writing a chapter on ALS would help to avoid the mistreatment of ALS patients, then one should write such a chapter.' 'But writing such a chapter would help to prevent the mistreatment of ALS patients.' 'Therefore, I should write such a chapter.' The deliberative insight's impulsion to value judgment, or the 'therefore' that follows from grasping (b) the conditioned 'if ..., then ...' link, and (c) the fulfilment of those conditions, stands out when one puts the foregoing pattern into bare logical form. Also, the deliberative insight grasps not just this latter link, but also the initial 'if ..., then ...' link.

23 Lonergan, *Method* 31, 48–52.

24 Hobbs Birnie and Rodriguez, *Uncommon Will* 138.

25 Sue seems to agree with others who fail to distinguish her ontic value from her qualitative values. Rather than challenging these views, she simply seeks to respond to them by expanding the legal options for persons facing end-of-life decisions. In contrast, Dennis seems to reject such an evaluation as a slight to persons, such as himself, or other ALS sufferers, such as Sue or Aleza.

26   I could press this same point further by tracing the links between this negative evaluation and Sue's core values. In broad outline, I would begin by
suggesting that one's core values come to light when they are challenged in
such a way that one experiences a personal crisis, as seems to have been the
case for Sue. The sort of core values that were challenged by this illness were
values such as power, independence, physical beauty, youth, and motherhood – core values that I suspect were widely shared by those most sympathetic toward her evaluation, if not also her decision. By contrast, although
Dennis surely suffered from the loss of similar values, his illness became for
him an opportunity to focus his attention on his cognitive life and family
relationships, and I would suggest that these emerged as his core values.

27   What I am assuming is that both Dennis and Sue are persons of *integrity*, as it
has been characterized by R. Hepburn. For Hepburn: 'To have integrity is to
have unconditional and steady commitment to moral values and obligations.
For such a person, the fundamental question whether to conduct life on the
plane of self-concern or of moral seriousness has been decisively resolved,
though particular life situations will doubtless continue to put that commitment to strenuous test.' See Honderich, ed., *Oxford Companion to Philosophy*,
s.v. 'Integrity,' by R.W. Hepburn.

28   This was the story of the elderly woman who fed Dennis one day when he
rested by the Shannon River during a cycling trip in Ireland. See Kaye,
Laugh, I Thought I'd Die 100.

29   Perhaps the clearest example of his position is his characterization of his
caring community as his true 'life-support system.'

30   Lonergan, *Method* 31.

31   For Lonergan, religious values are 'at the heart of the meaning and value of
man's living and man's world.' See ibid. 32.

32   Recall that the reason she would not agree to palliative care was her distrust
of physicians and her fear of losing control. She believed, to my dismay as a
physician, that palliative-care physicians would merely keep her alive in a
'drugged-out' twilight, which would be of no value to herself and would
make her an object of horror to others. See Hobbs Birnie and Rodriguez,
Uncommon Will 130–31.

33   It is important that one not confuse an aesthetic judgment and a moral
judgment, both of which are fourth-level evaluations for Lonergan. The
difference between the two arises when one asks whether a more aesthetically pleasing death is necessarily a better one. One might also wonder
whether, or to what degree, one's moral assessment of Sue's suicide would
change if one could eliminate any aesthetic difference between her natural
death from ALS and her death by physician-assisted suicide.

34   Again, to highlight the importance of certain cognitions that are characteristically affective, such as deliberative insights, as properly cognitive responses

that grasp values, in no way need diminish or undermine the importance of other intellectual cognitions, such as direct or reflective insights.

35 To express the same point in medical terms, my diagnostic performance as a general physician will doubtless be less than optimal if, for instance, I never physically examine patients. On the other hand, I may be very clear about the methodology of clinical practice, but still be rash or overly hesitant in my diagnoses.

36 The fact that this has not been identified as an ethical issue in the way that Sue's request for assistance in euthanasia was, suggests to me that the public, at least, does not think that Sue or Dennis were culpable for what I would label an 'allowing-to-die' decision. Nor does there seem to be any evidence from Dennis's story that this decision followed from any negative self-evaluation such as that his life was 'not worth living,' or that he in any way denied that his life was a 'basic good.' As I will point out later when treating some of the ethical and legislative discussion of the difference between killing and allowing to die, these reflections are curiously abstracted from concrete examples such as Sue's and Dennis's.

37 The reason why this evaluation is more difficult to assess is precisely because the issue is essentially an evaluative one, and so it involves the person who makes the evaluation. The other issues are matters of empirical judgments, which are easier to assess. Indeed, I think the main reason why the euthanasia debate is such a difficult one for people is that they, and even ethicists, have little appreciation for and critical control over evaluative judgments, at least by contrast with fact judgments.

38 For example, in chapter 2 I related another option suggested by a physician. He mentioned the possibility of respiratory support, such as a respirator, to relieve any sense of suffocating or choking. At some later point when Sue no longer felt her life was worthwhile, she could simply stop the respirator, which would make her case similar to Nancy B's, and hence involve an action that is within the law.

39 This is Tom Beauchamp's argument, which I will outline further in the next section.

40 Canada, Special Senate Committee on Euthanasia and Assisted Suicide, *Of Life and Death* 89.

41 One way into the debate is to force disputants to answer this question themselves. If they claim ignorance, then ask them about whether they think any life is worth living, including their own. The point of this is to challenge persons to locate the issue as one of making an evaluation, and then to press them to make at least one such evaluation in their own name.

42 Harvey Max Chochinov et al., 'Desire for Death in the Terminally Ill,' *American Journal of Psychiatry* 152 (1995) 1185–91.

43 On the legislative level of the debate, I have chosen to compare and contrast

the views of those holding the majority position with those holding the minority position in the Special Senate Committee, which I reported in chapter 2. The identity of the particular members on either side of this debate is not, to my knowledge, part of the public record. Although I suspect they have their reasons for not making their identities part of the public record, not knowing the identity of proponents and opponents adds to the slipperiness of the debate. This is not only because it is difficult to examine the underlying philosophical stances of individuals, but also because the pronouncements of a committee carry with them an air of authority, distinct from what Lonergan would refer to as authenticity. This semblance of authority is something of which members of an ethics committee will be well aware.

44 Richard McCormick, 'Killing and Allowing to Die: *Vive la Différence*,' *1997 Chancellor's Lecture* (Regis College, University of Toronto, 21 November 1997), published in *America* 177 (6 Dec. 1997) 6–12. Throughout the present discussion, I have sought to match opposing views on the euthanasia debate in order to compare and contrast the philosophical and empirical grounds of their positions. The point of this is to locate better where the differences lie between disputants on the evaluative issues at stake. This approach is in sharp contrast to James Rachels's methodology, in which he contrasts positions based on different decisions stemming from similar evaluations to conclude that there is no ethical difference between killing and allowing to die (see note 63 below).

45 To summarize, Beauchamp claims that 'persons in search of physician-assisted suicide, the person who seeks active euthanasia, and the person who forgoes life-sustaining treatment to end life are identically situated' (374). He also locates the key ethical issue underpinning these decisions at the cognitive level of deliberating on whether 'lingering in life is, on balance, worse than death' (371). As a further methodological point, he adds that it is *the person in question* who is best situated to decide whether bringing about one's own death 'causes them a loss or, rather, provides a benefit.' From this it seems clear, at least, that Beauchamp is prepared not only to admit the possibility of such an evaluation of one's own life, but also that it can be a normative evaluation, and hence, one that he would himself affirm. If this is true, then this places him in the awkward position of having to highlight the criteria that he thinks would condition such an evaluation (i.e., what kind of suffering does he think would make my life not worth living?). See Tom Beauchamp, 'Refusals of Treatment and Requests for Death,' *Kennedy Institute of Ethics Journal* 6 (1996) 371–74.

46 This is, of course, a somewhat tentative conclusion, given that Beauchamp does not label these personal elements as *feelings* or spell out their cognitive role in evaluations.

47 The difficulty of assessing evaluations, such as those made by Sue Rodriguez,

highlights the need to explore philosophically the role of affect. Philosophers and ethicists tend to emphasize the role of understanding and judgment in making decisions, and apply their critical tools to these cognitive
elements. But Beauchamp's stance on this issue reveals, I think, a general
neglect of the topic of affect among even contemporary ethicists who nevertheless seem to be convinced of its importance. Consequently, there are no
ready philosophical tools that would allow for some critical control of the
affective grounds of evaluations, and so one ends up with the Humean
position that values are merely personal feelings.

48 Recall Sue's surprise to learn that her predecessors' motto was 'I shall never
be content with idle stillness.' In this connection, her recurring dream was
about being held prisoner by some man for what seemed like years, unable
to escape, and in the company of others who were also being held captive.
Without claiming any expertise at dream interpretation, I wonder if these
images bear on the theme of the relation of the individual and social good.
Both are determined by cultural factors, including biases, that are often
beyond the capacity of most individuals even to recognize, much less to free
themselves successfully from. See Hobbs Birnie and Rodriguez, *Uncommon
Will* 136.

49 As McCormick puts it, 'I think Beauchamp is vulnerable to the accusation
that he confuses causality and culpability (this latter under the title of
authorization).' See McCormick, 'Killing and Allowing to Die' 10.

50 As I indicated in chapter 3, feelings have always been associated more closely
with *the body* than with *the mind* in the mind/body debate. In this regard,
Lonergan's view of affective cognitions as being, in some sense, more *spiritual* than intellectual acts places him within a distinct historical tradition that
I expect McCormick would also be sympathetic toward.

51 See McCormick, 'Killing and Allowing to Die' 12.

52 See Honderich, ed., *Oxford Companion to Philosophy*, s.v. 'Suicide,' by Tom
Beauchamp.

53 It is a 'generalized' empirical method because the data to which such a
method attends includes data of consciousness, and not just of sense.

54 To admit that feelings play a role in evaluations is not necessarily to endorse
them or the role they actually play. In fact, although Lonergan's stance on
the role of certain feelings in evaluations is a very positive one, I have found
that when I actually examine the role that others attribute to affective elements, such as compassion, there is such confusion about them that I risk
sounding overly critical of all feelings.

55 I refer the reader to my earlier discussion of this report in chapter 2. To
summarize, a minority of members recommended that 'the *Criminal Code* be
amended to permit voluntary euthanasia for competent individuals who are
physically incapable of committing assisted suicide' (88). In explaining this

381 Notes to pages 262–64

recommendation they appealed to several ethical notions. For instance, they thought that if they allowed assisted suicide, in favour of which they all argued, they would also have to allow euthanasia in order not to violate the *equality* argument in section 15 of the Charter of Rights. They also appealed to the principle of *autonomy*, which they interpreted as justifying the with-holding and withdrawing of life-sustaining treatment. From this, they reasoned that the same principle justifies permitting voluntary euthanasia on the basis of competent patients' wishes (where competence involves meeting intellectual criteria). This is because they denied any ethically important distinction between the status of acts of providing treatment to alleviate suffering that may hasten death, on the one hand, and voluntary euthanasia, on the other. The relevant point of similarity between these two acts, for them, was the foreseeable consequence of the death of the patient (87). Canada, Special Senate Committee Report, *Of Life and Death.*

56 See ibid. 86. Lonergan, I think, would use the language of *responsibilities* rather than *rights*, and in so doing challenge the presumption that the human good involves some essential opposition between the goods of the individual and those of the community.

57 Ibid. 87.

58 See the appendix, figure A.4, on the types of particular and general claims for Lonergan.

59 Note the strained logic of the equality argument. Because suicide has been removed from the Criminal Code of Canada (for obvious practical reasons), the assumption now is that society's physicians ought to help some people to commit suicide, even though this is still against the law. Hence, these same physicians are accused of treating others, like Sue, unfairly by not offering her similar help with her suicide plans.

60 Canada, Special Senate Committee Report, *Of Life and Death* 72.

61 Ibid. 87.

62 Ibid. 72.

63 Rachels's article first appeared in the *New England Journal of Medicine* 2 (1975) 78–80. In this very influential article, Rachels, who at the time was a professor of philosophy at the University of Alabama, takes on the medical establish-ment. He does this by criticizing the view common among physicians and endorsed by the House of Delegates of the American Medical Association. In Rachels's words, this mistaken view is that 'it is permissible, at least in some cases, to withhold treatment and allow a patient to die, but it is never per-missible to take any direct action designed to kill the patient' (385). He claims to refute successfully the underlying distinction between killing and allowing to die. He does this by appealing to invented cases, such as that of an unscrupulous uncle who plans to drown his six-year-old nephew in a bathtub in order to gain a large inheritance. The apparent ethical insight he

grasps in this case is that there is no ethical difference between the following two scenarios: in the first the uncle causes the death by deciding actively to drown the child; in the second the uncle decides not to rescue his nephew when he accidentally slips in the tub, is rendered unconscious, and begins to drown. He argues that in both cases the uncle is ethically culpable. Based on this case, Rachels rightly concludes that active causality, by itself, does not determine ethical culpability. But he then draws the non sequitur conclusion that, since the decision to 'allow to die' and 'killing' in this case both involve the 'intentional termination of life,' there is no ethical difference between these two decisions in any other case. See James Rachels, 'Active and Passive Euthanasia,' in Thomas Mappes and Jane Zembaty, eds, *Biomedical Ethics* (New York: McGraw-Hill Book Co., 1986) 385–88.

64 Canada, Special Senate Committee Report, *Of Life and Death* 87.

65 For instance, this treatment might bankrupt my family of its resources or, if everyone chose this treatment, society of its resources. Indeed, only a vitalist position would argue that I would always be culpable for not choosing some life-sustaining treatment, and this view is not well represented in the euthanasia debate.

66 See the appendix, figure A.4, for a set of increasingly general empirical claims that would be consistent with Lonergan's analysis.

Chapter 10

1 To be more precise, I would distinguish between the epistemic objectivity of value judgments for Kant and for John Finnis. If Kant's position on moral knowing is understood in the framework of the *Second Critique*, the objectivity of evaluations is merely practical. By contrast, for someone like Finnis, epistemic objectivity is genuine or speculative, and not merely practical. My point is that for both Kant and Finnis this moral objectivity is achieved by escaping the subjectivity of feelings, which puts them both at odds with Lonergan's view that at least some affective acts have cognitive significance.

2 Such a contribution to this debate, and to bioethics generally, is independent of whether thinkers agree with Lonergan's particular stances on these issues.

3 Lonergan, *Method* 37.

4 What I have labelled *philosophical* questions are actually also empirical inasmuch as they are answered by attending to the data of my own cognitive performance when I am engaged in knowing something. This is not to be understood in a Cartesian sense of the mind looking back at itself. Rather, it involves a heightened awareness of my own cognitive operations as I am engaged in knowing some object (i.e., a matter of objectifying my own subjectivity). Purely philosophical questions regard the transcendentals, which

my own cognitive processes presuppose. On the distinction between the approaches of Lonergan and the Idealist, see figure A.1 of the appendix.

5 In proffering any answer to such questions, one takes at least a performative stance on the cognitional and decisional issues Lonergan outlines. Making one's own performance explicit is a distinct task, and is also not a necessary condition for providing an adequate reply. What I have pointed out, however, is that this knowledge can certainly be of some advantage in distinguishing alternative replies, and even in formulating a better response oneself.

6 Some philosophers might label this as the *empiricist* family. I have decided not to use this label in order to avoid confusing it with how I have been using empirical in contrast to philosophical. On this account, 'empirical' has to do with objects but in no way is this in opposition to subjectivity. I also wonder if a similar perspective informs the previously mentioned view of the U.S. Ninth Circuit Court of Appeals, which rejected the reality of the distinction between killing and allowing to die. If what they mean by *real* is determined by sense experience, and the result in both cases is similar at the level of sense experience (i.e., a dead corpse), then they cannot be convinced that there is a real distinction.

7 I wonder if Beauchamp's view is not a more nuanced version of the same family. That is, I wonder whether the *person in question* for him is forever a question because, in principle, one cannot know another's foreign consciousness.

8 A better example of this third family is John Finnis, who expressly locates feelings as of just psychological importance. From the perspective of the euthanasia debate, this view is at odds with others on both sides of the debate in their answers to Lonergan's first question, 'Are feelings ever cognitively relevant.' On this issue, they seem to have few analytical tools to engage the problem on this level, or even to begin to appreciate 'the reasons of the heart.' From Lonergan's perspective, facility on these issues is the hallmark of the ethicist, whose task it is to bring to light all relevant features of the moral life.

9 I hasten to add that I am not the first to suggest that Lonergan's philosophical contributions have ramifications for designing a research program on an ethical issue, although I am perhaps the first to begin to work this out for studying the ethics of euthanasia from Lonergan's perspective. For instance, thinkers at the Woodstock Theological Center have devised a research program to study the business aspects of health care using Lonergan's methodology. James O'Connor, the director of the Center, distinguishes the four steps of this methodology, of which the reader will by now be familiar: experiencing, understanding, judging, and evaluating, deciding and doing. The Center developed a consensus statement on ethical considerations in

the business aspects of heath care during a business-ethics seminar involving about 40 participants chosen for their pre-eminence in their fields of health care. The seminar involved the group in addressing four distinct issues: (1) attending to the data, both in the realms of our experience (treating patients in this case) and in ourselves (what are we feeling, thinking, questioning, wondering, etc.); (2) understanding what is really going on (in the business of health care in this case); (3) passing judgment ('health care is ...'); and (4) discerning, deciding, and doing. This last step involved persons in an exercise of ranking maxims and reaching agreement on the more important goods. These were described in terms of the complementarity of virtues or values that health-care workers needed to cultivate in themselves. They then sought to decide what were the goods for which the health-care worker is most responsible. The doing step involved developing recommendations for courses of action. As I read this research program, the level of evidence is that which a medical person would identify as *expert opinion*. The ideal program, however, might strive for higher levels of empirical evidence, such as prospective quantitative and qualitative studies. See James Connor, 'Business Aspects of Health Care and Woodstock Methodology,' Woodstock Theological Center, Georgetown University, Washington, written for the Center's website, March 1996. The report is in Woodstock Theological Center Seminar in Business Ethics, *Ethical Considerations in the Business Aspects of Health Care* (Washington: Georgetown University Press, 1995).

10 The Special Senate Committee on Euthanasia and Assisted Suicide raised some of these questions in their recommendations. For instance, the majority recommended that 'research be undertaken into how many are requesting assisted suicide, why it is being requested, and whether there are any alternatives that might be acceptable to those who are making the requests.' Important though they are, answers to these questions would not address the further concerns of fact and of value about the proposed new situation. See Canada, Special Senate Committee, *Of Life and Death* 74.

11 An answer has already been agreed on in such policies as those regarding capital punishment, which is also an empirical, evaluative question.

12 The reason Beauchamp and others are so reluctant to make an evaluation about some *person in question* is, I think, because they recognize that such evaluations always involve one personally, and this makes them more insecure than when making mere fact judgments. What I have tried to point out, however, is that even in the latter case one is involved personally, though not affectively. The best response is not to flee from such evaluations for fear that one's evaluations are merely subjective because they involve one personally. Rather, the best response is to recognize such evaluations for what they are and to own one's evaluations as expressions of one's core values.

13 I think the Woodstock Center's research project in the area of health-care business ethics provides a very impressive model of research that illustrates the ramifications of Lonergan's philosophy. The Center has also demonstrated the practical effectiveness of such a project. The members of this project are clear about the underlying philosophical issues, have expressly faced and answered these questions individually and as a community of scholars, have devised a research methodology that addresses a comprehensive range of relevant questions in a certain order, and have explicitly integrated the answers to these questions to arrive at a decision and plan of action. To my knowledge, no other research project has had such an overall unity of vision, purpose, and objective ends and means. If this is truly the case, Lonergan's philosophy has huge ramifications not only for any particular research project, but even for the evaluative task of determining which projects are in most urgent need of research.

14 Note that the biblical story of the judgment of Solomon provides an illustration of *empirical* verification that does not involve an *empiricist* view of reality. In this story, Solomon was faced with the task of resolving a dispute over contested maternity. His hypothesis seems to have been that the genuine mother would not allow him to kill her son for the sake of settling a dispute. To test his hypothesis, Solomon ordered: '"Cut the living child in two ... and give half to one and half to the other.' At this the woman who was the mother of the living child addressed the king, for she burned with pity for her son. 'If it please you, my lord,' she said, 'let them give her the child; only do not let them think of killing it!' But the other said, 'He shall belong to neither of us. Cut him up.'" Solomon was able to verify empirically the genuine mother by noting her response to his proposal, and contrasting it with that of the other woman, who claimed to be the mother. The point is that although Solomon answered this question of maternity by appealing to empirical evidence – the two responses of the women to his proposal that the child be killed – this in no way implies that Solomon held what philosophers would regard as an *empiricist* view of reality. In fact, the empirical data he contrasts is that of distinct decisions and words, which correspond to distinct underlying evaluations of the life of the child. See Ted Honderich, ed., *The Oxford Companion to Philosophy*, s.v. 'Empiricism,' by Alan Lacey, and *The Jerusalem Bible*, 1 Kings 3:16–28. I am indebted to Frederick Crowe for pointing out this biblical example of empirical verification in private conversation.

15 My own explicit efforts to distinguish among four families of positions, and locate my own position in the fourth family with Dennis Kaye, illustrates a way of engaging one's own philosophical presuppositions, beginning with those of others.

16 Some of the research results that I mentioned in chapter 2 are surely

relevant to the deliberations of policy-makers. This might include important empirical research being done in medicine. See, e.g., Council on Scientific Affairs, American Medical Association, 'Good Care of the Dying Patient,' *JAMA* 275 (1996) 475; Harvey Max Chochinov et al., 'Desire for Death in the Terminally Ill,' *American Journal of Psychiatry* 152 (1995): 1185–91. As important as such research is to these questions, it is also important that policy-makers are aware of the types of claims such research can support, and of when researchers are venturing philosophical opinions that their empirical evidence might not support.

17 Most people agree that our society has a responsibility to provide adequate care for its members at the end of life. In fact, in 1995 the Special Senate Committee on Euthanasia and Assisted Suicide recommended that more resources be directed toward improving the care of the dying, especially through supporting palliative-care programs. Despite these good intentions, according to the director of one of Canada's longest-running and largest palliative-care services, not only has this promised support not yet arrived, but support has actually been withdrawn. This state of affairs makes one suspect that there are other issues and values at play behind the euthanasia debate, most obviously issues of distributive justice in health care.

18 I say *human* response to leave open the possibility of a shift in horizons that is more than the previously discussed shift from self-concern to moral serious-ness. What I have in mind is a story that Robert Doran reported during the discussion period following my presentation of Sue Rodriguez's life at an early stage in the development of my thought on the issue. He spoke of working with a young person with AIDS who, in the depths of despair and anxiety, decided he would end his life. His friends tried their best to help him, but to no avail. But some time before he actually turned his hand against himself, he had some deep experience that completely changed his outlook. After this experience and until his death he was a different person, at peace with himself and others. Spiritual guides might label such an ex-perience a *religious conversion*. Whatever this experience was, it illustrates that there are affective and spiritual dimensions of this problem that might not even be part of our contemporary vocabulary. It also highlights the theme of the *moving viewpoint* that was evident in both Sue Rodriguez's and Dennis Kaye's story. When deliberating about these issues, it might be important to remind ourselves that our own viewpoints on dying and living are apt to be challenged by these stories, as well as by our own experiences of our mor-tality. Discussion following Bill Sullivan, 'Lonergan and the Role of Feelings in Moral Knowledge,' Lonergan Research Institute Graduate Seminar, Regis College Toronto, 17 October 1991.

19 *Jerusalem Bible*, 1 Kings 3:28.

20 Honderich, ed., *Oxford Companion to Philosophy*, s.v. 'Justice,' by Edward Sankowski.

21 Reading some of the legal reasoning in Sue Rodriguez's case, a not uncommon view was that although Sue was proposing to commit an avoidable harm to herself, she would be neither *morally constrained* to avoid this nor would she (and her collaborators) be morally culpable for proceeding with this plan. Given this assessment of her request, it is understandable that some judges believed that *legally* constraining her (and others) from acting on this suicide plan would be without moral justification, and would therefore be unjust.

22 To link this discussion to the role of affect in evaluations, consider how self-transcending responses both conform to the demands of justice and also ground our notions of the structure of the human good. One example of this is the remarkable fund-raising success of institutions such as the Hospital for Sick Children, Toronto. I would suggest that their success is due, in part, to persons affectively responding to some unarticulated demand of justice with respect to dying or ill children. I would identify this as an instance of a self-transcending response to some important element of the invariant structure of the good. Some such response, I expect, also underpins the views of morally serious individuals on both sides of this debate. A key goal of a research program would be to identify systematically and relate the values to which persons are responding, and so help to ensure that our policies express not a moral idealism, but rather a concretely realizable human good.

23 Daniel Callahan, 'Professional Morality: Can an Examined Life Be Lived?' foreword to L.W. Sumner and Joseph Boyle, eds, *Philosophical Perspectives on Bioethics* (Toronto: University of Toronto Press, 1996) 9–17.

24 Lonergan, *Method* 76.

25 See, e.g., F.W. Hafferty, *Into the Valley: Death and Socialization of Medical Students* (New Haven, CT: Yale University Press, 1991).

26 James Christopher and Roderick Macleod, 'The Problematic Nature of Education in Palliative Care,' *Journal of Palliative Care* 9 (1993) 5–10, at 8.

27 Although describing them is beyond the scope of the present discussion, my own experience in applying these affective insights has been very positive. I think this is partly because I am convinced that it is not merely a matter of good manners to attend to the affective components of evaluations. Rather, it is crucial to understanding the values and concerns a person is expressing, even in their moments of despair.

28 See H. Thompson Prout and Randy Cole, 'Individual Counselling Approaches,' in Douglas Strohmer and H. Thompson Prout, eds, *Counselling and Psychotherapy with Persons with Mental Retardation and Borderline Intelligence* (Brandon, VT: Clinical Psychology Publishing Co., 1994) 136–37.

29 I have become convinced of the value of the final phase of one's life not from any arguments that I have heard, but from the experiences of persons for whom I have cared. I also expect that this is the reason that those physi-

cians who are most critical of the assisted-suicide movement are those who specialize in palliative care. Of all physicians, they are in a position to witness the remarkable personal growth of patients at the end of life, and the gift of healing that they can effect in others. Nevertheless, I am also aware that this experience is shaped by a number of factors, including one's ability to accept a series of losses. Despite the caregiver's best efforts to inspire hope, as Shavelson concludes, 'people tend to die the way they live.' See Lonny Shavelson, *A Chosen Death: The Dying Confront Assisted Suicide* (New York: Simon & Schuster, 1995) 38.

30 Since these objects are distinct, one's responses to them need never be in conflict. Still, it is one thing to make this distinction in the first place, and another to get the sufferer to grasp it. For example, an HIV-infected person might react to the news of their infection in several ways. For instance, the person might say that his or her life is over and they might as well commit suicide. Or that person might refuse to acknowledge their risk to others and fail to make any lifestyle changes or to inform prospective sexual partners of their HIV status. One might distinguish one's sympathetic and understanding response to this person from one's response to what they say or decide to do. A further challenge for a skilled counsellor is to help this person to grasp this distinction. And even if one is not successful in doing this, that does not undermine the validity of the distinction itself.

31 Sue's family doctor, Dr Donald Lovely, gave evidence in his affidavit that was later quoted at length in the dissenting opinion of Chief Justice Allan McEachern at the British Columbia Court of Appeal. Lovely mentions what I interpret him to consider to be 'morally obligatory care,' such as suctioning patients to remove oral secretions on which they might choke, turning patients to prevent pressure sores, and attending to their urinary and bowel care to keep them clean. Beyond these responses are more technical responses, such as feeding tubes, tracheostomies, and respirators, which he says are options that patients might elect to have. Given Lonergan's analysis, it is evident that even if Dr Lovely was simply reporting the facts of the disease and what is commonly done for it, all responses to the various medical problems involve a subsequent evaluation, some of which are widely judged to be appropriate (even obligatory), and others to be non-obligatory (hence, they are up to patients to accept or reject). See Hobbs Birnie and Rodriguez, *Uncommon Will* 61.

32 This case was similar, in some ways, to Tracy Latimer's case, except that both of Tracy's parents were opposed to the proposed surgical intervention.

33 A key point in the decision-making of someone at the end of life is when to forgo active medical treatment aimed at reversing the illness. In Sue's own story, she decided to end her life when it became clear that further therapies were ineffective. Perhaps her own thinking was constrained by the false

alternatives of deciding between 'doing' either x or y, without deliberating on the further possibility of simply 'allowing' z to happen. This distinction between 'doing' something and 'allowing' some process to unfold also has implications for the debate over the apparent moral equivalency of decisions to omit life-saving or life-sustaining treatments and decisions actively to kill oneself. The key issue is the underlying evaluation, such as whether a less than 'perfect' life is worth living. Although some decisions to forgo certain treatments might follow from such a negative evaluation of one's life, I would argue that they do not necessarily follow such an evaluation. Cardinal Bernardin illustrated this possibility in his own medical decision-making at the end of his life. He decided to forgo chemotherapy treatments for his cancer when it became clear that they were not helpful and were also quite burdensome. He expressed this decision as choosing 'life without the burden of disproportionate medical intervention,' and not as stemming from an evaluation that his life was not worth living. See Jan Crawford Greenburg, 'Affirm Life, Not Suicide, Bernardin Tells Justices,' *Chicago Tribune*, 12 Nov. 1996, web-posted 14 Nov. 1996 at http://www.chicago .tribune.com/news/bern/extras/suicide.htm.

Bibliography

Works by Bernard Lonergan

Collection: Papers by Bernard Lonergan, S.J. Vol. 4 of Collected Works of Bernard Lonergan. Edited by Frederick E. Crowe and Robert M. Doran. Toronto: University of Toronto Press, 1988.

'Critical Realism and the Integration of the Sciences.' Transcript of six lectures given at University College, Dublin, Ireland, May 1962. Toronto: Archives, Lonergan Research Institute. File 253.

Insight: A Study of Human Understanding. Vol. 3 of Collected Works of Bernard Lonergan. Edited by Frederick E. Crowe and Robert M. Doran. Toronto: University of Toronto Press, 1992.

Method in Theology. London: Darton, Longman & Todd; New York: Herder and Herder, 1972.

'Milltown Park Lectures on *Method in Theology*.' Transcript by N. Graham of lectures given in 1971 at Milltown Park, Dublin, Ireland. Toronto: Archives, Lonergan Research Institute. File 641.

'The Original Preface of *Insight*.' *Method: Journal of Lonergan Studies* 3 (1985) 3–7.

Phe.nomenology and Logic: The Boston College Lectures on Mathematical Logic and Existentialism. Vol. 18 of Collected Works of Bernard Lonergan. Edited by Philip J. McShane. Toronto: University of Toronto Press, 2001.

Philosophical and Theological Papers 1958–1964. Vol. 6 of Collected Works of Bernard Lonergan. Edited by Robert C. Croken, Frederick E. Crowe, and Robert M. Doran. Toronto: University of Toronto Press, 1996.

'Questionnaire on Philosophy.' *Method: Journal of Lonergan Studies* 2 (1984) 1–35. Reprinted in *Philosophical and Theological Papers 1965–1980.* Vol. 17 of Collected Works of Bernard Lonergan. Edited by Robert C. Croken and Robert M. Doran. Toronto: University of Toronto Press, 2004.

A Second Collection: Papers by Bernard Lonergan, S.J. Edited by William F. Ryan and
    Bernard J. Tyrrell. London: Darton, Longman & Todd; Philadelphia: West-
    minster, 1974.
Topics in Education: The Cincinnati Lectures of 1959 on the Philosophy of Education. Vol.
    10 of Collected Works of Bernard Lonergan. Edited by Robert M. Doran and
    Frederick E. Crowe from the unpublished text prepared by James Quinn and
    John Quinn. Toronto: University of Toronto Press, 1990.
A Third Collection: Papers by Bernard Lonergan, S.J. Edited by Frederick E. Crowe. New
    York: Paulist Press; London: Geoffrey Chapman, 1985.
Understanding and Being: An Introduction and Companion to Insight. Vol. 5 of Col-
    lected Works of Bernard Lonergan. Edited by Frederick E. Crowe, Elizabeth A.
    Morelli, Mark D. Morelli, Robert M. Doran, and Thomas V. Daley. Toronto:
    University of Toronto Press, 1990.
Verbum: Word and Idea in Aquinas. Vol. 2 of Collected Works of Bernard Lonergan.
    Edited by Frederick E. Crowe and Robert M. Doran. Toronto: University of
    Toronto Press, 1997.
'What Are Judgments of Value?' Typescript by Nicholas Graham of lectures given
    at the Massachusetts Institute of Technology, May 1972. Toronto: Archives,
    Lonergan Research Institute. File 695. Reprinted in *Philosophical and Theological
    Papers 1965–1980.* Vol. 17 of Collected Works of Bernard Lonergan. Edited by
    Robert C. Croken and Robert M. Doran. Toronto: University of Toronto Press,
    2004.

Works About or Influenced by Bernard Lonergan

Byrne, Patrick. 'Analogical Knowledge of God and the Value of Moral Endeavor.'
    Method: Journal of Lonergan Studies 11 (1993) 103–35.
Canadian Encyclopedia, 1988 ed. S.v. 'Lonergan,' by William Fennell.
Chambers Biographical Dictionary, 1996 ed. S.v. 'Lonergan,' by Magnus Magnusson.
Conn, Walter. 'The Desire for Authenticity: Conscience and Moral Conversion.' In
    The Desires of the Human Heart: An Introduction to the Theology of Bernard Lonergan,
    edited by Vernon Gregson. Mahwah, NJ: Paulist Press, 1988.
Crowe, Frederick. 'Complacency and Concern in the Thought of St. Thomas
    Aquinas.' *Theological Studies* 20 (1959) 1–39, 198–230, 343–95. Reprinted in *Three
    Thomist Studies,* ed. Michael Vertin, 71–203. Supplementary issue of *Lonergan
    Workshop,* vol. 16. Boston: Lonergan Institute of Boston College, 2000.
– 'Dialectic and the Ignatian *Spiritual Exercises.*' In *Appropriating the Longeran Idea,*
    edited by Michael Vertin. Washington: Catholic University of America Press, 1989.
– 'The Galilean World-view and Its Modern Echoes.' *Lonergan Review: A Multi-
    disciplinary Journal* 3 (1994): 113–143.
– 'Lonergan's "Moral Theology and the Human Sciences": Editor's Introduction.'
    Method: Journal of Lonergan Studies 15 (1997) 1–3.

- 'Lonergan's New Notion of Value.' In *Appropriating the Lonergan Idea*, edited by Michael Vertin, 51–70. Washington: Catholic University of America Press, 1989.
- 'Rethinking Moral Judgments: Categories from Lonergan.' *Science et Esprit* 40 (1988) 137–52.

Doran, Robert. *Theology and the Dialectics of History*. Toronto: University of Toronto Press, 1990.

Flanagan, Joseph. 'The Self-Causing Subject: Intrinsic and Extrinsic Knowing.' *Lonergan Workshop* 3 (1982) 33–51.

Morelli, Elizabeth. *Anxiety: A Study of the Affectivity of Moral Consciousness*. Lanham, MD: University Press of America, 1985.

Morelli, Mark, and Elizabeth Morelli, eds. *The Lonergan Reader*. Toronto: University of Toronto Press, 1997.

Omerod, Neil. 'Lonergan and Finnis on the Human Good.' In *Australian Lonergan Workshop*, edited by William Danaher, 199–210. Lanham, MD: University Press of America, 1993.

Tyrell, Bernard. 'Feelings as Apprehensive-Intentional Responses to Values.' In Fred Lawrence, ed., *Lonergan Workshop* 7 (1988) 331–60.

Vertin, Michael. 'Course Notes.' Philosophy 335S. University of Toronto, January 1994.
- 'The Doctrine of Infallibility and the Demands of Epistemology: A Review Article.' *The Thomist* 43 (1979) 637–52.
- 'Judgments of Value for the Later Lonergan.' *Method: Journal of Lonergan Studies* 13 (1995) 221–48.
- '"Knowing," "Objectivity," and "Reality": Insight and Beyond.' *Lonergan Workshop* 8 (1990) 249–63.
- 'Lonergan on Consciousness: Is There a Fifth Level?' *Method: Journal of Lonergan Studies* 12 (1994) 1–36.
- 'Lonergan's Metaphysics of Value and Love: Some Proposed Clarifications and Implications.' *Lonergan Workshop* 13 (1997) 189–219.
- 'Review: *Collection*: Vol. 4 of *Collected Works of Bernard Lonergan*.' *Toronto Journal of Theology* 6 (1990) 145–47.

Works on Affect and Cognition

Blackburn, Simon. *The Oxford Dictionary of Philosophy*. Oxford: Oxford University Press, 1994.

Buckman, Robert. *How to Break Bad News: A Guide for Health Care Professionals*. Toronto: University of Toronto Press, 1992.

Calhoun, Cheshire, and Robert Solomon, eds. *What Is an Emotion? Classic Readings in Philosophy and Psychology*. Oxford: Oxford University Press, 1984.

Chesterton, G.K. 'The Maniac.' In *Orthodoxy*. New York: Image Books, 1959.

de Souza, Ronald. *The Rationality of Emotion*. Cambridge, MA: MIT Press, 1990.

Drever, James. *A Dictionary of Psychology.* Middlesex: Penguin Books, 1955. S.v. 'Fear.'

Drost, Mark. 'Intentionality in Aquinas' Theory of Emotions.' *International Philosophical Quarterly* 31 (1991) 449–60.

– 'In the Realm of the Senses: Saint Thomas Aquinas on Sensory Love, Desire, and Delight.' *The Thomist* 59 (1995) 47–58.

Ferreira, M. Jamie. 'The Grammar of the Heart: Newman on Faith and Imagination.' In *Discourse and Context: An Interdisciplinary Study of John Henry Newman,* edited by Gerard Magill, 129–43. Carbondale: Southern Illinois University Press, 1993.

Finnis, John. *Fundamentals of Ethics.* Washington: Georgetown University Press, 1983.

Fortenbaugh, William W. *Aristotle on Emotion: A Contribution to Philosophical Psychology, Rhetoric, Poetics, and Ethics.* Worcester and London: Harper and Row Publishers, 1975.

Honderich, Ted, ed. *The Oxford Companion to Philosophy.* Oxford: Oxford University Press, 1995.

Kaplan, Harold, and Benjamin Sadock. *Comprehensive Glossary of Psychiatry and Psychology.* Baltimore: Williams & Wilkins, 1991.

Oxford English Dictionary, Unabridged Version, 1971.

Reid, John Patrick. 'Introduction,' in Thomas Aquinas, *Summa Theologiae* 19. London and New York: Blackfriars in conjunction with Eyre & Spotiswoode and McGraw-Hill Book Co., 1967.

Russell, Bertrand. *Skeptical Essays.* London: Allen and Unwin, 1977.

Scheler, Max. *Formalism in Ethics and Non-Formal Ethics of Values.* Trans. Manfred Frings and Roger Fung. Evanston, IL: Northwestern University Press, 1973.

Stein, Edith. 'On the Problem of Empathy.' In *The Collected Works of Edith Stein.* Trans. Waltraut Stein. Vol 3. Washington, ICS Publications, 1989.

Strasser, Stephen. *Phenomenology of Feeling, An Essay on the Phenomena of the Heart.* Pittsburgh: Duquesne University Press, 1977.

Vertin, Michael. *The New Dictionary of Catholic Spirituality.* Collegeville, MN: Liturgical Press, 1993.

von Hildebrand, Dietrich. *The Sacred Heart: An Analysis of Human and Divine Affectivity.* Baltimore: Helicon Press Inc., 1965.

Works on Ethics and Medicine

Albrich, Michael. 'Acute Myocardial Infarction: Comprehensive Guidelines for Diagnosis, Stabilization, and Mortality Reduction.' *Emergency Medicine Reports* 6 (1994) 51–60.

American Heart Association. *Textbook of Advanced Cardiac Life Support.* 2nd ed. Dallas, TX: American Heart Association, 1990.

Beauchamp, Tom. 'Refusals of Treatment and Requests for Death.' *Kennedy Institute of Ethics Journal* 6 (1996) 371–74.

Brock, Ira. *Dying Well: The Prospect of Growth at the End of Life*. New York: Putnam, 1997.

Canada, Special Senate Committee on Euthanasia and Assisted Suicide. *Of Life and Death*. Ministry of Supply and Services Canada, May 1995.

Chochinov, Harvey Max, et al. 'Desire for Death in the Terminally Ill.' *American Journal of Psychiatry* 152 (1995) 1185–91.

Christopher, James, and Roderick Macleod. 'The Problematic Nature of Education in Palliative Care.' *Journal of Palliative Care* 9 (1993) 5–10.

Cline, David, et al. *Emergency Medicine: A Comprehensive Study Guide*. 4th ed. New York: McGraw-Hill, 1996.

Council on Scientific Affairs, American Medical Association. 'Good Care of the Dying Patient.' *Journal of the American Medical Association* 275 (1996) 474–78.

Den Hartogh, Govert. 'Euthanasia: Reflections on the Dutch Perspective.' *Annals of the New York Academy of Sciences* 913 (2000) 174–87.

Doud, J. 'Use-effectiveness of the Creighton Model of NFP.' *International Review of Natural Family Planning* 9 (1985) 54.

Dworkin, Ronald, Thomas Nagel, Robert Nozick, John Rawls, Thomas Scanlon, and Judith Jarvis Thomas. 'Assisted Suicide: The Philosophers' Brief.' *New York Review of Books* 44:5 (1997) 41–42.

Finnis, John, et al. '"Direct" and "Indirect": A Reply to Critics of Our Action Theory.' *The Thomist* 65 (2001) 1–44.

Fleming, John. 'Hiding Reality behind Euphemisms.' Southern Cross Bioethics Institute publication on the website, www.adelaide.catholic.org.au.

Frame, Paul, Alfred Berg, and Steve Woolf. 'U.S. Preventive Services Task Force: Highlights of the 1996 Report.' *American Family Physician* 55 (1997) 567–76.

Ganzini, Linda, Wendy S. Johnston, and William F. Hoffman. 'Correlates of Suffering in Amyotrophic Lateral Sclerosis.' *Neurology* 52 (1999) 1434–46.

Gates, Thomas. 'Euthanasia and Assisted Suicide: A Family Practice Perspective.' *American Family Physician* 55 (1997) 2437–44.

Gilmour, Joan. *Study Paper on Assisted Suicide, Euthanasia and Foregoing Treatment*. Toronto: Ontario Law Reform Commission, 1996.

Gordijn, Bert, and Rien Janssens. 'New Developments in Dutch Legislation concerning Euthanasia and Physician-Assisted Suicide.' *Journal of Medicine and Philosophy* 26:3 (2001) 299–309.

Goroll, Allan, Lawrence May, and Albert Mulley. *Primary Care Medicine*. 3rd ed. Philadelphia: J.B. Lippincott Co., 1995.

Hébert, Philip. *Doing Right: A Practical Guide to Ethics for Physicians and Medical Trainees*. Toronto: Oxford University Press, 1996.

Hendin, Herbert. 'The Dutch Experience.' *Issues in Law and Medicine* 17:3 (2002) 223–46.

Hobbs Birnie, Lisa, and Sue Rodriguez. *Uncommon Will: The Death and Life of Sue Rodriguez*. Toronto: Macmillan Canada, 1994.

Hutchinson, Brian. 'Choice.' *Saturday Night Magazine* (Toronto), March 1995.

Jenish, D'Archy. 'What Would You Do?' *Maclean's Magazine,* 28 November 1994.

John Paul II, Pope. *Novo Millenio Ineunt.* Apostolic Letter of His Holiness Pope John Paul II to the Bishops, Clergy and Lay Faithful at the Close of the Great Jubilee of the Year 2000. Zenit News Agency, The World Seen from Rome, 6 January 2001.

Jonsen, Albert. 'What Is at Stake.' *Commonweal* 118 (1991) s2–s4.

Kaczork, Christopher. 'Distinguishing Intention from Foresight: What Is Included in a Means to an End?' *International Philosophical Quarterly* 41 (March 2001) 7–89.

Kant, Immanuel. *Foundations of the Metaphysics of Morals.* Trans. Lewis White Beck. 23rd ed. Indianapolis, IN: Bobbs-Merrill Educational Publishing, 1983.

Kaplan, Harold, and Benjamin Sadock. *Synopsis of Psychiatry: Behavioural Sciences, Clinical Psychiatry.* 6th ed. Baltimore: Williams & Wilkins, 1991.

Kass, Leon. '"I Will Give No Deadly Drug," Why Doctors Must Not Kill.' *Bulletin, American College of Surgeons* 77 (1992) 6–17.

Kaye, Dennis. *Laugh, I Thought I'd Die, My Life with ALS.* Toronto: Penguin Books Ltd., 1993.

Keown, John, ed. *Euthanasia Examined: Ethical, Clinical, and Legal Perspectives.* Foreword by Daniel Callahan. Cambridge: Press Syndicate of the University of Cambridge, 1995.

Knox, R. 'Poll: Americans Favor Mercy Killing.' *Boston Globe,* 3 November 1991, 1(A).

Lavery, James V., Bernard M. Dickens, Joseph M. Boyle, and Peter A. Singer. 'Bioethics for Clinicians: 11. Euthanasia and Assisted Suicide.' *Canadian Medical Association Journal* 156 (1997) 1405–8.

Lavery, J.V., and P.A. Singer. 'The "Supremes" Decide on Assisted Suicide: What Should a Doctor Do?' *Canadian Medical Association Journal* 157 (1997) 405–6.

Little, Miles. 'Assisted Suicide, Suffering and the Meaning of a Life.' *Theoretical Medicine and Bioethics* 20 (1999) 287–98.

McCormick, Richard. 'Killing and Allowing to Die: *Vive la Différence!*' *America* 177 (6 December 1977): 6–12.

McDaniel, Susan, et al. *Family-Oriented Primary Care: A Manual for Medical Providers.* New York: Springer-Verlag, 1990.

McWhinney, Ian. 'The Importance of Being Different: 1996 William Pickles Lecture.' *British Journal of General Practice* 46 (1996) 433–36.

Meilaender, Gilbert. 'The Point of a Ban: Or, How to Think about Stem Cell Research.' *Hastings Center Report* 31:1 (2001) 9–16.

Melchin, Kenneth. 'Revisionists, Deontologists, and the Structure of Moral Understanding.' *Theological Studies* 51 (1990) 389–416.

Meyer, Michael J., and L.J. Nelson. 'Respecting What We Destroy: Reflections on Human Embryo Research.' *Hastings Center Report* 31:1 (2001) 16–23.

Morgan, John, ed. *An Easeful Death? Perspectives on Death, Dying and Euthanasia.* Sydney: Federation Press, 1996.

Morris, C., John Niederbuhl, and Jeffrey Mahr. 'Determining the Capability of

Individuals with Mental Retardation to Give Informed Consent.' *American Journal on Mental Retardation* 2 (1993) 263–72.

Mullens, Anne. 'Just Getting Through the Day Was the Hardest Part.' *Toronto Star*, 14 February 1994, 19(A).

Pizarro, David. 'Nothing More than Feelings? The Role of Emotions in Moral Judgement.' *Journal for the Theory of Social Behaviour* 30:4 (2000) 355–75.

Rachels, James. 'Active and Passive Euthanasia.' *New England Journal of Medicine* 2 (1975) 78–80. Reprinted in *Biomedical Ethics*, edited by Thomas Mappes and Jane Zembaty, 385–88. New York: McGraw-Hill Book Co., 1986.

Rodriguez, Sue. 'To Die with Dignity.' *Vancouver Star*, republished in the *Toronto Star*, 4 March 1993, 1(B).

Ruff, Ronald, et al. 'Miserable Minority: Emotional Risk Factors That Influence the Outcome of a Mild Traumatic Brain Injury.' *Brain Injury* 10 (1996) 551–65.

Sack, Goldblatt Mitchell. 'The Sue Rodriguez Case: A Legal Perspective.' *Ontario Medical Review* 60 (1993) 79–85.

Sawa, Russell J., and H.A. Meynell. 'On Insight, Objectivity, and the Pathology of Families.' *Method: Journal of Lonergan Studies* 18 (2000) 145–60.

Scrivener, Leslie. 'MD's Often Give Drugs That Speed Up Dying.' *Toronto Star*, 10 May 1997, 29(A).

Shavelson, Lonny. *A Chosen Death: The Dying Confront Assisted Suicide.* New York: Simon & Schuster, 1995.

Steward, Moira. 'Effective Physician–Patient Communication and Health Outcomes: A Review.' *Canadian Medical Association Journal* 9 (1995) 1423–33.

Stewart, Moira, Judith Belle Brown, Wayne Weston, et al. 'The Second Component: Understanding the Whole Person.' In *Patient-Centered Medicine: Transforming the Clinical Method.* California: Sage Publications, Inc., 1995.

Sumner, L.W., and Joseph Boyle, eds. *Philosophical Perspectives on Bioethics.* Toronto: University of Toronto Press, 1996.

Tibbles, Patrick, and Peter Perrotta. 'Treatment of Carbon Monoxide Poisoning: A Critical Review of Human Outcome Studies Comparing Normobaric Oxygen with Hyperbaric Oxygen.' *Annals of Emergency Medicine* 24 (1994) 269–76.

Tollefsen, Christopher. 'Direct and Indirect Action Revisited.' *American Catholic Philosophical Quarterly* 74 (2000) 653–70.

Weithman, Paul J. 'Of Assisted Suicide and "The Philosophers" Brief.' *Ethics* 109:3 (1999) 548–78.

Williams, John, Frederick Lowy, and Douglas Sawyer. 'Canadian Physicians and Euthanasia: 3. Arguments and Beliefs.' *Canadian Medical Association Journal* 148 (1993) 1699–1702.

Wilson, Deborah, and Donn Downey. 'Obituary.' *Globe and Mail*, 14 February 1994, 4(A).

Wood, Daniel. 'Death Wish: Would You Choose Assisted Suicide?' *Chatelaine* 66 (July 1993), 25ff.

General Works of Philosophy and Ethics

Aquinas, Thomas. *Summa Theologiae.* Vol. 19: *Love and Desire* (1a2ae). Trans. Eric D'Arcy and John Reid. London and New York: Blackfriars, in conjunction with Eyre & Spottiswoode, and McGraw-Hill Book Co., 1967.

– *Summa Theologica of St. Thomas Aquinas.* Vol. 2 (1a2ae). Trans. Fathers of the English Dominican Province. New York: Benziger Brothers, Inc., 1948; repr. Westminster, MD: Christian Classics, 1981.

Aristotle. *On the Soul.* Trans. W.S. Hett. Cambridge, MA: Harvard University Press, 1936, reprinted 1986.

– *Metaphysics, Books I–IX.* Trans. Hugh Trendennick. Cambridge, MA: Harvard University Press, 1933; reprinted 1980.

– *Nichomachean Ethics.* Trans. Terence Irwin. Indianapolis, IN: Hackett Publishing Co., Inc., 1985.

Copleston, Frederick. *A History of Philosophy.* Vols. 1–8. *Greece and Rome; Augustine to Scotus; Ockham to Suarez; Descartes to Leibniz; Hobbes to Hume; Wolff to Kant; Fichte to Nietzsche; and Bentham to Russell.* New York: Doubleday, 1985.

Hunnex, Milton. *Chronological and Thematic Charts of Philosophies and Philosophers.* Grand Rapids, MI: Zondervan Publishing House, 1986.

Index

structure of, 292; what it is, 207–8, 265. *See also* goodness

Hume, David, 61–4, 78–9, 84–5, 199, 211–12, 216–17, 219, 260, 327n88, 329n98, 331n16

Hunnex, Milton, 10

Husserl, Edmund, 75, 77

Hutcheson, Francis, 64

ideology, 198–200

individualism: impact on community, 190–1; impossibility of, 14; relevance of social context, 192

insight: abstract intelligibility, 105; as authentic, 170–1; deliberate, 152–3, 156–8, 204–6, 220–1, 241–2, 273, 354–5n25, 357n49 (*see also under* evaluation, apprehension of value); direct insight, 99–101, 103–5, 109–10, 153–4; feelings as intentional responses, 12–13, 138; reflective insight, 107–10, 153–7; role in act of judgment, 161–2; subjective act of, 184; symbol for, 330n1. *See also under* cognitional structure

James, William, 62–3

judging: awareness of process of, 289–91; cognitional operations of, 146; deliberate insights, 152–3; evidence of a judgment, 109; hesitantly, 120; level of cognitional activity, 92; making the judgment, 105–11; of a medical diagnosis, 118–20, 347n5; rashly, 119; reasonably, 125–6; role of facts in, 109, 289–90

judgment: and achievement of knowledge, 111; clarity, 105; expression of, 110; false value, 182; negative, 163–5; subjective act of, 184; value *versus* fact, 162, 216–17. *See also* evaluation

Kant, Immanuel, 65–6, 71, 78, 84–5, 183, 199, 211–12, 218–19, 272, 332n27, 362n21

Kaye, Dennis: the act of choosing, 239–42; anger to righteous anger, 45–7; attitude to caregivers, 288; and community, 13, 48– 50, 242–4, 318n15, 326–7n83; empirical position of, 247–52; evaluations as subjective, 237–9; *Laugh, I Thought I'd Die*, 45; life as worthwhile, 244–5; philosophical position of, 245–7, 250–2, 277–8, 310; in relation to Lonergan, 250–4; role of feelings, 236–7, 260, 267; sense of humour, 47–8, 326n79; from vulnerability to love, 47–8. *See also* end-of-life stories

Kevorkian, Jack, 283

knowing: cognitive role of feelings in, 90, 204–6, 236–7, 331n16; definition, 127; as distinct from believing, 110–11; and doing, 167; of facts and values, 137, 150–1; the good, 197–8; group bias, 134–5, 187–8; in medical practice, 131–4; models of, 211–12, 229, 307, 336n97; in moral development, 180–2; as ocular, 211, 214, 285, 339n35; opposed to feeling, 138–9; performative norms for, 121–2, 134–5; unity of cognitional acts, 111–12, 114

knowledge: feelings sufficient for, 236–7, 267, 374n10; of the good, 180; moral, 271; more than subjective, 116–17, 206–7, 209, 214–17; of the real, 105, 109–11; of self, 91–3, 337n13; source of questions, 103–5, 107, 112, 236; subjective-objective distinction, 128–30; of values, 198–200, 209, 214–16

Latimer, Tracy, 21, 320n28